S0-APF-310

FIRST AID IN EMERGENCY CARE

FIRST AID IN EMERGENCY CARE

GUY S. PARCEL, Ph.D.

Assistant Professor of Pediatrics
and of Preventive Medicine and Community Health,
University of Texas Medical Branch,
Galveston, Texas

with 16 contributions and 194 illustrations

Williams Baptist College
FELIX GOODSON
LIBRARY
Walnut Ridge, Ark.

THE C. V. MOSBY COMPANY

Saint Louis 1977

Copyright © 1977 by The C. V. Mosby Company

All rights reserved. No part of this book may be reproduced in any manner without written permission of the publisher.

Printed in the United States of America

Distributed in Great Britain by Henry Kimpton, London

The C. V. Mosby Company
11830 Westline Industrial Drive, St. Louis, Missouri 63141

Library of Congress Cataloging in Publication Data

Main entry under title:

First aid in emergency care.

    Bibliography: p.
    Includes index.
    1. First aid in illness and injury.
2. Medical emergencies. I. Parcel, Guy S.
[DNLM: 1. Emergencies. 2. First aid.
WA292 P235f]
RC86.7.F57   614.8'8   77-322
ISBN 0-8016-3757-0

VH/VH/VH 9 8 7 6 5 4 3 2 1

66,494

CONTRIBUTORS

Sally Abston, M.D.
Director of Emergency Room, University of Texas Medical Branch Hospitals; Associate Professor, Department of Surgery, University of Texas Medical Branch, Galveston, Texas

Byron J. Bailey, M.D.
Chairman and Wiess Professor, Department of Otolaryngology, University of Texas Medical Branch, Galveston, Texas

John G. Bruhn, Ph.D.
Associate Dean of Medicine and Coordinator of Community Affairs, University of Texas Medical Branch, Galveston, Texas

Elton Dupree, M.D.
Pediatric Immunologist and Allergist; Clinical Associate Professor, Department of Pediatrics, University of Texas Health Science Center, Houston, Texas

Alexander Franco, M.D., F.A.C.O.G.
Gynecologist, Ritenour Health Center, Pennsylvania State University, University Park, Pennsylvania

Mary Dolores Hemelt, R.N., M.S., J.D.
Professor, Division of Allied Health, Essex Community College, Baltimore County, Maryland; Chairman, Board of Review, Department of Health and Men-

tal Hygiene of State of Maryland, Baltimore, Maryland

J. Maurice Mahan, Ph.D.
Assistant Professor of Preventive Medicine and Community Health, University of Texas Medical Branch, Galveston, Texas

Richard F. McConnell, Jr., M.D.
Assistant Director, Department of Pediatrics, John Peter Smith Hospital, Fort Worth, Texas

Rosemary K. McKevitt, R.N., Ed.D.
Associate Professor, School of Nursing, University of Texas Health Science Center at San Antonio, San Antonio, Texas

Robert H. Miller, M.D.
Assistant Professor of Medicine and Chief, Division of Emergency Medicine, Southern Illinois University School of Medicine, Springfield, Illinois

John N. O'Connor
Assistant in Emergency Medicine, Southern Illinois University School of Medicine, Springfield, Illinois

Guy S. Parcel, Ph.D.
Assistant Professor of Pediatrics and of Preventive Medicine and Community Health, University of Texas Medical Branch, Galveston, Texas

Charles Edwin Rinear, Ed.D.

Instructor, Emergency Care, Temple University, Philadelphia, Pennsylvania, and Bucks County Community College, Newtown, Pennsylvania

Edward L. Schor, M.D.

Assistant Professor, School of Health Services, Johns Hopkins University, Baltimore, Maryland

Barbara E. Williams, M.S.W.

Director, Adolescent Inpatient Unit, Division of Child Psychiatry, University of Texas Medical Branch, Galveston, Texas

James A. Williams, M.S.W.

Coordinator, Educational Planning and Community Affairs, Office of The Dean of Medicine, University of Texas Medical Branch, Galveston, Texas

J. Robert Wirag, H.S.D.

Director of Health Education, University Health Services, The Pennsylvania State University, University Park, Pennsylvania

Coordinator of artwork
Mark Weakley, M.A.

Medical Illustrator, University of Texas Health Science Center at San Antonio, San Antonio, Texas

To the memory of
Ralph C. Parcel

FOREWORD

Murphy's first law, "Whatever can go wrong, will," has found in the field of injury control routine substantiation. Trauma is the leading cause of death into middle age, a leading cause of suffering throughout the span of life, and has been awarded the dubious status of "society's most neglected disease."

Recent legislative attention to injury control, however (for example, the Highway Safety Act), has been accompanied by a variety of intensified educational efforts. Orthopedic surgeons, anesthesiologists, and other physicians are helping to upgrade the competence and use of emergency medical technicians by specially structured courses. Physicians not only increasingly are opting to confine their practice to the emergency department of a hospital, but a new medical specialty with such focus is now recognized. The Emergency Medical Technician, who has completed a nationally standardized course of study, has replaced the ambulance attendant of the past. The American Heart Association and the National American Red Cross have reorganized their efforts to upgrade the public's abilities to recognize and manage effectively an emergency situation. What one decade ago, for example, was too controversial to put into any layman's first aid program (closed cardiac massage) is now being advocated for high school students as a fundamental life-support skill. The layman remains the first link in the emergency medical service system.

This sudden respectability of first aid and emergency care as an educational focus has not emerged without its problems. Standards and recommendations for handling particular emergencies are shifting rapidly as scholarly attention to these matters becomes more sophisticated. The Red Cross programs must be designed to accommodate any interested member of the general public regardless of educational background, whereas athletic trainers, nurses, and emergency medical technicians are receiving preparation of advanced nature. A profoundly worrisome residual has been the blurring of both the distinction between first aid and emergency care and the authority for expressed principles of emergency attentions.

This book attends to this residual. Current textbooks tend to address two extreme groups—general public or professional emergency medical personnel. In most cases neither of these kinds of textbooks is appropriate for a college first aid course. This book is written for the college student, who can be expected to absorb tangible and abstract concepts for judgmental as well as mechanical skills.

It is consistent with the latest concepts of first aid management as advanced by the National American Red Cross, yet it broadens and deepens the understandings for application in variable contexts.

This book will be of special interest to college students with career goals that will require responsibility for the welfare of others, such as teachers, physical educators, coaches, recreation leaders, safety educators, and administrators. Moreover, it is hoped that the users of this book will come to connect emergency care and injury control as a formidable component of health education. To gain health, one must risk it. It is safe to sit in a corner, but such is hardly living a full and rewarding life. To risk one's health for a targeted goal requires planning both to contain the risk by preventive actions and to contain the consequences of Murphy's law when it is invoked. To plan requires an anticipation of principles that could apply and a resourcefulness for competent execution in variable settings. To anticipate and be resourceful requires an educational preparation that is enabled by this book.

Kenneth S. Clarke

Professor and Chairman, Health Education,
Pennsylvania State University,
University Park, Pennsylvania

PREFACE

First Aid in Emergency Care is a textbook written for advanced courses in first aid. It is designed primarily to meet the needs of students enrolled in college courses covering first aid and emergency care. Most colleges and universities today offer such courses. Students take these courses as an elective or as a requirement of degree programs such as teaching, physical education, safety, health education, recreation, child care, and allied health.

The project that eventually led to the publication of this book grew out of my own frustration as an instructor of first aid and emergency care courses at three different universities. I felt the need for a text that went beyond the step-by-step information presented in first aid manuals. It seemed that college students were seeking more information about why to do certain procedures rather than just how to do them. With the emergence of the new paramedical professionals, emergency medical technicians (EMTs), new texts have been published for training the professional first aider. However, these texts tended to go beyond first aid for the lay person. What was needed was a textbook that utilized established first aid guidelines for lay personnel and presented information that would be interesting and challenging to college students. In addition, the book should address the special role of the nonmedical professional who has responsibility for the welfare of other people.

This book has been developed for and is offered as an alternative to meet these needs. The approach is to include first aid procedures within the context of the total sequence for emergency care. The distinction between first aid and emergency care is clarified. Procedures presented in this book are appropriate for nonmedical personnel.

The content of the book is the combined work of seventeen contributing authors. In addition to writing their own chapters, many of the authors reviewed and made suggestions for other chapters. The authors include health educators, an emergency medical technician, nurses, physicians, a lawyer, a community organizer, a social worker, and a sociologist. The authors bring to the book a wide range of experience in all components of emergency care. Their combined expertise far exceeds that of a single author.

It is hoped that this text will contribute to the education and training of students participating in first aid and emergency care instruction. The ultimate goal is to provide the best possible first aid care for those stricken by injury or sudden illness.

Sincere appreciation is expressed to the contributing authors. Without their efforts this book would not have been possible. Also, appreciation is extended to Margaret Canavan, Judi Godwin, and Mary Ann Mabry for their assistance with preparation of the manuscript. Finally, special thanks go to Mark Weakley for completing an extensive art program within a short time period.

Guy S. Parcel

CONTENTS

Section II   CARDIOPULMONARY EMERGENCIES

7   MANAGEMENT OF WOUNDS AND HEMORRHAGING, 83
Charles Edwin Rinear and Guy S. Parcel

8   POISONING AND TOXIC REACTIONS, 97
Richard F. McConnell, Jr., Elton Dupree, and Guy S. Parcel

14 HEAT-RELATED ILLNESSES AND EMERGENCIES, 186

J. Maurice Mahan

15 PSYCHOLOGICAL EMERGENCIES, 197

Rosemary K. McKevitt

Section V APPLICATION OF EMERGENCY CARE SKILLS AND PRINCIPLES

INTRODUCTION TO FIRST AID IN EMERGENCY CARE

Guy S. Parcel and Barbara E. Williams

*First aid is the immediate and temporary care given to a person who has been injured or becomes suddenly ill.**

Injury or sudden illness becomes an emergency when life is threatened, suffering occurs, or problems develop that endanger physical or psychological well-being. Injured or ill individuals involved in emergency situations become dependent on others for their well-being. Health professionals (physicians, nurses, psychologists, and technicians) are trained to deal with these emergencies and to provide the necessary care. However, a health professional is unlikely to be the first person to attend to the needs of an injured or suddenly ill person. The concept of first aid grew out of the recognition that *immediate* care was the necessary first step in an emergency.

Emergency care is the full range of procedures and services administered to a person who has been injured or becomes suddenly ill. It begins with first aid and includes emergency transportation, emergency medical care, and follow-up care. Each of these components is essential to the effective management of trauma and sudden illness. Different individuals and professionals will be involved in each component. First aiders, emergency medical technicians (EMTs), nurses, physicians, physician's assistants, nurse practitioners, and allied health professionals all play a role in the total sequence of events in providing emergency care.

The figure on p. 2 shows the interrelationship of these different groups in providing emergency care. Four major groups are located on the chart where each has a major responsibility for a particular component of emergency care. However, the arrows show how there is an overlapping of responsibility into other components for each group. The trained first aider is primarily involved in the first aid component, but responsibility can extend into emergency transportation and follow-up care. There may be times when transportation services provided by EMTs are not available or not necessary and the first aider will provide transportation. Follow-up care is care provided once the emergency condition or problem has been stabilized.

---

*Adapted from the definition of the American Red Cross.

1

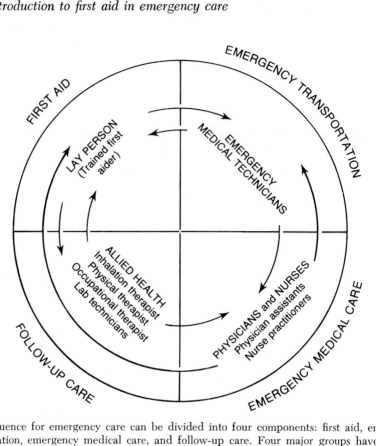

Total sequence for emergency care can be divided into four components: first aid, emergency transportation, emergency medical care, and follow-up care. Four major groups have responsibilities within each component. Arrows show how responsibilities overlap for different professionals and first aider.

In some cases, first aid intervention may stabilize a condition, and the first aider may direct attention to some basic follow-up care procedures.

All three of the other groups are shown as having responsibility for first aid. The EMT in many cases is the first trained person to arrive at an emergency situation and will provide the first aid care. In other cases the EMT will take over responsibility for first aid after a first aider has provided initial care. Physicians, nurses, and other health care professionals will at times be called on to administer first aid. This might happen because they are the first to arrive at the scene of an emergency. In many cases it is because there was no first aider to initiate emergency care.

Emergency care can be viewed as a sequence of events involving many individuals to resolve a threatening condition or problem. The essential first component in the sequence is the administration of first aid. The key to this first component is the availability of a person trained in administering first aid care. Despite advancements in medical technology, first aid in emergency care is still the first critical link in the management of trauma and sudden illness.

DIMENSIONS OF THE PROBLEM

Each year many people sustain substantial financial losses and endure a burden of suffering that ultimately touches every household. Medical emergencies, inappropriately handled, contribute to the spiraling incidence of disability and death. In this last quarter of the twentieth century, statistics have forced the attention of the medical and lay public alike to focus on the emergence of a new type of response—immediate, knowledgeable, adequate, and *at the scene.* The full impact and cost of inadequate training within the citizen group is recognized. Lives are lost or saved due to luck: Was there someone on the scene who knew the correct response? All too often the answer has been No.

Trauma

In terms of human suffering and financial loss, preventable accidents rank second only to ancient plagues and modern world wars. In one year alone, there were more persons killed on the streets and highways of the United States than were lost on the battlefields of Korea. In the last 60 years, more Americans have died from accidents than from all combat wounds of all our wars. Accidents are the leading cause of death among persons between the ages of 1 and 37 and the fourth leading cause of death for all ages. In addition, accidents are the number one disabler, accounting for over 11 million permanently physically impaired Americans. The estimated cost of accidents in the United States for the year 1965 was $18 billion; it had risen to $37 billion in 1973 and continues upward.

Each year one out of four Americans receives a significant injury. The National Center for Health Statistics (HEW) reports that an average of 63.4 million Americans a year are hurt seriously enough to seek medical attention or restrict their activities for at least a day. Over 2.6 million are hospitalized. More Americans receive disabling injuries in their own homes than any other place. In polling all accidents, 43% occur in private residences with children, adolescents under 17, and persons over 65 as the most frequent victims. Children miss 15.1 million school days a year, the majority due to accidents, and thousands of children suffer permanently disabling accidents in their own homes. The American home is becoming more dangerous as technology increases. Although electric hazards are decreasing at work, they are increasing at home with the advent of power tools. In 1973, power lawn mowers alone accounted for 1846 accidents.

In fatality statistics, the automobile holds first place as the most lethal weapon Americans own. Despite development and promotion of various safety devices, drivers and passengers continue to die and be maimed. Of all accidents, 34% occur in public places—recreational, commercial, and on streets. The vast majority of fatalities involve vehicles. Motor vehicles constitute the leading cause of accidental death for all age groups. Over 2 million deaths have been attributed to automobile accidents. Children, although chiefly passengers, are at high risk for automobile injury and death. Automobiles accounted for 6000 deaths to children under 14 in 1970 alone, and there were 2670 deaths and 145,500 injuries to children actually riding in the cars.

At high risk as drivers are adolescent and young adult men. Not only is the mortality rate for this group twice as high as for women in the same group, but morbidity figures are equally alarming. For example, 85% of all patients with spinal cord injury, a serious crippler, are men between 18 and 25 years of age. Of all spinal cord injuries, 50% result from automobile accidents, affecting 10,000 young people each year. The crucial period for this group of injuries is the first 4 hours after trauma. Of particular importance are (1) proper care at the scene and (2) proper transportation from the scene. These two variables mean the difference between minimum or no disability and severe lifelong impairment.

Medical conditions

Since the turn of the century, medical science has made giant strides in controlling infectious diseases, virtually eliminating some, such as smallpox and polio, and greatly reducing others, including malarias, measles, diphtheria, and tetanus. Now new killers have risen to take their place, many with precipitous crises associated with death. Heart attacks are the single leading cause of fatalities in this country, with 650,000 deaths a year. Of those individuals who die from heart attack, half never reach the hospital alive, and two thirds are dead within 2 hours. Diabetes, despite the use of insulin, continues at the same incidence and mortality rate as it did three quarters of a century ago. Diabetic coma, undetected and untreated, remains as consistently fatal as ever. Stroke victims, seizure cases, and certain types of acute respiratory distress patients all represent chronic diseases that have sudden onset crises, requiring immediate care. With the heart attack victim the crucial first 5 minutes spell the difference between life and death, between adequate recovery or permanent impairment. This slender margin of time depends on one variable: the availability of adequate and immediate care.

Psychological problems

Mental illness has emerged as one of the leading disablers of the twentieth century. One in every three hospital beds in the United States is filled with an emotionally disturbed patient. Americans have a one in ten chance of becoming mentally ill during their lifetime. It is the rare family indeed that does not need to have some understanding of mental illness and the ability to cope with crisis in that context. This may range anywhere from the slow deterioration of the patient to a violent and sudden display, possibly with fatal results. For instance, the 1960s was a period of rising death rates for teenagers and young adults. This was primarily due to increases in behavioral causes, including suicide, homicide, and accidents. The homicide and suicide rates have doubled since 1960, both as an absolute and as a percentage increase. Drug abuse, an increasingly frequent companion to mental illness, has steadily increased the number of overdosed patients requiring intervention. Of growing national concern are the thousands of abused children, victims of problems within the parent and family systems. These children experience physical and emotional trauma requiring sophisticated management techniques so as not to increase the damage. Inept treatment could result in present or future death of the child or severe psychological and/or physical damage for life. In addition to the danger to the patient, the treatment person in a psychological emergency may himself become a victim of a situation he does not have the training to cope with.

Environmental risks

There are numerous environmental factors that impinge on health. The pace of modern living contributes to heart attacks, increased use of the automobile accelerates everyone's accident risk, deteriorating support systems for families jeopardize the individual members, and power tools produce new hazards.

In considering the natural history of disease, there are certain predictable aspects that can be attributed not to individuals and their behaviors but to group situations, societal demands, or cultural factors. For example, there is twice the injury death rate for males as for females; poor people suffer according to their participation in high-risk jobs, their residence in substandard housing, and the use of hazardous appliances such as space heaters; the differential rates for populations correspond directly to the differences in access to adequate medical care.

Until the present time, almost exclusive concentration on the individual in the disease process has resulted in labeling him as culpable due to human error, which is a usual ingredient. Error is simply defined as a missing or inappropriate response, either psychological or physiological, and the person's behavior should not be viewed as necessarily culpable or delinquent. It may, in fact, be so intertwined with the other factors of environment that it would be difficult to separate the component parts. Because of the assumption of host culpability, prevention too often has been exclusively concerned with educating or changing the host. It is no longer feasible to shrug off the victim as solely responsible for his medical emergency. Professionals and informed lay citizens are beginning to stress the responsibility of the total environment, including the development of adequate response to the whole range of problems.

Emerging responses

Until recently, the prevailing attitude of the medical profession and the health care system was that responsibility for the trauma victim began at the door of the hospital. The cause of the illness or injury, the circumstances surrounding the event, and how the patient was cared for and transported from the scene to the hospital remained secondary considerations at best. In the 1960s this began to change. Figures indicating that at least 20% of all accident and coronary deaths were directly avoidable with prompt medical attention at the scene and en route to the hospital indicated an unnecessary and expensive waste of human life. These figures translated into an average city with a population between 50,000 and 60,000 would result in the saving of between twenty and forty lives, the prevention of hundreds of disabilities, and the avoidance of a $6 million annual loss to the economy. The impact of these statistics has been forcing a reappraisal of the total picture, arguing for fresh approaches and utilization of a wide variety of techniques.

Prevention and safety have taken on new meaning. Four possible considerations have been suggested.[4] First would be modification of the environment, which has large areas of untapped potential, including everything outside the individual—clothing, occupation, housing, and cultural factors such as the social use of alcohol. A second approach would be intellectual or skills changes in the individual, including education, training in various areas, driver instruction, swimming lessons, and education of consumers. A third target area would be actual physiological strengthening with emphasis on diet and exercise. The fourth would entail the establishment of adequate emergency response systems. Increasing numbers of programs are being established with various aspects of this scheme emphasized.

Industry has taken innovative and concrete steps to reduce trauma. Despite increasing amounts of mechanization, involving complex machinery, death rates from work accidents in manufacturing have decreased in the last 40 years. Efforts directed toward education, training, surveillance of the workers, and improving the design of hazardous machinery have been responsible for a significant rate reduction. Deaths have fallen from 37 per 100,000 population in 1933 to the present 20 per 100,000. One of industry's basic tenets has been emphasis of safety and prevention. In addition, the industrial worker has been taught how to deal with emergencies promptly and correctly.

In 1966, the Committee on Trauma, the Committee on Shock, the Division of Medical Sciences, the National Academy of Sciences, and the National Research Council joined forces to call attention to the national health problems surrounding the paucity of appropriate and adequate emergency health care. They believed that the general public was insensitive to the magnitude of the problem and that millions lacked even basic instruction in first aid. In 1970, a national survey of cities with populations of over 100,000 was conducted to obtain some idea of the quantity and quality of emergency services that were being provided. Only 23% of the responding cities reported municipal provision of emergency ambulance service. This serves to emphasize strongly that Americans are at risk for future disabling injury after trauma due to several factors. First, in the majority of cases, hospitals are remote from the scene of the accident. Add to this the haphazard spectrum of ambulance service across the nation. Second, professional medical personnel are rarely at the scene. There is a delayed availability in the vast majority of cases. Third, at the present time, the statistical probability of a trained first aider being on the scene is low.

WHY FIRST AID?

The average individual will receive first aid care many times in his lifetime. The majority of times it will involve the application of a topical antiseptic, a bandaid, or a thump on the back. Usually the inexperienced administrator has sufficient knowledge to adequately apply the healing touch. However, the high probability of serious injury, as indicated by current statistics, makes the absence of a trained first aider a prelude to tragedy. Folk wisdom does not suffice when induced vomiting for specific poisons ensures further injury or death. Good intentions and prompt action do not save the choking victim when no one knows the correct procedure for dislodging food particles. Drowning victims are not revived by appalled onlookers. What despair the victim must feel if he consciously realizes that his life ebbs away with his blood because there is no immediate help available. What bitterness is the lot of a permanently disabled person whose plight was the direct result of hasty mismanagement after trauma.

Teachers and other professionals in human care and services have added dimensions in their job. Assumption of the professional role entails an obligation that assumes responsibility for other people. The care of human beings presumes a basic investment in maintaining the best environment for learning, growing, and safety. It also ensures that the professional will equip himself or herself with the basic tools necessary to maintain an optimum of care for his or her charges. For example, the teacher who takes children on a picnic or a field trip without having adequate first aid training would be culpable and could be a major factor in serious consequences.

The ultimate goal for all Americans is adequate health care. Trauma- and crisis-oriented medicine has become increasingly important. The AMA is presently in the process of establishing guidelines and training programs in emergency medicine. But doctors are not the only ones moving into the broadening horizons of emergency medical services. Increasing numbers of health administrators, allied health personnel, government officials, hospitals, fire fighters, police officers, ambulance and rescue workers, and an informed public are becoming involved. The field of allied health professionals is expanded with training for emergency medical technicians and paramedics. First aid courses are more sophisticated and detailed. Responsibility for the injured now extends to the patient wherever he is located.

The first link in the chain of medical care is not the health care professional. It is impossible to have adequate medical personnel to cover every possible scene at all times. And yet, time is of the essence in crisis medicine. The transportation of adequate medical care to the scene in time is frequently impossible. The allied fields in injury control are coming of age. The focus must move increasingly to the group and the community. Expanding scientific knowledge is of little value unless it is used effectively in planning and implementing programs to reduce injuries and their consequences.

FIRST AIDER'S ROLE

The *trained* first aider has an essential role to play in a system for providing emergency care. It is important to emphasize the meaning of *trained*. A first aider is more than just a person willing to help. Anyone who assumes responsibility for first aid care assumes the responsibility for the life and well-being of another person. This requires making decisions that are based on a knowledge of what to do and based on established guidelines for administering first aid care. Becoming trained means more than reading a book on first aid. Training should be done through certified courses under the direction of qualified instructors. This becomes the first responsibility of the first aider: preparation for administering first aid care. This responsibility continues in the form of keeping current and up to date. It is important to practice first aid skills as well as to continue periodic training.

When assuming the responsibility for providing care for another person, the first aider is entering into a provider-patient relationship. A patient is an injured or ill person who is being cared for by another person. In a provider-patient relationship, the patient gives verbal or implied consent to be helped by the first aider. The first aider agrees to do everything within his or her ability to provide assistance. This means that once assistance is begun, the first aider will follow through until more qualified assistance can be obtained. This is a relationship of trust. The patient is placing his or her well-being into the hands of another person. It is critical that the first aider does not violate this trust. Once care is assumed, the primary responsibility is to the well-being of the patient.

The first aider is restricted to his or her defined role in emergency care. He or she must stay within established guidelines for the administration of first aid care. First aiders should perform only those procedures that they have been trained to do. These will vary according to different levels of training. For example, a basic first aid course does not include external cardiac compression, but an advanced course would include this procedure. The first aider needs to know his or her limitations. Limitations are determined by the type and level of training as well as self-awareness of what one does not have the ability to do.

First aid by definition is restricted to immediate and temporary care. This means that the care must follow an acute injury, sudden illness, or emergency situation. Also, it implies that the first aid care is not meant to resolve the problem and that additional care by medical professionals always follows first aid care.

First aiders can never assume the role of independent care providers. They must follow guidelines established by health care professionals. They function to provide care only until the services of medical personnel can be obtained. First aiders should readily request and rely on the guidance and advice of trained medical personnel.

When medical services and advice are obtained, it is important for the first aider to communicate his role in caring for a patient. Medical personnel will need to know the qualifications of the first aider as well as what has been done for the patient.

The trained first aider is the first link in providing emergency care. Much of what happens further down the chain of events in providing emergency care may depend on the actions of the first aider. Nonmedical personnel can play a vital role in responding to the problems of trauma and sudden illness by becoming trained in administering first aid care. For those professionals such as teachers and recreation leaders who have responsibility for the welfare of others, first aid training is essential. For anyone entering into a first aid training course or program, it is important to be aware of the responsibility that will accompany that training.

REFERENCES AND RECOMMENDED READINGS

1. Accident facts, Chicago, 1970, National Safety Council.
2. Accidental death and disability: the neglected disease of modern society, Public Health Service Publication No. 1071-A-13, Public Health Service, Rockville, Md., 1970, U.S. Department of Health, Education, and Welfare.
3. Arena, J. M.: Testimony before the Senate Commerce Committee: S. 2162—the Poison Prevention Packaging Act of 1969, Clinical Toxicology 3:289-290, 1970.
4. Baker, S. P.: Determinants of injury and opportunities for intervention, American Journal of Epidemiology 101:98-102, 1975.
5. Burke, D. C.: Spinal cord injuries and seat belts, Medical Journal of Australia 1973:801-806, 1973.
6. Canada, A. T.: The drug information center movement: some correlations with poison control, Clinical Toxicology 3:277-280, 1970.
7. Cochrane, B. M.: What can we do to reduce deaths from asphyxiation due to choking? Canadian Medical Association Journal 111:460, 1974.
8. Daniel, M. C.: Special programs on

health and safety, Occupational Health Nursing **22**:14-15, March, 1974.

9. Developing emergency medical services—guidelines for community councils, Chicago, 1973, American Medical Association.

10. Emergency medical services systems: program guidelines, Public Health Service, Rockville, Md., 1975, U.S. Department of Health, Education, and Welfare.

11. The emergency physician: a new specialist moves into "the pit," Medical World News, February 1, 1974.

12. Flanagan, P., and Fortuna, J.: Emergency health services, American Journal of Public Health **64**:402-405, 1974.

13. Hammond, G.: The nurse's contribution to health and safety at work, Physiotherapy **61**:144-145, May, 1975.

14. Jamisson, K. G.: Of man, machine and malady, Medical Journal of Australia **1973**:1137-1142, 1973.

15. Korcok, M.: Conferences view auto deaths: the neglected disease, Canadian Medical Association Journal **111**:847-849, 1974.

16. Neumann, C. G., Neumann, A. K., Cockrell, M. E., and Banani, S.: Factors associated with child use of automobile restraining devices: knowledge, attitude, and practice, American Journal of Diseases of Children **128**:469-470, 1974.

17. Park, W. H., and DeMuth, W. E., Jr.: Wounding capacity of rotary lawn mowers, Journal of Trauma **15**:36-38, January, 1975.

18. Schwenger, C. W.: Injuries and injury control, Canadian Journal of Public Health **66**:221-233, 1975.

19. Smull, N. W., Wise, G. W., and Green, V.: Improved delivery of health care to children through poison control information, including data processing and clinical toxicology laboratory services, Clinical Toxicology **3**:281-288, 1970.

20. Verhulst, H. L.: Toward better utilization of federal and state resources in the communication of poison information, Clinical Toxicology **3**:275-276, 1970.

21. Werner, J. L.: Providing emergency medical services, Management Information Service Report **6**:1-17, August, 1974.

22. Westaby, J. R.: Injury control, American Journal of Public Health **64**:394-401, 1974.

Parameters for administering first aid in emergency care

WILLIAMS BAPTIST COLLEGE LIBRARY

1

GENERAL PROCEDURES FOR
EMERGENCY CARE

Guy S. Parcel

*Each emergency situation has its unique problems and charac-
teristics, all of which cannot be fully anticipated ahead of time. To
prevent as much as possible oversights or errors, it is necessary to
apply a standard set of general procedures to every emergency situation.*

At the time of an emergency involving an injury or sudden illness, everyone
involved, including the first aider, is under severe emotional stress and pressure
to take action and quickly find solutions to pressing problems of suffering and
threat to human life. Under these circumstances, it is absolutely essential that the
first aider be prepared to proceed in a calm, orderly, organized approach to the
administration of emergency care. The following general procedures are designed
to provide a framework for providing care for any type of emergency. The first
aider should proceed by following each general procedure step by step and plug-
ging in specific emergency care procedures as priorities are systematically determined. The following five general procedures provide the general framework
for administering emergency care:
1. Survey the situation.
2. Determine the nature and severity of injuries, illness, or presenting problem.
3. Administer appropriate first aid.
4. Notify appropriate authorities and arrange for transportation.
5. Complete follow-up care.
Each of these five procedures will be discussed in greater detail within this
chapter. Each step should be kept in mind while proceeding to offer care in an
emergency. For most emergencies one will be able to follow the procedures in
the order presented. However, circumstances surrounding a given emergency
may require a change in the sequence of the procedures. For example, if there
is someone to assist, it may be possible to have them notify authorities before
completion of the administration of first aid. Also, when the emergency is life
threatening, it is necessary to follow through emergency procedures for the most
serious problems before attending to non–life-threatening problems.

13

SURVEY THE SITUATION

A systematic approach to the administration of emergency care begins with the collecting and processing of pertinent information. This includes direct observation, collection of a history, and evaluation of the patient. The more complete the knowledge is about a given situation, the better one will be able to make the right decisions about the administration of emergency care. The amount of time that should be spent performing this first step (surveying the situation) will vary greatly depending on (1) how obvious are the presenting problems, (2) how life threatening are the presenting problems, (3) how much is already known about the patient, and (4) how threatening are the dangers within the immediate environment.

The following examples will serve to illustrate some possible implications of these factors. A driver involved in an automobile accident is thrown through the windshield and is lying on the pavement with a large gaping wound in the neck that is bleeding profusely. The bleeding is obvious, and it is immediately known that there are only seconds to control the bleeding. Therefore, the correct action is to quickly, without wasting time, apply first aid procedures. In contrast, a man is found lying on a department store floor, breathing, with no visible injuries. In this case the first aider must obtain certain information before it would be correct to apply specific first aid procedures.

Observation

The first task of the first aider when arriving on the scene of an accident or sudden illness is to size up the situation by carefully scanning the environment. This can be accomplished in a minimal amount of time if the first aider observed the cause of the emergency or if the underlying cause is apparent. Quickly look around for clues to the following questions:

1. How many people are involved?
2. Who has an emergency presenting problem?
3. What factors led up to the problem?
4. What were the basic mechanisms causing the problem?
5. What immediate dangers exist to the patient or to the first aider?

The emergency situation may involve more than one person. An accident, such as an automobile wreck, may cause injuries to several people. Food poisoning may affect a whole group of people. The parent of an injured or ill child may become emotionally upset, faint, or go into shock and become part of the emergency situation. Onlookers to an emergency may overreact and disrupt control of the situation. All of these factors can be observed and quickly taken into consideration.

Observation focused on mechanisms of cause will enable the first aider to begin to categorize the type of emergency. Falls and impacts will most likely lead to muscular skeletal injuries, head injuries, or internal bleeding. Situations involving sharp objects will cause primary concern for external bleeding. Electric shock, drowning, water accidents, or poisonous gases will focus attention on respiratory emergencies. Empty containers of toxic substances lead to suspicion of internal poisoning. Fire or hot objects precipitate concern for burns. Through quick observation the first aider can begin to narrow down the type of emergency and can begin to prepare for appropriate action.

History of the event

Not all injuries or illness problems will be easily observable. The process of surveying the situation continues by collecting a history of immediate past events and current complaints. If the patient is conscious, the history can be collected by direct questioning. The purpose of questioning at this point is to find out what happened so that major types of concern can be identified. Ask questions so that the patient provides you with the information rather than leading questions that may confuse the patient. For example, ask, "What happened?" or "How did it happen?" rather than, "Did you fall off the roof and break your arm?"

If the patient is unconscious or unable to respond to questions, a history can be collected from anyone who may have observed the incident. Guide the observer to focus on pertinent information. There is no need at this point to go into what might have happened, a similar accident they saw last year, or other irrelevant information.

History of the patient

Knowing the information associated with the events surrounding the injury will enable you to direct more specific questions related to the current status of the patient. In some situations it may be possible or necessary to move directly to history regarding the patient. The situation may be so obvious or the patient in such great distress that you may need to be concerned immediately with the patient's status.

Ask questions that are not leading and in a way that the questions will not upset the patient. Ask, "How do you feel?" rather than "Do you think you are going to faint?" Ask about major discomforts, and note the patient's chief complaints. Collect some baseline data so that you can get a picture of the patient as a particular type of person. Important data include age, sex, previous known health problems, name and location of personal physician, recent medications taken, members of the immediate family, and who to contact in regard to this emergency.

Time factor

Surveying the situation is important, but an unreasonable amount of time should not be spent that would delay essential first aid procedures. What is considered a reasonable amount of time will be determined by the circumstances of each individual emergency situation. The first concern is to recognize life-threatening problems and to intervene with appropriate first aid procedures. A careful survey of the situation will help to make decisions about priorities and prevent neglecting important considerations.

DETERMINE NATURE AND SEVERITY

During the second step in the standard procedures, the task is to determine the specific problem by considering the *nature* and the *severity* of the emergency. Nature is the classification of the type of emergency. Notice that this text broadly classifies emergencies into (1) cardiopulmonary, (2) trauma, and (3) medical emergencies and devotes a section of the text to each type. There is an overlap in that trauma or illness may lead to cardiopulmonary emergencies. This organization is intentional to emphasize the critical importance of maintaining adequate breathing and circulation of blood in all emergency situations.

The seriousness of an emergency is the estimated immediate risk to life or a graduation of a problem from mild to severe. An injury may be severe, such as a severe sprain, but it is not a threat to life; therefore it would not be as serious as severe shock, which would be a threat to life. Each chapter within Sections II, III, and IV in the text deals with specific emergencies that are subcategories of the major types of emergencies. The relative seriousness of the specific emergencies will be discussed within each chapter. After the completion of all three sections, one should be able to determine both the nature and severity of any emergency situation. Once this determination has been made, the first aider will be in a position to make effective decisions concerning appropriate first aid procedures.

Examination of the patient

The determination of the nature and severity of the emergency is based on careful evaluation of the patient. This process must not be done in a haphazard, disorganized fashion. There is too great a risk that critical information may be overlooked before action is taken. To determine both nature and severity of the emergency, examine the patient using the following sequence of procedures.

Check for vital life signs. First, is the patient breathing? Listen for air passing in and out of the mouth and/or nose. For laryngectomees (individuals who have had an operation that allows breathing through an opening in the neck), check for passage of air through the neck opening (Fig. 1-1). Observe the chest for rise and fall of the ribs as air moves in and out. Is skin color normal? A bluish color is an indication of a lack of adequate oxygen supply. For individuals with black or dark skin a change in skin color will be more difficult to determine. More subtle changes can be observed in the palms of the hands, soles of the feet, eyelids, and lips.

Second, is there effective circulation of blood? Examine for presence or absence of pulse at the radial artery (thumb side of wrist) or carotid artery (side of the neck). Observe the pupils of the eyes. Ineffective circulation will result in dilated (expanded) pupils that do not respond by constricting when exposed to light.

Checking the vital life signs will tell the first aider if there is cardiac arrest (stoppage of the heart) and/or pulmonary arrest (stoppage of breathing). Conditions involving cardiac and/or pulmonary arrest are given highest priority because of the immediate threat to life. Prompt action and first aid intervention must be taken at once.

Check for severe bleeding. It is usually possible to quickly observe severe bleeding from external wounds. However, be careful not to overlook severe bleeding from covered-up body parts or parts not visible because they are facing the ground or floor. Carefully examine the patient's entire body and look under clothing and debris for severe bleeding. Also, consider the possibility of serious internal bleeding when signs and symptoms of severe shock follow any type of trauma. Severe bleeding is given a high priority because it is possible to bleed to death, or excessive loss of blood can cause life-threatening shock in just a few minutes after injury. If severe external bleeding is immediately apparent, it may be necessary to intervene before taking any additional action or to attempt to control bleeding while checking for vital life signs.

Check for internal poisoning. Depending on the type and amount of chemical taken, internal poisoning can affect vital life functions and lead to death in a short period of time. In many cases, prompt intervention with emergency care means the difference between life and death. Specific signs and symptoms will vary depending on the ingested chemical; however, general indications of poisoning include empty containers, burns or stains in and around the mouth, and depressed breathing and circulation.

Check for shock. Shock is a depressed condition of the circulatory system resulting in insufficient flow of blood to the brain. Shock always has the potential to be life threatening, and severe shock requires rapid medical intervention. A patient in shock will appear pale, cold, and clammy, will have a weak and rapid pulse, may have depressed respiration, and may be unconscious.

Check body parts. After examining the patient for the above four conditions, examine the body parts by proceeding in the following order: (1) head, (2) neck, (3) chest, (4) abdomen, (5) back, (6) external genital organs, (7) arms, hands, and fingers, (8) legs, feet, and toes. Look for the following conditions when examining the patient: (1) internal damage to organs (for example, con-

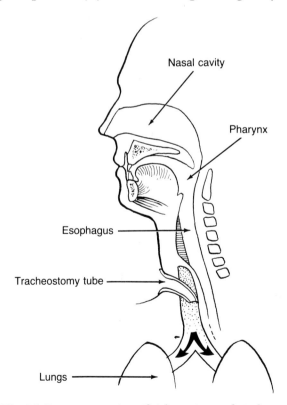

Fig. 1-1. Laryngectomy is artificial opening made in larynx.

cussion, collapsed lung, or ruptured spleen), (2) burns, (3) wounds, (4) fractures, (5) dislocations, (6) sprains, (7) strains, (8) contusions.

Check for sudden illness and nontraumatic problems. The foregoing procedures are primarily concerned with emergencies involving trauma. Emergency conditions may also arise from a variety of causes other than apparent trauma. These conditions may range from mild to life threatening. In emergencies that do not involve any apparent trauma, the first aider may proceed to examine the patient for types of sudden illness and nontraumatic problems. Specific conditions are presented in Chapters 13 to 16. When the specific presenting problem is not apparent, the first aider should proceed by reviewing the body systems, making note of patient's complaints and normal and abnormal functioning. Systems include nervous, cardiopulmonary, vascular, urinary, endocrine, digestive and excretory, reproductive, musculoskeletal, and skin.

Important signs and symptoms

A *symptom* is a departure from normal function in a patient that indicates disease, illness, or injury. Pain, dizziness, numbness, and nausea are examples of symptoms. A *sign* is an objective symptom, that is, a change in normal functioning that can be observed or measured, such as skin color, pulse rate, breathing rate, and deformity.

Types of medical emergencies caused by trauma, illness, or other abnormal functioning will produce physiological changes, some of which can be observed as symptoms and in some cases measured and therefore can be identified as specific signs. The remaining chapters in the text will present signs and symptoms for specific types of medical emergencies. In an emergency, it is the task of the first aider to examine the patient for signs and symptoms that will enable him or her to determine both the nature and severity of the problem or problems. Once this is accomplished, the first aider is in a position to administer the appropriate emergency care.

Following is a description of signs and symptoms that will assist the first aider in arriving at a determination of the type and severity of the emergency problem(s). Specific interpretations of the signs and symptoms will be discussed in the remainder of the book dealing with the different types of emergencies.

State of consciousness. State of consciousness is the status of the patient in terms of general wakefulness and responsiveness to the environment. Levels of consciousness may include:

1. *Alertness:* can communicate and respond to questioning and other stimuli
2. *Lethargy:* awake but responding slowly; may be confused about surroundings and recent events
3. *Drowsiness:* sleepy; unable to maintain attention; confused
4. *Semiunconsciousness:* difficulty in communicating and answering questions; little reaction to stimuli
5. *Unconsciousness:* noncommunicative; no response to stimuli; no controlled movement

Skin color. Look for major changes—red, white, or blue. (Check lips, palms, soles, and eyelids of black patients.)

Respiration. Rate is the number of breaths a minute, which can be fast or slow. The normal respiration rate is approximately 12 to 15 breaths a minute for adults and about 20 breaths a minute for children. Other descriptions of respiration may include shallow, deep, labored, or gasping respiration and absence of respiration.

Pulse. The pulse rate is an indirect measurement of the heart contractions per minute. As the heart pumps blood through the body, a corresponding beat can be felt in the larger arteries. The normal pulse rate is 60 to 80 beats a minute for adults and 80 to 100 beats a minute for children. The usual sites for taking a pulse are at the radial artery in the wrist and the carotid artery in the neck. As shown in Fig. 1-2, the correct technique is to use the fingers (never the thumb) to count the number of beats a minute.

In addition to the pulse rate it is important to monitor pulse intensity (strong versus weak). A strong pulse feels full and forceful, and in contrast a weak pulse may be thready and difficult to feel. The intensity of the pulse can be used as a rough indication of blood pressure, which is the pressure that circulating blood exerts against the walls of the arteries. A strong pulse may indicate elevated blood pressure, and a weak pulse may indicate lowered blood pressure.

When taking a pulse, both factors—rate and intensity—should be considered. Various types of emergencies will have specific effects on these two factors. For example, shock usually results in a weak and rapid pulse caused by lowered

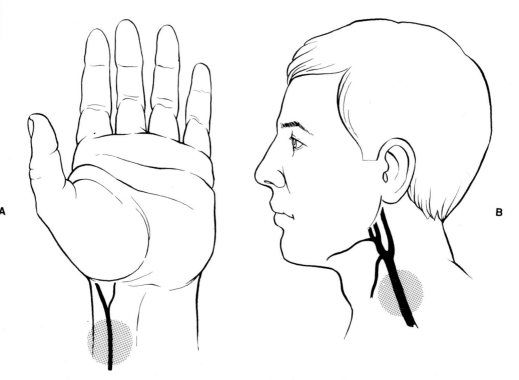

A   B

Fig. 1-2. Locations of **A**, radial, and **B**, carotid, pulse.

blood pressure and an increased heart rate. Other changes in the pulse will be discussed in the remaining chapters dealing with specific injuries.

Pupils. The circulation of blood to the pupils of the eyes is sensitive to changes in blood pressure and to brain injury resulting in pressure on the blood vessels. When exposed to light, the pupils normally constrict (opening narrows). If the pupil does not constrict and remains dilated (fixed open) when exposed to light (Fig. 1-3), this is usually an indication of insufficient circulation of blood. Together with an absence of breathing, this pupil dilation indicates cardiac failure (stoppage of the heart function).

Normally the pupils of both eyes respond in the same manner. If they are unequal (one constricted, one dilated), this is an indication of brain damage or abnormal pressure on blood vessels in the head. Possible causes include injury such as concussion, skull fracture, or cerebral vascular accidents (stroke).

An overdose of certain drugs may also affect the pupils of the eyes. For example, narcotics such as heroin produce pinpoint constriction of the pupils. Other drugs, depending on their effect on the circulatory system, may produce dilated pupils. The major first aid concern when observing dilated pupils would be depressed circulatory function.

The possibility of a glass eye should be considered whenever one is examining the eyes. Always examine both eyes and carefully compare the two eyes.

Pain. There are several factors to consider regarding pain as a symptom of illness or injury. The determination of pain requires a conscious patient and systematic questioning and observation by the first aider.

Ask: Where does it hurt?
Observe: General body area
          Specific anatomical structure
          Extent of the area that feels painful
Ask: How does it feel?
Observe: Sharp pain
          Dull pain
          Radiating pain
          Slight pain, tolerable
          Severe pain, intolerable
Ask: When does it hurt?
Observe: All the time
          Intermittent
          Only when part is moved
          Only when touched
Ask: How long has it hurt?
Observe: Sudden onset
          Gradual onset
          Time: day, hours, minutes
          Since injury

Individual patients will respond differently to pain. If the patient is frightened or hysterical, the pain may seem worse than it really is. In some cases such as severe shock, depression, or excessive alcohol or drug usage, the pain may be masked or not apparent. The absence of pain is not an indication of severity. Injuries involving nerve damage may disrupt the sensations of pain.

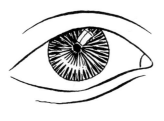 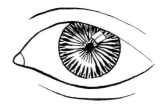

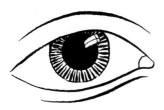 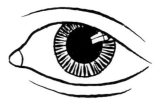

Fig. 1-3. Top: pupils constricted; bottom: pupils dilated.

Ability to move. Normal movement of body parts is dependent on normal functioning of muscular, skeletal, and nervous systems. Paralysis (inability to move) should be considered as an indication of damage to nerves, the spinal cord, or the brain. This may be caused by direct injury to the nerve fibers, fractured spine, head injury, cerebral vascular accident, tumors, certain illnesses, or prolonged use of some drugs.

Partial movement or painful movement may indicate injury to the musculoskeletal system. Extreme caution must be taken when examining a patient for ability to move body parts. If there is a fracture or spinal cord injury, movement can cause serious damage. Do not ask the patient to demonstrate movement unless you are sure that the movement will not cause further injury. Specific procedures relating to movement will be discussed in some of the remaining chapters.

Numbness. A loss of sensation to touch will produce a feeling of numbness in affected body parts. The patient may have difficulty feeling touch or pain induced by the first aider. This may result from disruption of nerve impulses or circulation of blood to the body part.

Swelling. A collection of blood, lymph, or other body fluid may produce a swelling of body tissues. This is usually more apparent in tissues close to the surface of the body. Swelling may result from injury, infection, allergic reaction, or disruption of normal blood flow.

Deformity. Injury to body parts may produce an abnormal positioning or appearance. Dislocated joints and sometimes fractures will produce deformities. Deformities can usually be determined by comparing the injured part to the corresponding uninjured part.

Discharge from body openings. Blood, mucus, or other fluid coming from body openings without apparent injuries to the opening is usually an indication of injuries to connecting internal organs or structures. Openings include ear, nose, mouth, urethra, anus, and vagina. It is important to make note of the color, consistency, and amount of the discharge.

Nausea and/or vomiting. Nausea is a general feeling of upset stomach, and vomiting is an expulsion of the contents of the stomach. Nausea and vomiting may indicate direct involvement of the upper gastrointestinal tract as caused by infection or poisoning. Also, general body reactions to stress, trauma, or illness may produce nausea and vomiting. The amount, contents, odor, color, and consistency of the vomited material should be noted.

Convulsions. A violent involuntary muscular contraction is referred to as a convulsion. Extremely high body temperature, epilepsy, brain damage, and poisoning with certain toxic agents are examples of conditions that might result in convulsions. The intensity and duration of the convulsions should be noted.

Interpretation. The signs and symptoms listed in this section are major clues the first aider can use to determine the type of emergency situation being presented by a patient. The detection of these symptoms requires observation of, listening to, and feeling body parts and body functions. The interpretation of these and more specific signs and symptoms will be presented in the remaining chapters.

ADMINISTER FIRST AID

The selection of appropriate first aid procedures is based on the interpretation of the data collected in the preceding steps: surveying the situation and determining the nature and severity of the emergency. The examination of a patient began with an evaluation of vital life signs and proceeded from the most serious conditions to the least serious. The same priority system must be applied to the administration of first aid. As soon as life-threatening conditions are detected, appropriate first aid must be applied. Administration of first aid for life-threatening emergencies must precede further examination for less serious conditions. Once the serious conditions have been cared for, then the first aider can continue examination and care for less serious conditions.

Cardiopulmonary arrest and profuse bleeding are given the highest priority. Time is a critical factor, and a few minutes are all that the first aider has to intervene in these emergencies. Internal poisoning and severe shock must also receive a high priority for administering first aid.

Next in priority are medical emergencies that require immediate medical intervention to resolve the threat to life. Medical emergencies include coma, heart attack, cerebral vascular accident, heat stroke, and surgical emergencies such as internal bleeding, appendicitis, and ruptured spleen. Serious and extensive burns also require rapid medical attention. Difficult or complicated childbirth should also be considered a medical emergency.

Injuries or conditions that are a threat to life must receive immediate first aid. Once these conditions are stabilized, then the examination should be continued and care provided for less serious problems. This approach is emphasized to prevent delay and possible oversight when administering first aid.

NOTIFY AUTHORITIES AND ARRANGE FOR TRANSPORTATION

All first aid emergencies must be referred to medical personnel and the appropriate authorities informed of the incident. First aid by definition is only *immediate* and *temporary* intervention. The first aider must never assume complete responsibility for the resolution of an emergency situation. In regard to emergency care, the first aider acts as a lay person and can act only within the limits of his or her first aid training. Referral means that the responsibility for a patient is turned over to higher authority who can assume medical and/or legal responsibility. This must be done to protect not only the patient but also the first aider.

When to notify

If someone else is present to assist the first aider, this step may be implemented before any other procedures. The first aider may instruct someone to call for assistance and arrange for transportation. If alone, it is necessary to first stabilize the patient and provide first aid for any problem that is a threat to life. If the patient is not in danger, all appropriate first aid may be carried out before notification and a referral is implemented. In some cases, transportation to medical care is the first and most important procedure.

Who to notify

This will depend on the nature of the emergency and the availability of emergency medical services. Serious life-threatening emergencies will require the most rapid assistance as well as the most qualified medical personnel. In a community with coordinated emergency medical services, this assistance is provided by a team of professionals. The first contact point is the established emergency telephone number. In many communities this number is 911. If there is no specific number, call the operator, police, or nearest hospital.

The first person to provide assistance may be a trained emergency medical technician (EMT). An EMT is trained to provide emergency care and to provide rapid transportation to a medical facility. It is appropriate for the first aider to turn over responsibility for the patient to the EMT. Not all ambulance drivers are trained emergency medical technicians. If the ambulance driver is not trained in emergency care, it may be appropriate for the first aider to remain with the patient during transportation and to turn over responsibility for the patient to emergency room personnel at the nearest hospital.

In most cases, it is best to rely on professional transportation (ambulance) rather than private vehicle. An ambulance is usually better equipped to transport the patient safely to a medical facility. If it is necessary to transport the patient in a private vehicle, do not speed or ignore traffic regulations. Many accidents have occurred as a result of someone attempting to speed to a hospital. If possible, contact the police to provide an escort to the hospital. When rapid transportation is not necessary, take the time to provide the safest, most comfortable means of transportation.

The police must be notified in any incident that involves violence, a criminal act, or a motor vehicle accident. The fire department should be notified if any emergency involves fire, smoke, threat of fire or explosion, escaping gas, or the need for rescue equipment. Special rescue squads may be needed for extrication and removal of entrapped victims. If the patient has a private physician, attempts should be made to contact the physician. The patient's physician may have valuable information or knowledge about the patient that will greatly contribute to providing emergency care.

The notification of the patient's relatives is usually not the responsibility of the first aider. This responsibility is usually assumed by the medical personnel who are providing care for the patient. In some cases the first aider may become involved in notifying the relatives. The patient may request that someone be notified before referral to medical personnel, or there may be a delay in transporting to a medical facility. If action is taken to notify relatives, it is important to calmly explain who you are, what happened, and what is being done. Do not go into extensive detail attempting to make a diagnosis or prognosis concerning the problem. Let the relatives know where they can see the patient or indicate where the patient is being transported.

Information to be provided

Regardless of who is being notified of an emergency, certain essential information must be provided. It is important to emphasize that one should clearly think through the sequence of information items to make sure that a critical item is not left out. The following essential information should always be provided:

1. *Identification:* your name, telephone number, and location where you are calling from
2. *Nature of emergency:* kind of emergency (accident, drowning, illness), number of people injured or ill, and seriousness of injuries or conditions
3. *First aid instructions:* what has been done and what type of assistance or equipment is needed
4. *Directions* for locating the site of the emergency (if possible, have someone waiting in the street to flag down the ambulance and lead to the patient)

Try to be calm and talk clearly. Do not hang up until the person you notified has had an opportunity to ask questions and it is clear that he has the correct information, and wait until he hangs up the phone.

FOLLOW-UP CARE

Follow-up care consists of procedures to support, supplement, and follow first aid. These procedures range from general care provided by the first aider to technical procedures performed by medical personnel. In most emergencies, the first aider should consider these general follow-up care procedures:

1. Maintain an open airway and check vital life signs.
2. Make the patient comfortable: loosen clothing and support limbs and body parts.
3. Maintain body temperature: keep warm and prevent excessive loss of body heat.
4. Provide emotional support and reassurance.
5. Provide fluids unless contraindicated by the type of injury or illness.

6. Maintain crowd control: keep bystanders from interfering with the administration of first aid or the comfort of the patient.
7. Complete arrangements for referral: for minor injuries or nonserious illness, advise the patient of the importance of obtaining follow-up medical care. More serious emergencies will require direct referral to medical personnel.

More specific follow-up procedures will be outlined in the remaining chapters as they apply to specific types of emergencies. Many follow-up procedures require the experience and training of emergency medical personnel. The role of the first aider is to recognize the need for medical care and to obtain that care as efficiently as possible.

SUMMARY

An orderly approach to emergency care is most likely to be achieved if the first aider has a predetermined framework for approaching emergency situations. The general procedures outlined in this chapter are intended to serve as a framework for approaching most emergency care situations. This framework should be applied when studying the remaining text material and practicing specific emergency care procedures. Although the general procedures are not mentioned in each chapter, it is important that the first aider keep these procedures clearly in mind and apply them to each emergency care situation.

FIRST AIDER COMPETENCIES

After studying the material presented in this chapter, the student should be able to:
- List in order the five general procedures for administering emergency care.
- Describe how to survey an emergency situation.
- Explain the difference between the nature and the severity of an emergency.
- Outline procedures for examining a patient, indicating the priorities that must be considered.
- List and describe major signs and symptoms that can be used to assist in determining the nature and severity of an emergency problem.
- Explain how priorities are established for the administration of first aid procedures.
- Describe procedures for notifying authorities and list essential information to be provided by the first aider.
- List general follow-up procedures for administering emergency care.

2

▲▲

LEGAL CONSIDERATIONS INVOLVED IN EMERGENCY CARE BY NONMEDICAL PERSONNEL

Mary Dolores Hemelt

RESPONSIBILITY FOR PROVIDING EMERGENCY CARE

The traditional common-law rule holds that there is no legal duty to provide emergency aid to another human being who is in danger. Therefore any individual may legitimately refuse to supply first aid in an emergency. The refusal assumes that there is no legal requirement to provide emergency care under certain circumstances. A person cannot be charged with negligence when there is no legal obligation to act. Although there is no legal obligation to provide emergency care, most individuals realize there is a moral duty to provide care, and they are also aware of the public disapproval that would follow from refusal to give basic emergency care that could save a life.

One must clearly understand that there is no legal duty to act in an emergency situation. But if one undertakes to assist a person in an emergency and the aid negligently causes injury, then legal liability may be incurred. The legal principle is that when one undertakes an affirmative course of conduct, then a duty of reasonable care is owed and becomes the standard by which the law will measure and evaluate the aid provided. Generally, any individual who gives reasonable emergency care under existing emergency circumstances will be protected from any liability that might arise.

The Good Samaritan law

Beginning in 1941, forty states enacted legislation that has become known as the Good Samaritan law. Generally the statute provides that a doctor or nurse who renders emergency care to accident victims shall be immune from civil damages as a result of ordinary negligence in giving such care. In some states the Good Samaritan statute covers only roadside accidents, other states include emergencies, and still others are moving to grant immunity to resuscitation teams. In some states only doctors or nurses are covered by the statute, whereas other states have extended the statute to cover policemen, firemen, and other paramedical personnel. The intent of this legislation was to encourage health personnel to give lifesaving care to victims of accidents by providing immunity from civil liability to those persons rendering emergency care. The immunity is automatic unless the emergency care was grossly negligent. Despite myth and misunderstanding surrounding the purpose of the law, there is no recorded instance in which a medical person has been found liable for assisting a victim at the scene of an accident and giving emergency medical care.

The State of Vermont[1] is unique in imposing a duty on all its citizens to give reasonable aid to other citizens exposed to grave physical harm. The Vermont statute imposes a positive duty on all persons and imposes criminal sanctions for failure to give reasonable aid and does not limit this duty to roadside accidents.

The Secretary's Commission on Medical Malpractice[9] studied this emergency care issue and recommended that all states enact legislation that would provide qualified immunity to health care personnel responding to emergencies arising from unexpected complications arising while giving medical treatment such as resuscitation.

Care by nonmedical personnel

The giving of first aid by a nonphysician constitutes the *administration* of medical treatment. It *does not* constitute the practice of medicine.[11] In Smith vs. City of Lexington,[10] a 1957 Kentucky case, the Court of Appeals of Kentucky held that a first aid and emergency service operated by the municipal fire department was a proper exercise of governmental function.

There are no known cases to date in which a teacher or teachers' associates have been sued and found liable in giving first aid or emergency care to children in their charge. If such cases would begin to develop and result in teachers or teaching personnel failing to act for fear of litigation, then, it appears, they as a body would need to seek appropriate legislation to protect themselves. Anyone who has dealt with the legislature knows that only after the fact and after a need is demonstrated is legislation enacted. There is no data base at present to support an argument for or against teacher emergency immunity statutes. As everyone becomes more proficient and more knowledgeable in giving first aid and emergency care, legislation to protect those who perform their job in a reasonable and conscientious manner should quickly follow.

A case of a District Court of the United States, decided in 1964,[2] illustrates the doctrine of respondeat superior ("let the master respond") and how an agent or employee of an institution can involve the employer in a lawsuit.

Thomas Downie, an electrician aboard a ship owned by U.S. Lines Company, complained of sharp pain in the chest that radiated down his arm. He was sent to the Ship's Purser by his immediate supervisor. The Ship's Purser, Pomerleau, also served as a Pharmacist's Mate. Pomerleau gave Downie a note requesting treatment addressed to the medical officer at the Albert Dock Hospital. He directed Downie to the hospital, which was a mile away, and made no arrangements for transportation. Downie proceeded to walk the mile to the hospital. He suffered a heart attack and was confined to a hospital for 3 weeks. Downie sued Pomerleau and contended that Pomerleau knew, or should have known, that Downie may have been suffering a heart attack and should have put him on strict bedrest. Downie said that the book *The Ship's Medicine Chest and First*

Aid at Sea was required to be aboard the vessel and in fact was aboard the vessel and that Pomerleau did not make use of the book. On cross-examination, Pomerleau admitted the first aid treatments indicated for the symptoms demonstrated by Downie were bedrest and call a doctor. The book clearly verified this was the case. The court found Pomerleau negligent in this instance.

OBLIGATIONS OF TEACHERS, TEACHER'S AIDES, AND GUARDIANS IN EMERGENCY AID SITUATIONS

Traditionally the education of children was considered a duty and obligation of the state. Consequently the student was perceived as a ward of the state. It became acceptable to refer to the state as acting in loco parentis, that is to say, "in the place of parents." It was then axiomatic that teachers were considered to be in loco parentis during the time students were under their jurisdiction.

The state has always perceived certain classes of persons as being under a liability or handicap. Some examples of such persons are the mentally retarded, the aged, children, and the sick and infirm. These classes of persons who often are unable to protect themselves are the object of special solicitude on the part of the state. Professionals or individuals dealing with such handicapped persons generally owe them a higher degree of care. The standard in dealing with the ordinary, average person is that of the duty of ordinary care. It is assumed that the average person is capable of protecting himself or herself and making adequate judgments in his or her own regard, hence the state imposes no special duty unless there are other extenuating circumstances.

Teachers or persons employed in agencies that give care in any capacity to the young have a special obligation or a duty of higher care. Because of the special relationship of teacher to student, the teacher is considered to be in loco parentis. The younger the child in age or the more diminished his faculties, the higher the duty of care or responsibility. The teacher would be obligated to anticipate that a child of tender years such as a kindergarten student would need more observation than a junior high school student.

But does the teacher have a legal obligation to render medical care in emergency situations? The principles of law would be the same as outlined before. The teacher would have no legal obligation to give medical emergency care unless (1) he or she were qualified to render such care, (2) he or she had contracted to render such care, or (3) state statutes imposed or mandated the rendering of such care.

Does the teacher have a moral or ethical obligation to render the best emergency care possible under the circumstances? Most members of the teaching profession and members of the general public would say that teaching is a profession of public trust and teachers and their associates have a definite obligation to those entrusted to their care.

CONCEPTS OF LIABILITY

Law is the sum total of rules and regulations by which society is governed. It reflects society's needs, ethics, attitudes, and mores. The law is not a rigid, inflexible set of rules. The law is a composite of court decisions, state and federal statutes, and administrative regulations. Interpretations of laws by different courts in different states may lead to different conclusions in what appear to be the same factual situations. The courts apply certain principles of law to a particular set of facts. Because reasonable men can differ as to the inferences and conclusions to be drawn from the same set of facts, so too can reasonable men perceive that different principles of law are appropriate to the same circumstances.

The general category of law concerned here is called *torts*. A tort is a legal wrong committed against the person or property of another. It involves unreasonable interference with the interests and rights of others; it is conduct that is socially unreasonable. It is the inherent right of every individual to expect individuals to use reasonable care in their dealings with one another.

Doctrine of personal liability

At law every person is responsible for conducting himself or herself in a reasonable and prudent manner, regardless of whether he or she is a layperson or a professional. *Liability* refers to the state of being held legally responsible for the harm one causes another individual.

A fundamental rule of law is that everyone is responsible for his or her own negligent acts. This is known as the rule of personal liability. This rule of law says a wrongdoer cannot avoid legal liability for wrongdoing even though another is equally liable.

Doctrine of respondeat superior

Another related legal doctrine is the doctrine of respondeat superior, "let the master respond." This doctrine holds an employer liable for the negligent acts of his employees that occur while the employee is working within the scope of his authority and in the employer's interests. Since few, if any, teachers are self-employed, the doctrine of respondeat superior is of paramount importance. Two things must be present before the employer can be held liable for the negligence of the employee: (1) there must be an employer-employee relationship, and (2) the employee must be functioning within the scope of his or her job parameters when the negligent act is committed. For example, if the school policy states that a teacher is not to transport students in his or her private car but may use only a school or college car, if a teacher transports a student he or she does so at his or her own risk. In the event of an automobile accident, the school or agency employing the teacher would not be liable for any negligent acts of the teacher because the act was outside the policies of the school. The teacher if negligent would be personally liable.

Doctrine of the reasonably prudent person

The main standard or criteria on which all of our actions are measured is reasonableness. The law refers to it as the reasonably prudent person theory. This standard requires an individual to function as any reasonable person of ordinary prudence, with comparable education, skills, and training under similar circumstances would act in a comparable situation. Although a simple concept, everything is relative to the particular set of circumstances at a particular time. For example, if a student were injured on school property or while participating in school activities, it would be reasonable to expect that a teacher would do what any reasonable person would do in the circumstance. The teacher would examine the injury and determine whether medical care or hospitalization is necessary. If the need for care is determined, the teacher would see that the student gets appropriate medical attention.

I extend a caveat (warning). The brief review of a limited number of principles serves only for illustration of the concepts of liability and does not purport to be an extensive study of the law. These main concepts are hopefully sufficient for the purposes of this text.

WAYS TO PREVENT AND LIMIT LIABILITY

No matter how sophisticated many of us as professionals would like to perceive ourselves, each is concerned about the possibility of being sued and, worse, being found liable as a result of our actions while performing our job or related activities. No one can guarantee immunity from suit, but some means to limit or diminish the potential for litigation are the following.

Recording the incident

During an emergency situation, the person providing assistance is not primarily concerned with documenting the incident. After the assistance is given, the events preceding care, the type of care itself, and any observations after the care should be written down as soon as possible. No one should rely on memory for recalling any significant facts. The most important thing to remember in recording events is to record facts, not opinions. Record what your senses tell you, that is, what you see, hear, smell, or palpate (such as a lump or swelling). For example, if an individual is staggering and talking funny, or seeming to act drunk, your record might read, "victim or individual swaying when walking, speech was slurred, odor of alcohol was on breath." It is up to the doctor or other interested persons to draw the appropriate or educated conclusions.

Some experts may disagree as to the necessity of nonmedical personnel making a record. Although not legally required, it would appear to be the wiser course of action. The main purpose of the record is to provide a means of communication between the health professionals contributing to the patient's care and the individual who gave first aid emergency care. It would serve the patient's best medical interest because it would relay to the doctor important symptoms initially demonstrated by the patient to which he or she was privy. The record serves as that of an objective eyewitness, assists the doctor is either diagnosing or treating the patient's symptoms, and may serve as a legal document for the patient if proof for insurance, workmen's compensation, criminal charges, or other purposes is necessary for the patient's benefit. It would also give a measure of protection to the individual giving the emergency care in the event there was a conflict of testimony during any litigation that might arise. There is no question a memo of events has both medical and legal value, but its value depends on the accuracy and objectivity of the recorder. The medical record is a confidential document. It would become the legal property of the doctor or hospital treating the patient. The patient would have the right to authorize access to the record to any appropriate persons or agencies.

Confidentiality

The development of the common-law right to privacy is for the protection of an individual who desires to live free from undesired publicity. The principle is the weighing of the individual's right to privacy against the public's right to know.

An individual who has been injured and is in need of emergency care or first aid submits himself or herself to the integrity of the person providing the care. Strictly speaking, there is no legal obligation of confidentiality imposed on a nonmedical individual rendering emergency care. In absence of a confidentiality statute, common law recognizes only the fiduciary relationship (relationship of confidence or trust) of the psychiatrist, attorney, and clergyman.

It is conceivable that an individual rendering emergency care may be involved in caring for persons under the influence of drugs, alcohol, or other conditions that are not for publication. The patient receiving care is entitled to a certain degree of privacy. Ethics require than an individual may not reveal the confidences entrusted to him in the course of a relationship unless required by the law or to protect the welfare of the patient or the community. The communication, though not privileged under the law, would still require the consideration of moral and ethical responsibilities. Most legal and health experts stress the confidentiality of patient's records and verbal information under such circumstances as a basic right. It comes under the constitutional right to privacy under the U.S. Constitution enunciated in the decisions of the U.S. Supreme Court.

Policies and procedure guidelines

The importance of emergency care cannot be minimized. Colleges, schools, and public institutions, where emergencies are likely to occur, should provide guidelines for nonmedical, uninitiated persons to follow before, during, and after an emergency. The policies and procedure guidelines should include instructions to be followed, persons to be contacted, and records to be prepared for the institution. The policies and practices should be modified to meet the needs of the institution and the students or employees of the institution. A manual should be developed and maintained continuously to assure that those who properly follow the established policies shall have the support of the administration whenever appropriate.

Another aspect of the policy factor dictates that the institution carry adequate liability insurance, workmen's compensation insurance, and other appropriate insurance in accordance with the specific requirements of the laws of the state and sound business practices.

Permission or consent to treatment

There should be some attention devoted to the issue of permission or consent to treatment. The general rule of law is that consent of the individual to be treated must be obtained unless an emergency exists. An emergency is defined as an unforeseen combination of circumstances or the resulting state that calls for immediate action. Any treatment performed on an individual without a valid consent is generally construed to be a trespass. An emergency situation is an exception. But the problem is in determining what is and what is not a true emergency. Consent may also be implied from the circumstances. It would be implied by law that an unconscious individual who was hemorrhaging would consent to having someone stop the bleeding to save his or her life.

In many states, minors 18 years or older may donate blood without consent of parents if they are not paid for the blood. The majority of the states also permit minors who are pregnant, who are thought to have a venereal disease, or who are emancipated by marriage to accept clinical or medical services without parental permission. Each person should know the age of minority held by their particular state, since some states hold an individual reaches the age of majority at 18 years of age, and other states hold 21 years of age is majority.

The unlicensed or nonmedical person who renders aid in an emergency situation without the expressed consent of the individual being aided is considered to be benefiting the public at large or society as a whole by the action. It is because of this overriding public interest that the law condones the care given to a patient in an emergency. This is the priority, and unless there is gross and wanton negligence, the law will protect the individual who assists another at such a critical time.

Therefore, it should be evident that although there are some risks in rendering first aid or emergency care, if done in a reasonable manner considering all the circumstances, one has little fear of litigation and even less fear of being found liable for negligent behavior.

SUMMARY

- No one has a legal obligation to render emergency care.
- One who assumes the obligation by a positive act of rendering care owes the patient a reasonable degree of care and skill under the existing emergency circumstances.
- The Good Samaritan statute enacted in most states confers immunity from liability unless the provider was grossly negligent.
- Any individual rendering emergency care should know his or her own limitations and act only within the parameters of his or her own abilities.
- A record of any care rendered should be documented with any appropriate observations.
- Everyone is responsible for his or her own negligent acts.
- The employer can be held vicariously liable for the employee's negligence.
- Everyone is required to act in a reasonable manner under the specific circumstances.
- A patient or individual receiving emergency or first aid care is entitled to an ethical duty of confidentiality.
- Guidelines to be followed in providing emergency care should be developed and made available to all appropriate personnel.
- Teachers by professional calling have a higher ethical and moral obligation to their students.
- Legislation to protect teachers by granting immunity from liability similar to the present Good Samaritan statutes may be warranted in the immediate future.
- Consent to treatment is implied in certain circumstances.

REFERENCES AND RECOMMENDED READINGS

1. Annotated code of Vermont, 12 section 519 (Supp. 1971).
2. Downie vs. U.S. Lines Co., 231 F. Supp. 192 (1964).
3. Goldsmith, L., editor: Liability of hospitals and health care facilities (H4-2894), New York, 1973, Practicing Law Institute.
4. Hay, E., and Hayt, J.: Law of hospital, physician and patient, ed. 3, Berwyn, Ill., 1972, Physicians' Record Co.
5. Lasagna, L. C.: Life, death, and the doctor, New York, 1968, Alfred A. Knopf, Inc.
6. Medical malpractice: report of the Secretary's Commission on Medical Malprac-tice, (0573-88), Washington, D.C., 1973, U.S. Department of Health, Education, and Welfare.
7. Practicing Law Institute: Doctor and hospital liability today (H4-2874), New York, 1972.
8. Professional negligence in hospital emergency rooms, Journal of the American Medical Association **208**:231, April 7, 1969.
9. Report of the Secretary's Commission on Medical Malpractice ([OS] 73-88), Washington, D.C., U.S. Department of Health, Education, and Welfare.
10. Smith vs. City of Lexington, 307 S.W. 568 (1957).
11. State vs. Medcraft, 9 P2d 84 (1932).

Cardiopulmonary emergencies

3

▲▲

CARDIOPULMONARY ARREST AND RESUSCITATION

Guy S. Parcel

If an accident or condition results in the cessation of breathing and/or the absence of functional circulation, the patient will die in 4 to 6 minutes unless effective cardiopulmonary resuscitation techniques are immediately applied by the first aider.

Clinical death occurs when a person's heart stops beating and he ceases to breathe. The various cells and tissues of the body do not immediately die but begin to deteriorate as the oxygen supply ceases. Many organs remain biologically alive for a short time after clinical death has occurred. If the patient can be documented to have been without oxygen for over 10 minutes, then resuscitation is unlikely to restore the victim to normal central nervous system functioning. The period of 4 to 6 minutes after clinical death offers the first aider the best opportunity to reverse conditions leading to death and perhaps save a human life.

CARDIOPULMONARY FUNCTION

The human body requires various processes to maintain life. Among these processes are the intake of oxygen and the corresponding elimination of the waste product, carbon dioxide. The exchange of these gases between the human body and its environment is referred to as respiration. It is important to understand the fundamental principles of the process of respiration so that accurate and rapid decisions are made when cardiopulmonary emergencies occur. A brief summary of normal basic respiratory function is presented in the following paragraph. For detailed information, refer to the anatomy and physiology texts listed among the references at the end of the chapter.

Respiration can be divided into two types: *external,* the exchange of gases in the lungs; and *internal,* the exchange of gases at the cellular level. Air moves from the surrounding environment through the nose, the pharynx (throat), the larynx (voice box), the trachea (windpipe), the bronchi, and into the lungs by means of the development of negative intrathoracic pressure (Fig. 3-1). This is accomplished by the contraction of the diaphragm and the chest-elevating muscles, which increase the diameter of the thorax, thereby creating a reduction in intrathoracic pressure resulting in lung expansion. Air flows into the alveoli (air

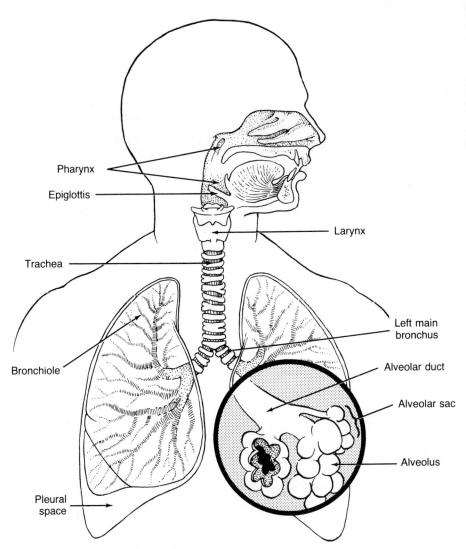

Fig. 3-1. Respiratory system structures.

sacs) of the lungs because the pressure in the lungs becomes less than that of the atmosphere. Oxygen is then passed into the bloodstream, and carbon dioxide is passed into the lungs. Expiration occurs when the inspiratory muscles relax, raising the intrathoracic pressure, creating a positive pressure gradient from alveoli to the atmosphere.

The circulatory system carries out the function of internal respiration. Four pulmonary veins (two from each lung) carry oxygenated blood back to the heart, which then pumps it through the arterial tree of the body. Throughout the body oxygen diffuses from the capillaries to cells, and carbon dioxide diffuses from cells to the capillaries. Deoxygenated blood returns to the heart by the veins. The heart pumps the blood to the lungs through the pulmo-

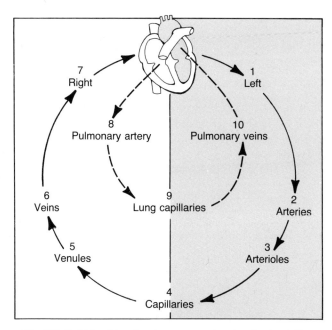

Fig. 3-2. Relationship of pulmonary and systemic circulation.

nary arteries to complete the cycle of internal and external respiration. (See Fig. 3-2.)

Both types of respiration are essential for human life, since one cannot function without the other for any significant period of time. With this in mind, the first aider will be able to better understand the role and function of cardiopulmonary resuscitation. If a person suddenly stops breathing, the first aider must supply air to the lungs to carry on external respiration. If the heart stops beating effectively, the first aider must supply artificial circulation (external cardiac massage) so that internal respiration may take place.

Many conditions or types of traumas may lead to an interruption or interference of normal breathing and circulation. Most common among small infants are respiratory obstructions from foreign objects and accidental poisoning from toxic substances such as aspirin. During middle childhood and adolescence, drowning is often the cause of cardiopulmonary failure. Heart disease is the leading cause of death among adults, and heart attacks will frequently lead to ineffective circulation. Other causes of respiratory failure include anaphylactic reaction, such as sensitivity to insect bites; lack of oxygen, such as suffocation in a plastic bag or abandoned refrigerator; electric shock; depression from drugs, such as sleeping pills; or compression of the chest cavity.

Special problems may be created by each particular cause of cardiopulmonary failure. Special considerations with which the first aider may be required to cope will be presented in the next two chapters. The following material is a presentation of techniques and skills necessary for successful cardiopulmonary resuscitation.

CARDIOPULMONARY RESUSCITATION TECHNIQUES

The probability of successful resuscitation rapidly decreases with time. Therefore it is critical that the first aider immediately check for the presence of breathing in all patients.

Indications for resuscitation

The first aider may recognize the stoppage of breathing by the following procedures: (1) look for absence of the rise and fall of the chest (movement of the chest and abdomen may occur in the presence of an obstructed airway); (2) listen and feel for the movement of air at the mouth and nose; and (3) observe the skin color, since blue skin will usually indicate a lack of oxygen supply.

Establishment of an open airway

As shown in Fig. 3-3, the muscles at the base of the tongue will usually fall back against the pharynx, blocking the air passage to the lungs. The opening of the airway can be easily and quickly accomplished by extending the neck and tilting the head backward (Fig. 3-4). The first aider should place the patient in a supine position, place one hand under the neck and lift upward, and place the other hand on the forehead and push downward. An unconscious patient should never be left with his head elevated by a pillow. In many cases the establishment of an open airway may be all that is needed for the patient to resume breathing. If the establishment of an open airway does not result in effective breathing, ventilation by mouth to mouth is indicated.

Ventilation by the mouth-to-mouth method

Since biological death will occur in 4 to 6 minutes, little time should be wasted before beginning artificial ventilation. No more than 10 seconds should be needed to prepare the patient for mouth-to-mouth resuscitation. This includes the establishment of an open airway.

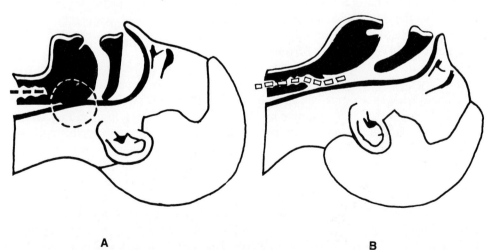

A   **B**

Fig. 3-3. A, Position of tongue muscles blocking airway. **B,** Airway opened by extending neck and pulling tongue muscles away from airway.

With the fingers of the hand pushing on the forehead, pinch the nose and maintain the upward lift of the neck with the other hand to keep an open airway throughout resuscitation. Then open your mouth widely, take a deep breath, make a tight seal with your mouth around the patient's mouth, and blow into the airway, watching for the chest to rise (Fig. 3-5). Then remove your mouth and allow passive exhalation.

Determine whether sufficient air is reaching the lungs by (1) observing the rise and fall of the chest, (2) feeling resistance of the lungs as they expand, and (3) listening for air to pass out during exhalation. If these three conditions do not occur, double-check your procedure: extend the neck, pinch the nose, and make an airtight seal with your mouth. Sometimes it is necessary to further open the air passages by displacing the lower jaw forward. This can be done by grasping the jaw with the fingers and pulling forward or by pushing the jaw forward at the angles of the jaw (Fig. 3-6).

If efforts to get air into the lungs are still unsuccessful, there may be an obstruction in the airway. For an unconscious patient with a respiratory obstruction use the following procedures:

1. Administer four back blows. Kneel and roll the patient onto his or her side, facing you with the chest against your knee(s). Deliver sharp blows to the back with the heel of your hand over the patient's spine between the shoulder blades. Place your other hand on the chest to provide support.
2. Administer eight manual thrusts. Abdominal thrust is performed by placing the patient face up, with your knees close to the hips. Place the heel of one hand against the patient's abdomen between the tip of the sternum

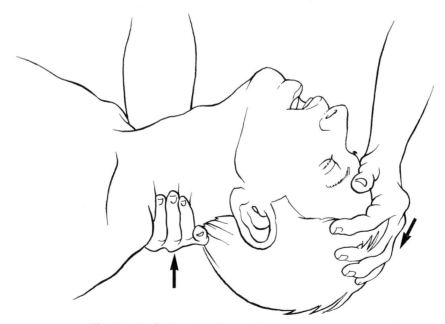

Fig. 3-4. Head tilt method for establishing open airway.

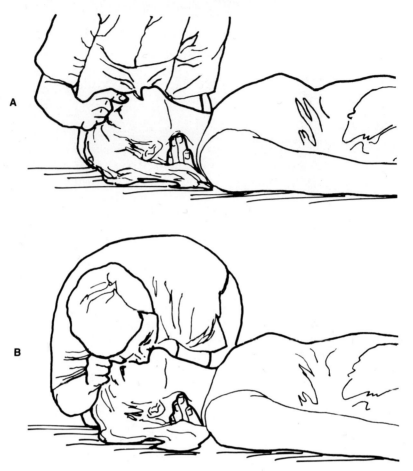

Fig. 3-5. Mouth-to-mouth resuscitation. **A,** Position for pinching nose closed. **B,** Position for making seal around patient's mouth.

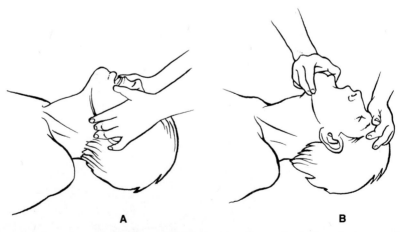

Fig. 3-6. Supplemental methods for establishing open airway. **A,** Pushing lower jaw forward. **B,** Pulling lower jaw forward.

and the umbilicus (navel). Place the second hand on top of the first. Press into the patient's abdomen with a quick upward thrust.

3. Open the mouth using the jaw lift technique. Insert your index finger down the inside of the cheek, deeply into the throat to the base of the tongue. Then use a hooking action to dislodge the foreign body and maneuver it into the mouth. Sometimes it is necessary to use the index finger to push the foreign body against the opposite side of the throat. Be careful not to force the object into the airway. Grasp the foreign object and remove it.

4. Reposition the head with extended neck and attempt to ventilate the patient.

5. If this is unsuccessful, repeat the preceding steps.

Efforts are continued because the muscles may relax, making it easier to remove the obstruction. If only a partial dislodging of the object is possible, a slow, full, forceful ventilation may keep the patient alive by bypassing the obstruction. If there is vomitus in the mouth or throat, turn the head to the side, wipe it out, and proceed.

Mouth-to-mouth procedures should be repeated twelve times a minute except for the first four inflations, which should be somewhat faster. Ventilate the lungs four times and then palpate the carotid pulse. If there is a pulse, continue ventilation. No pulse indicates the need to go to the procedures for external cardiac compression and artificial ventilation. The procedures for mouth-to-mouth resuscitation are the same for children except that the child's mouth and nose should be covered with your mouth. Also increase the rate of inflations to 15 to 20 times a minute for children and 20 plus for infants. The lungs of a baby are much smaller and will require only small puffs of air to inflate.

An alternative method for the mouth-to-mouth method is mouth-to-nose. This is accomplished by keeping the mouth closed and blowing directly into the nose. However, allow the mouth to open for exhalation. It may be necessary to use the mouth-to-nose method if the structures of the mouth have been damaged to the extent that an airtight seal cannot be formed. The mouth-to-mouth method is considered to be a more effective method than the mouth-to-nose method.

External cardiac compression

Both external and internal respiration must occur to supply the required oxygen to the individual cells so that the functions of the vital organs may continue. Therefore, if after four lung inflations the patient has not started breathing independently, quickly determine the status of circulation. This is accomplished by checking for the presence of the carotid pulse. If the pulse is *absent,* breathing is absent, and victim has a deathlike appearance, then effective circulation has ceased, and external cardiac compression must be started immediately. External cardiac compression does involve a certain amount of risk and should be administered only when indicated by cardiac failure. Cardiopulmonary resuscitation (CPR) correctly performed can provide approximately a third the normal carotid blood pressure. To protect against damage to internal organs and to achieve maximum benefit, it is essential to follow the established procedures as closely as possible.

Precordial thump. In some cases cardiac arrest is characterized by abnormal contractions of the heart that result in ineffective pumping of the blood. These conditions are explained in Chapter 6 and may include sudden ventricular fibrillation, ventricular tachycardia, or asystole. In cases in which there is witnessed cardiac arrest with suspected arrhythmia, a thump delivered to the chest within a minute of arrest may restore regular heart contractions (Fig. 3-7). The precordial thump is performed by elevating the hand 8 to 12 inches above the sternum and delivering a strong blow of about 100 pounds to the patient's midsternum with the fleshy side of the fist. The thump must be delivered within a minute of cardiac arrest. Take a pulse before and after giving the thump. Give the thump only once; if there is no pulse, go into procedures for CPR. The precordial thump is not effective for established cardiac failure in which generalized hypoxia (oxygen deficiency) of the heart muscle occurs. It is also not recommended for children.[22]

CPR procedures for adults

1. Place the patient on a firm surface (floor, board, or firm object).
2. Position yourself at either side of the patient. Do not straddle the patient.
3. Locate the lower half of the sternum (breastbone) and place the heel of one hand about an inch above the xiphoid process (tip of the sternum) with the long axis parallel with the sternum. Place the other hand over

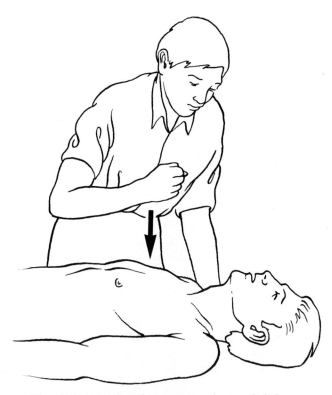

Fig. 3-7. Position for administration of precordial thump.

the first. Keep your fingers up, and apply pressure only at the point where the heel of the hand contacts the sternum (Fig. 3-8).

4. Apply pressure downward, keeping the arms straight and using the body weight for compression. Press a half second down and a half second up, using a smooth, uninterrupted rhythm.

5. Depress the sternum 1½ to 2 inches at a rate of once a second for adults. This requires 80 to 120 pounds of pressure. The action should be regular, avoiding sudden or jerking movements, maintaining contact on the sternum, but not on the chest wall.

6. If alone, first inflate the lungs three to five times and follow with 15 compressions. Then continue by alternating two deep, rapid inflations of the lungs with 15 compressions (a ratio of 2:15) at a rate of 80 compressions a minute.

7. If two operators are present, continue closed-chest compression at a rate of once a second while the other operator rapidly inflates the lungs after

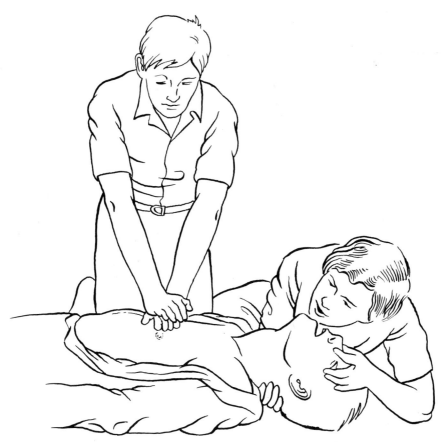

Fig. 3-8. Position for two-rescuer cardiopulmonary resuscitation. The two rescuers are on same side of patient for illustration purposes. In practice the two rescuers should be on opposite sides of patient.

every fifth compression without interrupting compression (a ratio of 1 inflation to 5 compressions).

It is important throughout external cardiac compression to maintain an open airway to continue ventilation of the lungs.

CPR procedures for children and infants. Modifications of the preceding techniques are necessary for children and infants. For children, depress the sternum about an inch at a rate of 80 to 100 times a minute using the heel of one hand. For babies, use only two fingers and depress the sternum approximately a half inch at a rate of 100 to 120 compressions a minute. Because of the smallness of the chest, the pressure should be applied on the midsternum rather than the lower half of the sternum.

The carotid pulse and the pupils of the eyes should be checked periodically to determine the effectiveness of cardiopulmonary resuscitation. It is important that cardiopulmonary resuscitation be a continuous process and should not be interrupted for more than 5 seconds at a time for any purpose.

Definitive therapy

The ABCD steps of cardiopulmonary resuscitation as outlined by the American Heart Association stand for Airway, Breathing, Circulation, and Definitive therapy. The trained first aider, with practice, can save a life by properly applying techniques to perform the first three steps, ABC. The fourth step, *definitive therapy,* requires the knowledge and skills of medical personnel. For example, if the heart is in ventricular fibrillation (rapid ineffectual contraction of the heart), the first aider can only supply artificial respiration and circulation but cannot resolve the problem. The heart will have to be defibrillated by medical personnel using special equipment. In other cases it is necessary to administer drugs, fluids, or oxygen to save the patient. This does not mean that you as a first aider have no role in the fourth step of cardiopulmonary resuscitation, but it does indicate your limitations. Your role is a critical one and must not be overlooked. Your responsibility is to take measures to call for help as soon as possible. Do not interrupt artificial ventilation or artificial circulation, but call for assistance. Send a bystander or another first aider to call for emergency medical care and transportation to the hospital.

All cardiopulmonary emergency patients should be transported to a hospital. It is essential that ventilation and compression continue without interruption during transportation unless normal heart-lung action has returned. Competent rescue squads and medical emergency units are extensively trained, have more experience, and are better equipped to handle these emergencies than the first aider. Attempt to obtain their services as soon as possible.

WHEN TO START AND STOP CARDIOPULMONARY RESUSCITATION

Cardiopulmonary resuscitation should be administered to most patients who have stopped breathing or have ineffective circulation (Fig. 3-9). The first aider should keep in mind the following guidelines established by the American Heart Association:

Anyone who is trained in resuscitation should be familiar with the problem of the proper selection of patients. . . . the rescuer suddenly confronted with a non-

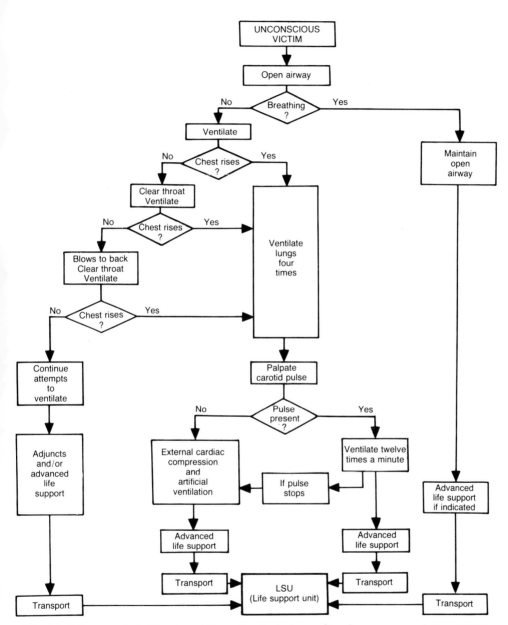

Fig. 3-9. Life support decision tree. (From Standards for cardiopulmonary resuscitation [CPR] and emergency cardiac care [ECC], American Heart Association, Inc., Dallas. Reprinted with permission.)

breathing, pulseless victim usually does not know the duration of arrest. Therefore he should initiate resuscitation efforts with all victims in cardiac arrest, with the following exceptions:

1. Patients known to be in the terminal states of a fatal disease (as determined by a physician)
2. Patients reasonably known to have been dead for over 10 minutes

Nonmedical trainees should be advised that it is the responsibility of a physician to make the decision whether or not to discontinue resuscitation, depending on his assessment of the cerebral and cardiovascular status.[6]

THE PHYSIOLOGY OF CARDIOPULMONARY RESUSCITATION

Expired-air ventilation (mouth-to-mouth or mouth-to-nose) is considered to be the most effective method of artificial respiration. Manual methods of artificial respiration are less effective and should not be considered for use by the first aider unless it is impossible to use expired-air ventilation.

How does it work and why is it effective? The air we breathe in contains approximately 21% oxygen, 79% nitrogen and rare gases, and less than 0.1% carbon dioxide. The air we breathe out contains 16% oxygen, 79% nitrogen and rare gases, and 5% carbon dioxide. Thus the air provided for a patient during expired air ventilation has enough oxygen to be effective for external respiration. Expired-air ventilation actively inflates the lungs, thereby providing nearly a normal volume of air. An important feature of expired-air methods is that cardiac compression can be accomplished without interfering with artificial respiration.

The heart is located in the space between the sternum and the spine almost in the middle of the chest (Fig. 3-10). The sternum is attached to the ribs by means of costal cartilages, which are flexible and capable of allowing limited movement of the sternum. Artificial circulation is accomplished by forcing the sternum downward and compressing the heart against the backbone. This action forces the blood out of the heart and through the arteries to the capillaries where oxygen diffuses into the cells of the body. When the pressure on the sternum is released, the heart

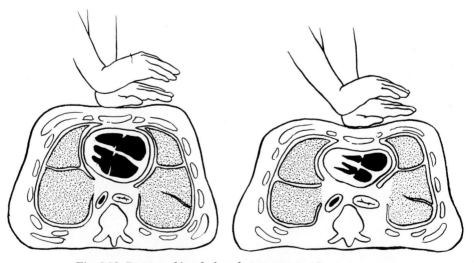

Fig. 3-10. Position of hands for administering cardiac compression.

returns to its normal position and fills up with blood. The blood pressure obtained from cardiac compression is lower than normal, but it is sufficient to keep a patient alive until normal heart action returns.

SPECIAL CONSIDERATIONS

Laryngectomees. Because of cancer or other causes, some individuals must have their larynx surgically removed. This operation makes it impossible for air to flow through the nose and mouth into the lungs. Therefore the surgeon makes a new airway to sustain life. The windpipe is shortened and a permanent small opening in the front of the neck is made to allow ventilation. Most laryngectomees wear a small tube in the neck opening. The American Cancer Society estimates that there are more than 25,000 laryngectomees living in the United States. The first aider should be aware of this condition and be prepared to aid the laryngectomee in an emergency condition. If a laryngectomee has stopped breathing and there is no other apparent cause, the tube in the neck may be blocked. An open airway may be established by removing the tube. If removal of the tube leads to the return of breathing, keep the patient quiet and seek medical care. If artificial respiration is necessary, do not apply mouth-to-mouth or mouth-to-nose methods. Use the same procedure used in mouth-to-mouth, exhaling air into the opening in the patient's neck, keeping the neck in a straight position.

Accessory devices. Various devices have been designed to assist resuscitation efforts. Unless the first aider is properly trained to use this equipment and unless it is readily available, he or she should not attempt to use it. Artificial airways are usually not available in an emergency situation and should not be depended on by the first aider. The first aider should obtain the assistance of emergency medical personnel who are expertly trained to use such equipment. Examples of mechanical equipment used by emergency medical personnel may include manually operated self-inflating bag-valve mask units, oxygen-powered manually triggered ventilation devices, and external cardiac compression machines. The conventional pressure-cycled automatic resuscitators should not be used with the administration of external cardiac compression because the pressure from compression will stop the inflation cycle.

PREPARATION OF THE FIRST AIDER FOR CARDIOPULMONARY RESUSCITATION

Cardiopulmonary resuscitation is an effective but potentially dangerous emergency procedure. Serious complications may result from the improper application of external cardiac massage. Such complications include rib fractures, liver damage, fracture of the sternum, damage to the lung tissue, bone marrow emboli, and heart damage. Studies have shown that the effectiveness of CPR is related to the quality of training. To promote a high standard and uniform quality of training, all training programs should adhere to the standards of the American Heart Association. Training of the first aider in cardiopulmonary resuscitation should include:

1. Lectures, films, slides, and demonstrations of proper procedures
2. Practice sessions conducted in smaller groups in both ventilatory and circulatory aspects of cardiopulmonary resuscitation on lifelike manikins

3. Demonstration of ability to correctly apply cardiopulmonary resuscitation procedure on lifelike manikins
4. Refresher training and retesting of first aid personnel at frequent intervals

SUMMARY

In the event of an accident or sudden illness that causes the cessation of breathing or the interruption of normal circulation, the first aider should be prepared to properly administer cardiopulmonary resuscitation. The following ABCD steps of cardiopulmonary resuscitation should be followed by the first aider:

Airway opened
    Place in supine position
    Tilt head back
    Extend neck
    Clear and remove obstructions
Breathing restored
    Pinch nose
    Form seal with mouth
    Inflate lungs
    Check circulation

Circulation restored
    Locate lower half of sternum
    Compress sternum
    Alternate with ventilation
Definitive therapy
    Get medical help

FIRST AIDER COMPETENCIES

After studying the material and practicing the techniques presented in this chapter, the student should be able to:

- Identify and explain the signs and symptoms of a patient who has stopped breathing.
- Explain under what circumstances external cardiac massage should be applied.
- Explain the first aid procedures for a respiratory obstruction.
- Describe the steps for mouth-to-mouth resuscitation.
- Indicate some special considerations presented by laryngectomees.
- Describe the procedures for administering external cardiac massage to babies, children, and adults.
- Explain some of the complications involved with transportation of nonbreathing cardiac arrest patients.
- Demonstrate the ability to administer cardiopulmonary resuscitation on a lifelike manikin.

REFERENCES AND
RECOMMENDED READINGS

1. Anthony, C. P., and Kolthoff, N. J.: Textbook of anatomy and physiology, ed. 9, St. Louis, 1975, The C. V. Mosby Co.
2. Baringer, J. R., et al.: External cardiac massage, New England Journal of Medicine **265:**62-65, 1961.
3. Boyd, D. R., and Folk, F. A.: The resuscitation and initial management of the severely injured, Journal of Occupational Medicine **12:**262-266, 1970.
4. Braun, P., et al.: Closed-chest cardiac resuscitation, New England Journal of Medicine **272:**1-6, 1975.
5. Cardiopulmonary resuscitation, Journal of the American Medical Association **198:** 372-379, 1966.
6. Cardiopulmonary resuscitation: a manual for instructors, Dallas, 1967, American Heart Association.
7. Cardiopulmonary resuscitation tech-

niques, Washington, D.C., 1965, U.S. Government Printing Office.

8. Curry, G. J., editor: Immediate care and transport of the injured, Springfield, Ill., 1965, Charles C Thomas, Publisher.

9. Emergency measures in cardiopulmonary resuscitation, Dallas, 1969, American Heart Association.

10. First aid for laryngectomees, 1962, American Cancer Society.

11. Gillespie, L., Jr., et al.: Successful external cardiac resuscitation in myocardial infarction, Journal of the American Medical Association **185**:44-47, 1963.

12. Gordon, A. S., editor: Cardiopulmonary resuscitation conference proceedings, Washington, D.C., 1967, National Research Council.

13. Gordon, A. S., et al.: Mouth-to-mouth versus manual artificial respiration for children and adults, Journal of the American Medical Association **167**:320-328, 1958.

14. Imburg, J., and Hartney, T. C.: Drowning and the treatment of non-fatal submersion, Pediatrics **37**:684-697, 1966.

15. Jude, J. R., et al.: Cardiac arrest, Journal of the American Medical Association **178**:1063-1070, 1961.

16. Kouwenhoven, W. B., et al.: Closed-chest cardiac massage, J.A.M.A. **173**:1064-1067, 1960.

17. Lillehei, C. W., et al.: Four years' experience with external cardiac resuscitation, Journal of the American Medical Association **193**:85-92, 1965.

18. The nurse and closed-chest cardiopulmonary resuscitation: special memo from the Committee on Nursing Practice, New York, American Nurses' Association.

19. Quarrell, E. J.: Artificial ventilation: normal respiratory mechanism and function, Nursing Times, Oct. 8, 1970.

20. Safar, P.: Recognition and management of airway obstruction, Journal of the American Medical Association **208**:1008-1011, 1969.

21. Safar, P., et al.: Ventilation and circulation with closed-chest cardiac massage in man, Journal of the American Medical Association **176**:574-576, 1961.

22. Shapter, R. K.: Cardiopulmonary resuscitation: basic life support, Clinical Symposia **26**:5, 1974.

23. Standards for cardiopulmonary resuscitation (CPR) and emergency cardiac care (ECC), Journal of the American Medical Association (Suppl.) **227**:833-868, 1974.

24. Stephenson, H. E., Jr.: Cardiac arrest and resuscitation, ed. 4, St. Louis, 1974, The C. V. Mosby Co.

25. Tuttle, W. W., and Schottelius, B. A.: Textbook of physiology, ed. 16, St. Louis, 1969, The C. V. Mosby Co.

26. Wilder, R. J., et al.: Cardiopulmonary resuscitations by trained ambulance personnel, Journal of the American Medical Association **190**: 531-534, 1964.

27. Winter, P. M., and Lowenstein, E.: Acute respiratory failure, Scientific American **221**:23-29, Nov., 1969.

4

⁕⁕

RESPIRATORY EMERGENCIES

Elton Dupree, Richard F. McConnell, Jr., and Guy S. Parcel

Although death may result from primary failure of any of several body organs, compromise of lung and cardiac function with resultant brain injury leads to rapid demise. Consequently, the prime concern of the first aider must be to maintain respiratory, cardiovascular, and, indirectly, central nervous system function.

First aid measures must have as a primary aim the reestablishment and maintenance of these functions. Therefore the initial examination should yield a rapid but accurate evaluation of these systems. The sequence of physical examination should move quickly from the head, face, neck, and upper airway to the chest. A rapid estimate can be made of the rate and character of respiration. In addition, the first aider must look for signs of obstruction of the airway during either inspiration or expiration or for signs of ineffective movement of the chest wall due to a crushed chest or penetrating wound.

CHEST INJURIES

Trauma to the chest wall may produce pulmonary lacerations and contusions as well as other life-threatening injuries. Automobile accidents are the leading cause of serious chest injuries. Other accidents responsible for chest injuries are stab wounds, gunshot wounds, and falls.

Flail chest

Flail chest and *crushed chest* are terms used to describe the phenomenon in which critical respiratory distress results from multiple rib fractures, usually in more than one place. This results in an unsupported area of chest wall that moves freely inward with inspiration and outward with expiration. These paradoxical excursions of part of the chest wall lead to ineffective ventilation and dyspnea (shortness of breath).

This injury most often results from steering column injury, impact with blunt objects such as furniture, and crush injury from heavy objects or cave-ins of earth.

Signs and symptoms. The clinical picture includes local pain that is aggravated by motion. Tenderness and crepitation (which feels like the crinkling of tissue paper) can be elicited by applying gentle pressure on the fractured ribs.

The site may be swollen and bruised, and the affected area may often be seen to move inward as the chest wall moves outward with inspiration.

First aid procedures. Emergency care is aimed at minimizing altered breathing mechanics by stabilizing the chest wall as quickly as possible. The most efficient first aid procedure is application of a wide elastic bandage around the chest wall to keep it from ballooning outward. This also helps stabilize the diaphragm so that it can function more efficiently. The injury may also be effectively managed by stabilizing the affected side by sandbags or rolled blankets until medical aid can be obtained. Moving a patient with fractured ribs or flail chest should be done with extreme caution, since the sharp ends of the ribs can perforate the pleura and lung, leading to a pneumothorax or hemothorax.

Pneumothorax

Wounds to the chest from knives, bullets, and other missiles may result in puncture of the pleura or lung itself, allowing air to escape into the surrounding space. Broken ribs may directly puncture the lung without any obvious penetration of the chest wall. Blunt chest injuries, too, may disrupt the bronchi or trachea, allowing air to escape. When air leaks into the pleural space (the space between lung and chest wall) from any of these conditions, the lung collapses, a condition called *pneumothorax* (Fig. 4-1).

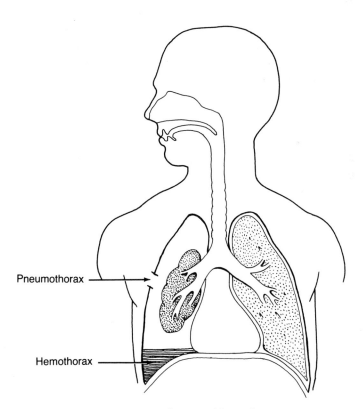

Fig. 4-1. Pneumothorax and hemothorax.

Signs and symptoms. Difficulty in breathing, shortness of breath, and chest pain aggravated by breathing or coughing suggest pneumothorax. Often when air escapes through tears in the bronchi or trachea tissue, it dissects through the tissues and can be felt under the skin in the upper chest and neck areas.

First aid procedures. Medical intervention is necessary, and the role of the first aider is to recognize the seriousness of the problem and arrange for transportation. Keep the patient quiet and as comfortable as possible during transportation. In penetrating wounds of the chest with pneumothorax, air may move to and fro through the wound and can often be heard. This is referred to as a *sucking* wound. The size of the defect that can be tolerated varies somewhat, and when symptoms are severe, immediate covering and occlusion of the wound is life saving.

The wound should be immediately covered with any available material such as a coat or wadding of cloth. A credit card or driver's license also makes a suitable cover and may be taped in place. If the covering is placed at the end of expiration, maximal use of the lung will be preserved. The dressing or covering should not be removed until immediate surgery is available. Signs and symptoms of shock and circulatory compromise should be looked for, since serious bleeding may also accompany such injuries.

Hemothorax

Hemothorax results from bleeding into the pleural cavity. In most patients with an injury to the chest, variable amounts of blood will escape into the pleural cavity. Difficulty in breathing, shortness of breath, and chest pain on the affected side are the most obvious symptoms. If internal bleeding is significant, low blood pressure and symptoms of shock may develop (see Chapter 7 for specific symptoms).

The major first aid concerns are to care for shock and transport to a medical facility as soon as possible. Immediate therapy is to remove the blood by needle as necessary for comfort. Therefore medical intervention is necessary.

Laryngotracheal injuries

Blunt trauma to the neck or face may compromise the airway due to the collapse of the larynx (voice box) or trachea (windpipe). This collapse will lead to variable degrees of airway obstruction. Usually the site of injury will be apparent due to swelling and bleeding into tissues. Air may also be felt under the skin in the neck and upper chest. The integrity of the larynx or trachea will be lost. Signs of inadequate ventilation include air hunger (gasping for air) and cyanosis (a blue coloration of the lips) if the airway is obstructed.

If the respiratory distress is evident, then prompt establishment of an airway is necessary. The neck should be hyperextended to lengthen the trachea and open the airway. If this is not successful, transport at once to a hospital, since an emergency tracheotomy must be performed by medical personnel for the relief of respiratory obstruction. The first aider should never consider doing a tracheotomy.

Follow-up care for chest injuries

Follow-up care for chest injuries includes (1) continual monitoring of vital life signs, (2) taking steps to maintain an open airway and being prepared to begin

CPR if necessary, (3) caring for shock, (4) providing constant reassurance and as much comfort as possible, and (5) transporting the patient without delay.

RESPIRATORY OBSTRUCTION

Airway obstruction is one of the most common life-threatening emergencies and may be caused by foreign objects such as food, trinkets, vomitus, mucus, or even water blocking air passages after entering the trachea. Airway obstruction with respiratory compromise should be suspected in all emergencies presenting with difficulty in breathing or cessation of respiration.

Aspiration of foreign body

A common type of respiratory obstruction that leads to death occurs in restaurants when the patient's larynx or trachea becomes blocked by a piece of food, usually meat. The victim chokes on a piece of food too large to swallow. In many cases, the blood alcohol level has been found to be significantly elevated, which may have led to depression of normal reflexes.

Foreign body aspiration in children most often occurs in toddlers (1½ to 3 years of age). They tend to aspirate peanuts, popcorn, beads, safety pins, coins, or other small objects that they can pick up with the thumb and forefinger. Fortunately, most foreign bodies that children aspirate do not entirely occlude the airway.

Signs and symptoms. A chunk of meat, a marshmallow, or inhaled vomitus may quickly block the airway. Effective steps must be taken or death will occur. Signs of airway obstruction can be easily recognized. There is a great effort to breathe. The stomach and lower part of the neck may be sucked in, the head is thrown back, the eyes bulge and the face becomes blue. In partial obstruction, some air can be felt or heard coming from the patient's mouth. In complete obstruction, however, nonmovement of air is evident.

First aid procedures. Respiratory obstruction must be relieved quickly and followed immediately by artificial respiration if there is no spontaneous effort to breathe. No attempt to remove the foreign body with the fingers should be made unless the object can be removed without pushing it further down the airway. Frequently, patients can expel the foreign object by an explosive expiratory effort with the head lower than the body. If this fails, the neck should be hyperextended in an attempt to partially relieve the obstruction. If obstruction persists, then mouth-to-mouth aspiration should be tried while the nose is occluded by pinching the nostrils together. Place your mouth tightly over the patient's mouth and attempt to suck out the obstructing material. This creates a negative pressure that may dislodge the object.

Other measures include the following procedures. If the patient is a child, hold the child upside down and strike one or more hard blows on the back between the shoulder blades (Fig. 4-2). This may cause the trapped air to act as a ram to force the object out. If the patient is an adult, place on a table or other elevated area with the head and body down and strike sharply between the shoulder blades. Objections have been raised to this procedure because the patient may attempt to inspire, thereby creating a negative pressure, which may suck the object further down the trachea.

Recently, an effective method of dislodging foreign bodies from the larynx has

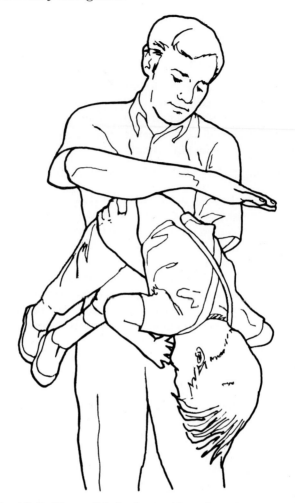

Fig. 4-2. Position to dislodge foreign object from child's airway.

been developed[5] (Fig. 4-3). One should stand behind the subject and wrap his arms around the patient, just below the rib cage, grasping one wrist with the other hand and pulling sharply inward. This compresses the upper abdomen, pushing the diaphragm up and creating a force that may expel the object.

If these measures fail, try mouth-to-mouth resuscitation in the hope of getting some air past the obstruction. If this fails, the only recourse is rapid transportation to a medical facility.

It is important that the first aider be familiar with all of the above procedures so that each of these may be carried out expediently. Time is most important; only 4 to 5 minutes can elapse before irreversible brain damage or death occurs.

Near-drowning

Drowning ranks as the fourth most common cause of accidental death, with about 7000 occurring in the United States annually. When an individual cannot

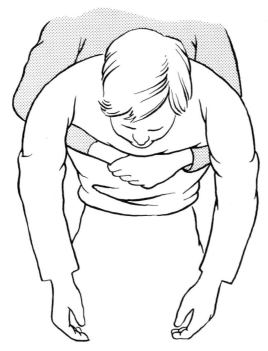

Fig. 4-3. Procedure for dislodging aspirated chunk of food.

stay afloat and begins to submerge, the urge to breathe is so great that water is taken into the lungs by involuntary swallowing movements. As water is taken into the larynx (voice box) and spasm of the larynx occurs without adequate oxygen, unconsciousness ensues, which causes relaxation of the larynx, allowing water to flow into the lungs. In about 10% of cases, laryngeal spasm prevents significant intake of water into the lungs, and these victims die of asphyxiation (lack of oxygen) alone.

In freshwater drowning, water diffuses into the blood vessels of the lung and may make the blood so dilute that rupture of red blood cells occurs. Death may also occur due to imbalance of chemical elements in the blood, which affects the heart. In saltwater drowning, the salt content of the water is higher than that in the blood, and fluid is drawn from the bloodstream into the lungs. This causes a condition called *pulmonary edema,* which may occur minutes or hours later.

First aid procedures. Irrespective of the type of drowning, as soon as a drowning victim is removed from the water, immediately prepare for mouth-to-mouth resuscitation. Even during rescue, before the patient has been removed from the water, mouth-to-mouth resuscitation should be done so that air is forced into the lungs without delay. The most critical factors are restoring oxygen to the bloodstream and reestablishing adequate cardiac circulation. If the patient has some spontaneous respiration with adequate heartbeat at the time of rescue, survival is likely. However, if there is no effort to breathe, no pulse, and dilated pupils, then CPR should be started. Efforts to remove water from the lungs are usually a waste of time.

Follow-up care. Any patient with respiratory obstruction from any cause should be transported to a hospital rapidly. Many of the procedures required to save a life must be done by a physician and other medical personnel. Delay could result in death or permanent brain damage. Even if the patient does begin to breathe on his own, follow-up medical care is necessary to care for possible undetected complications.

ASTHMA

This disease, which afflicts from 3% to 5% of the population, is caused by multiple factors, specifically allergies, infections, emotional stresses, and environmental conditions, occasionally air pollution.

The asthmatic attack is a result of these stimuli on hyperreactive airways (bronchi) and mucus-secreting glands. There is bronchial constriction and increased mucus production, which produces wheezing. This interferes with oxygenation. As the asthmatic attack proceeds progressively, more air becomes trapped in the lungs, leading to hyperinflation. The chest wall becomes distended, and the patient is seen struggling to breathe, using neck and shoulder muscles and exhaling forcibly through pursed lips.

It is important to recognize that many diseases can produce wheezing. In addition to asthma, heart failure, emphysema, bronchitis, pulmonary emboli (clots in the lung), and upper airway obstruction can all produce shortness of breath and audible wheezing. Although it is at times difficult even for a physician to distinguish between these causes of wheezing, a brief history from the patient may be helpful. Generally speaking, it is unusual for middle-aged people to suddenly get asthma; heart failure is more frequent. Aspiration of foreign bodies usually occurs during or after eating and is frequently characterized by inspiratory noises as well as expiratory wheezing.

Signs and symptoms. Initially, in early asthma, only prolonged expiratory wheezes are heard. As the asthma worsens, both inspiratory and expiratory wheezing are present. With accumulation of mucus in the lungs, the breath sounds become harsher. An ominous sign in asthma is extreme respiratory distress with little air exchange. These individuals are in grave danger and must have immediate medical care.

Air trapping occurs because it is easier to move air into the alveoli (air sacs) than out because of collapse of the bronchioles in expiration. This air trapping flattens the diaphragm and results in little useful respiratory activity. The asthmatic patient inspires by lifting the rib cage with accessory muscles (the neck muscles and shoulders).

First aid procedures. The first aider should make the patient comfortable and give reassurance. There is nothing more frightening than air hunger; therefore reassurance to the patient can be of much benefit. In mild attacks, the asthmatic may simply take oral medications that have been prescribed by a physician. In more severe attacks, medical assistance must be obtained because it is unlikely that oral medication alone will be sufficient. These severe attacks nearly always require medical therapy, including drugs, which should be given by a physician or experienced nurse. If a patient has been wheezing for several hours or if there have been recurrent attacks within a few days, it is unlikely that home therapy will be sufficient. Help should be obtained at the nearest medical facility.

EMPHYSEMA

Emphysema is defined as overdistention of terminal air passages associated with destruction of alveolar walls. This condition is usually associated with heavy smoking in individuals with predisposition to the disease. Emphysema is a chronic condition but may present as an emergency if the patient becomes distressed, develops a lung infection, or experiences undue exertion.

Signs and symptoms. There is an increased respiratory rate and a prolonged expiratory effort. However, the movement of the lungs with respiration is decreased due to overdistention of the alveoli and their inability to empty normally. Overaction of the accessory muscles of respiration results in retraction between the ribs as well as below or at top of the rib cage, similar to that seen in asthma. The rib cage usually appears barrel-shaped in these patients. In severe respiratory distress these patients may appear anxious, sweaty, and cyanotic (turning blue). At times they may be comatose or difficult to arouse. This represents a medical emergency, and they should be immediately transferred to a hospital.

First aid procedure. There is little that the first aider can do except to recognize the seriousness of the situation and arrange for transportation. Generally encouragement to slow the breathing rate and to breathe through pursed lips will help the emphysematous patient feel more comfortable.

Oxygen should not be administered in an *uncontrolled* manner to these patients. These patients are frequently sensitive to oxygen, and administration of large doses of oxygen may lead to total cessation of respiration. Provide reassurance and make the patient as comfortable as possible. Having the patient lie on one side usually results in more efficient respirations than the sitting position, which limits diaphragm motion.

ANAPHYLACTIC SHOCK

Swelling occurs when there is acute dilation of the small blood vessels of the larynx because of an acute allergic reaction. Swelling may also occur in other areas of the body such as the eyelids, lips, or tongue. Occasionally, anaphylactic shock is associated with the swelling. Cardiovascular collapse accompanies anaphylactic shock. Anaphylaxis can produce death if appropriate first aid measures are not taken immediately. An example of this type of reaction is that which occurs when a bee venom–sensitive person is stung. Reactions range from a mild local response to serious anaphylaxis. The extent of the reaction is due to several factors, including the amount of venom injected and the degree of sensitivity of the individual.

Signs and symptoms. Various parts of the body, such as the eyelids, lips, or tongue may be swollen. If the vocal cords are involved, there will be hoarseness or inability to talk. If the larynx is swollen, there will be varying degrees of air hunger (gasping for air). If anaphylactic shock occurs, the pulse will be thready or absent. In extreme shock, the person will be unconscious.

First aid procedures. When difficulty in breathing occurs, medical aid must be sought immediately even though the initial symptoms may not seem serious. Maintain an open airway by keeping the neck extended, and transport to medical care. For a bee sting, the stinger should be flicked out with a fingernail. Caution must be taken not to pinch the stinger, since this may inject more venom from the sac. If the person has a bee sting kit, the antihistamine should be administered, and epinephrine (Adrenalin) should be injected from the preloaded syringe into the fatty tissue of the leg or arm. If necessary, perform cardiopulmonary resuscitation while transporting to a hospital.

HYPERVENTILATION

Hyperventilation is a condition in which breathing too deeply and rapidly occurs because of emotional stress. This may be due to stress from any cause (such as anxiety on the job). Breathing rapidly and deeply creates a situation in which there is light-headedness, weakness, and tingling and numbness of the fingers and lips. The light-headedness is due to the decrease in blood flow to the brain. Voluntary hyperventilation may lead to fainting or convulsions. These individuals have a feeling of air hunger.

In the hyperventilation syndrome, immediate treatment includes rebreathing into a paper bag and reassurance. The paper bag prevents blowing off too much carbon dioxide, which resulted in the initial symptoms. Prevention requires further investigation of the person's life situation by a physician to determine the cause of the emotional stress.

TOXIC GASES
Carbon monoxide poisoning

Carbon monoxide is odorless and is present in automobile exhaust fumes, sewer gas, and smoke from fires and furnaces. Sufficient carbon monoxide may be inhaled within a few minutes to cause death. Carbon monoxide has 250 times the affinity that oxygen does for the hemoglobin of red blood cells. This reduces the amount of oxygen that can be transported to the tissues and organs. Death results from lack of oxygen supply to the brain.

There are usually no symptoms until the individual collapes, but headache or dizziness may occur. The skin has a cherry-red color, especially noticeable in the lips. Failing respiration eventually develops if poisoning continues.

It is critical to get the patient into fresh air immediately. If breathing has stopped, begin mouth-to-mouth resuscitation and transport immediately to a medical facility.

Smoke inhalation

Inhalation of smoke, such as occurs in a burning house, is responsible for bronchial irritation and edema (swelling). In addition to persons trapped in burning buildings, this is a common problem for fire fighters and forest fire fighters.

If the patient is not unconscious, severe coughing will be the main symptom. Occasionally sooty sputum may be coughed up. If some time has elapsed in severe smoke inhalation, shortness of breath or rapid respiration will be present. Pulmonary edema is a frequent complication.

The first procedure is to get the patient into fresh air. If respiration has ceased, begin artificial respiration immediately. Oxygen should be administered if available. The patient should be taken to a medical facility because bronchial edema and lung congestion of varying degrees can occur within minutes or hours later.

SUMMARY

When an accident or illness precipitates a respiratory emergency, the first aider must evaluate respiration quickly. If signs of obstruction are present, the airway must be cleared quickly to prevent permanent brain damage or death. Once the airway is functional and the cardiac status has been evaluated or established, medical aid must be obtained in most situations.

FIRST AIDER COMPETENCIES

After studying the material in this chapter, the student should be able to:
- Identify and explain signs and symptoms of respiratory distress.
- Describe methods of emergency care of chest injuries.
- List and describe methods of relieving obstruction of the airway.
- List and describe methods to be taken in emergency care of near-drowning.
- Identify and explain signs and symptoms of asthma, emphysema, and hyperventilation.
- Describe how to recognize and care for anaphylactic shock.
- Identify signs, symptoms, and emergency care of toxic gas poisoning.

REFERENCES AND RECOMMENDED READINGS

1. Cleveland, R. J., and Rheinlander, H. F.: Diagnosis and care of chest trauma, Post-graduate Medicine **55**:115, 1974.
2. Crews, E. R., and Lapuerta, L.: A manual of respiratory failure, Springfield, Ill., 1972, Charles C Thomas, Publisher.
3. Cumming, G., and Semple, S. J.: Disorders of the respiratory system, Oxford, England, 1973, Blackwell Scientific Publications, Ltd.
4. Ellen, W. C., and Haugen, R. K.: Food asphyxiation—restaurant rescue, New England Journal of Medicine **289**:81, 1973.
5. Heimlich, H. J.: A life-saving maneuver to prevent food-choking, Journal of the American Medical Association **234**:398-401, 1975.
6. Naclerio, E. A.: Chest injuries: physiologic principles and emergency management, New York, 1971, Grune & Stratton, Inc.
7. Oppenheimer, R. P.: Airway—instantly, Journal of the American Medical Association **230**:76, 1974.
8. Shires, G. T.: Care of the trauma patient, New York, 1966, McGraw-Hill Book Co.

5

◆◆◆

CARDIAC EMERGENCIES

Elton Dupree and Richard F. McConnell, Jr.

When either the pulmonary or cardiovascular system fails to function properly, the heart itself may fail to beat effectively because of either an abnormal rate or cardiac standstill. This type of emergency requires prompt action from the first aider because failure of the heart to provide tissue perfusion and oxygenation will result in rapid cell death if not quickly reversed.

Heart disease and cardiac emergencies have a serious and ever-growing impact on American society today. Deaths from cardiovascular disease claim more American lives than all other diseases combined. Heart attacks alone result in more than a half million deaths annually. Consequently, it is important for everyone to be familiar with the signs and symptoms of a heart attack and first aid care for the victim.

MECHANISM OF HEART ACTION

The heart is a muscular pump about the size of a fist, which serves as the center of the cardiovascular system. Its prime function is to transport blood throughout the body. As blood moves through the arteries, it carries nutrients as well as oxygen to tissues and organs. Veins carry blood back to the right atrium of the heart (Fig. 5-1). From there, blood flows into the right ventricle and is pumped into the lungs where carbon dioxide is exchanged for oxygen. Oxygenated blood flows from the veins of the lung into the left atrium and then is returned to the left ventricle, which pumps it into the aorta and arteries. The cardiovascular and pulmonary systems are intimately related, both anatomically and physiologically. If one system fails to function properly, the other is often affected also. Lung diseases often present identical symptoms to those of primary cardiovascular disorders and may lead to some confusion in determining the specific cause of an emergency.

At the beginning of each cardiac cycle the two atria contract and pump blood into the ventricles. Both ventricles then contract, forcing blood into the aorta and pulmonary arteries. Closure of the valves separating the major vessels (aorta and pulmonary arteries) from the ventricles and the atria from the ventricles prevents the backflow of blood and consequently assists in maintaining blood pressure. Closure of the two valves separating the atria (upper chambers) from the ventricles (lower chambers) occurs immediately after the onset of contraction of the heart (systole) and produces the first heart sound. Closure of the aortic and pulmonic valves occurs at the beginning of relaxation of the heart (diastole) and results in production of the second heart sound.

As the force of the heart contraction is transmitted to the arteries, the pressure in these vessels rises rapidly. This pressure is not only determined by the force of the contraction but also by resistance in the vessel walls and the viscosity (thickness) of the blood. As the heart contracts, the pressure rises, resulting in the *systolic pressure*. The normal mean systolic pressure is 120 millimeters of mercury (mm Hg) but can usually be estimated for adults by adding 100 to the subject's age in years. (Example: 100 + 50 years = 150 mm Hg, the upper limit acceptable for a 50-year-old subject.) At the end of a beat the heart relaxes, allowing the pressure to fall. This lower pressure is known as the *diastolic pressure*. The average normal diastolic pressure is 80 mm Hg in the adult and should not normally exceed 90 mm Hg.

Determination of the blood pressure with a sphygmomanometer (blood pressure cuff) is a standard clinical procedure. First aiders normally will not have a blood pressure cuff available during emergencies. However, it may be helpful in appreciating the importance of blood pressure to practice in first aid class with a blood pressure cuff. (See Chapter 6 for additional information concerning the cardiovascular system.)

There are numerous abnormalities that lead to malfunction of the heart and

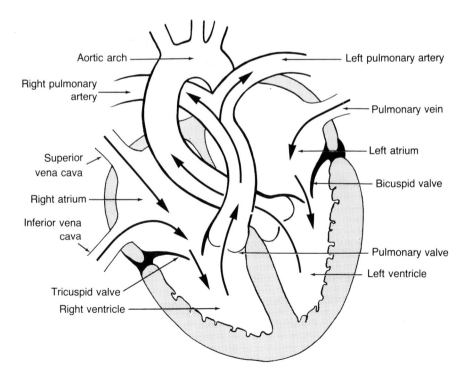

Fig. 5-1. Structures of heart showing direction of blood flow through heart.

create emergency situations. Among these, defects involving the conduction fibers of the heart may lead to abnormal heart rates or rhythms. Other conditions that lead to cardiac emergencies include pulmonary embolism (blood clot in the lung), insufficient blood through the coronary arteries (coronary insufficiency), and direct trauma to the heart and great vessels.

ABNORMAL HEART RHYTHMS

Cardiac arrhythmias are varied in presentation, with a spectrum ranging from an occasional extra beat (extra systole) or slow rate (bradycardia) to an abnormally rapid rate (tachycardia). A slow heart rate may be found in many athletes, in instances of narrowing of the coronary arteries because of atherosclerotic heart disease, in congenital defects of the heart, and in certain drug ingestions.

Heart rate is determined by taking a pulse rate. For an adult, a normal range for pulse rate would be 70 to 90 beats a minute. A normal range for children would be 90 to 110. A careful history and examination should be made to determine any previous history of cardiovascular disease, complaints of chest pain, and signs of circulatory insufficiency.

Bradycardia

An abnormally slow heart rate resulting in a pulse less than 60 beats a minute is defined as *bradycardia*. Bradycardia can result from heart blockage because of atherosclerotic disease (narrowing of the arteries of the heart), congenital defects, or the effect of certain drugs.

Signs and symptoms. The pulse rate will be abnormally slow (less than 60 beats a minute). If low blood pressure accompanies bradycardia, the pulse may be weak or undetectable, and the patient may experience dizziness and weakness.

First aid procedures. There is actually little the first aider can do to correct the underlying cause of bradycardia. Once bradycardia is suspected, the most important procedure is to arrange for transportation to medical care. The patient must receive medical attention to determine the cause and severity of the bradycardia. Medication may be needed to increase the heart rate, or improper dosage of a cardiac drug may have to be adjusted by a physician.

Until medical attention is obtained, the first aider should make the patient comfortable and continue to monitor vital life signs (breathing, pulse, and pupils of the eyes). If the pulse rate becomes so faint that it is difficult to detect, cardiac arrest may be imminent. It is then necessary to administer cardiopulmonary resuscitation to maintain circulation.

Tachycardia

This condition is defined as an excessively rapid heart rate and is usually applied to rates above 100 beats a minute under resting conditions in the adult. Tachycardia may be due to abnormal stimulation of the conducting fibers in the heart or to an abnormality in the heart muscle itself. *Sinus tachycardia* occurs in shock, fever, anxiety states, hypotension (low blood pressure), hyperthyroid conditions, certain drug ingestions, excessive exercise, and after the use of alcohol and stimulants such as tobacco and coffee.

Atrial tachycardia results from stimulation arising in the atrial wall and may be caused by emotional stress, excitation, fatigue, and the use of stimulants. Atrial tachycardia results in a more rapid heart rate than sinus tachycardia and may range as high as 220 beats a minute. *Ventricular tachycardia* results from stimulation of the conducting system of the ventricles or irritation of the muscle of the ventricular wall itself. It is often associated with underlying heart disease or digitalis intoxication. (Digitalis is a drug used to increase the pumping efficiency of the heart in congestive heart failure.)

Signs and symptoms. In sinus tachycardia the heart rate will be greater than 100 beats a minute, but usually less than the 200 or more beats a minute seen in atrial tachycardia. With atrial tachycardia the patient may experience discomfort accompanying a rapid rhythm and may have a vague sensation of fluttering in the chest. If coronary or cerebral circulation is compromised, there may be chest pain or neurological symptoms, such as confusion, disorientation, or even unconsciousness. In ventricular tachycardia symptoms range from an awareness of a rapid heartbeat to an observable picture of shock with pallor, cyanosis, cold extremities, and mental dullness.

First aid procedures. The patient should be made comfortable and reassured. If the patient is dizzy or weak he should be placed in a reclining position and the knees or legs elevated. If tachycardia converts to ventricular fibrillation, CPR efforts must be made. Follow-up treatment of the underlying cause of the tachycardia must be provided by a physician, therefore transport the patient at once to medical care.

HEART ATTACKS

Over 500,000 people die of heart attacks each year. Predisposing factors include obesity, lack of exercise and conditioning, cigarette smoking, high blood pressure, high levels of blood cholesterol, diabetes, and a family history of heart attacks. Myocardial infarction, commonly referred to as heart attack, is a frequent occurrence in our society, primarily because of eating habits, sedentary life-styles, and stress. Professional and business groups are said to be more prone to heart disease. If a man is in the age range of 50 to 60 years, he has a 35% chance of having a heart attack. Also, men in general have a higher incidence of heart disease than women, the ratio being about 2:1 or 3:1.

Angina pectoris

The commonly used term *angina pectoris* means simply pain in the chest. This chest pain is due to an insufficient blood supply to a portion of the heart muscle. The decrease in blood flow is due to narrowing of the coronary arteries. If there is an increased demand for oxygen because of excitement or exercise, the narrowed artery will be unable to provide increased blood flow.

Signs and symptoms. The resulting pain is usually described as "crushing" or "squeezing" and is located in the lower chest or upper abdomen. Frequently there is referred pain to the left shoulder and down the left arm. Just as frequently, however, the pain is felt radiating into the neck and angle of the jaw. The patient may turn pale and sweat during a severe attack. Respiration may be shallow and the patient reluctant to move. Often there is a sense of impending death and, indeed, death may occur. If the pain persists longer than a few minutes, myocardial infarction (heart attack) should be suspected.

First aid procedures. The patient should be placed in a comfortable sitting position and protected from exertion and emotional stress. Reassurance should be given. The patient should not be moved until the pain subsides. Often the patient may carry a glass ampule of amyl nitrite or nitroglycerin tablets. The glass ampules of amyl nitrite should be cracked in a handkerchief and the patient allowed to inhale the contents to relieve the pain. Nitroglycerin tablets should be placed under the tongue, not swallowed. Such medications should be given only if they have been prescribed by the patient's physician.

Follow-up care. Do not delay referral to a physician, and do not leave the patient unattended. On recovery from the episode, the patient should avoid any exertion and stress.

Acute myocardial infarction

Acute myocardial infarction results from occlusion (blockage) of a coronary artery due to the formation of a clot. This results in death of the heart muscle supplied by the involved vessel. The pain is similar to that of angina pectoris except that it is more prolonged. Acute myocardial infarction is frequently followed by sudden death from abnormal rhythms. The majority of these deaths occur within the first 2 hours after an attack.

Signs and symptoms. The patient usually has a severe, viselike pain in the chest. Frequently, the pain is referred to the left shoulder and down the left arm, but it may also radiate into the neck and jaws as in angina pectoris. The patient is often ashen gray and may collapse and lose consciousness. Urine and feces may be passed. Shock from cardiovascular collapse can occur and is shown by the absence of the pulse and unresponsiveness of the patient.

First aid procedures. Establish an open airway for the patient and make him comfortable. Give oxygen if it is available, and provide reassurance to reduce anxiety. Exertion of any kind must be avoided. If the pulse or heartbeat is absent, begin CPR immediately. Obtain medical care as quickly as possible.

Follow-up care. The patient must be transported as quickly as possible to the nearest medical facility. Monitor the heartbeat and the other vital signs en route, and if necessary maintain CPR during transportation. The patient should be in a semireclining position (Fig. 5-2) during transportation unless it is necessary to administer CPR.

Complication of myocardial infarctions. When an area of the heart muscle dies from loss of its blood supply, several complications may ensue. Among these, the more severe include shock, congestive heart failure, arrhythmias (abnormal rhythms), and embolism (blood clot) to the lung, either from the heart itself or from the peripheral veins of the lower extremities. The clinical signs of shock include a drop in blood pressure, weak or absent pulse, cold, moist skin, pallor, or cyanosis. In congestive heart failure, shortness of breath and an inability to lie flat are prominent manifestations. Arrhythmias are most often detected as an irregularity of the pulse. Embolism usually occurs later and does not concern the first aider. The first aider can do little for congestive heart failure, arrhythmias, or an embolism but must be prepared to care for the shock or cardiac arrest that may result. Since the first aider is limited in his ability to treat these conditions, transportation to a medical facility as soon as possible is essential.

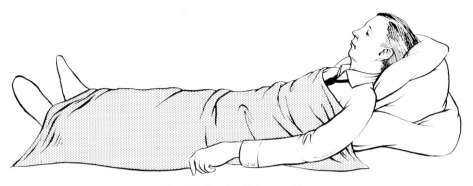

Fig. 5-2. Semireclining position.

HYPERTENSIVE CRISIS

Hypertension refers to abnormal elevated blood pressure. There usually are no apparent symptoms to indicate chronic elevated blood pressure. Hypertension is detected primarily by means of measuring blood pressure with a pressure cuff. When a patient experiences the abrupt extreme elevation of blood pressure (diastolic pressure of 150 mm Hg or greater) or if symptoms of heart failure, convulsions, or disturbances of consciousness occur associated with elevated pressure (diastolic blood pressure of 120 mm Hg or greater), a hypertensive crisis is said to be present.

One should maintain a high index of suspicion when a known or suspected hypertensive patient manifests any of the signs or symptoms mentioned in the following paragraph. A hypertensive crisis may occur with or without symptoms of central nervous system involvement. It may be due to kidney disease, adrenal gland tumors, abuse or overdose of such drugs as amphetamines, or it may have no clearly definable cause, as in cases of essential hypertension.

Signs and symptoms. The patient may have severe pounding headaches, nausea, vomiting, irritability, confusion or disorientation, convulsions, or frank coma. Other neurological signs include blurred vision, paralysis of the facial muscles, or paralysis of one side of the body. Bleeding into the brain may occur during a hypertensive crisis and result in a stroke.

First aid procedure. Other than making the patient comfortable, the only thing that the first aider can do is to seek prompt medical attention. The patient should be placed in a position of comfort, preferably a supported sitting position, and should be reassured and kept quiet, since anxiety tends to further exacerbate blood pressure elevation.

CARDIAC INJURIES

Direct or indirect trauma to the heart itself may be serious and result in rapid deterioration. Most frequently these injuries result from gunshot wounds or stab wounds to the chest that involve the heart. They are also seen after blunt trauma to the chest in persons involved in high-speed automobile accidents. Stab wounds to the heart with knives or other sharp instruments often allow blood to accumulate in the pericardial sac surrounding the heart. Since the hole in the pericardium

(Fig. 5-3) may be small and self-sealing, the accumulating blood will result in what is known as a *cardiac tamponade.* Contusions of the heart may occur after blunt trauma to the chest. In these cases if the heart muscle is damaged sufficiently, serious arrhythmias may result, and death of the heart muscle may occur resulting in a traumatic myocardial infarction.

Signs and symptoms. In contusions of the heart there may be little or no evidence of external injury. In these cases a high index of suspicion for cardiac injury is the best course of action. Shock out of proportion to the other injuries present should suggest this possibility. In penetrating wounds to the heart overt signs of shock may rapidly ensue. In those cases in which cardiac tamponade is the prominent feature, the pulse may be slow and weak with a low blood pressure. Veins of the head, neck, and upper extremities may be distended, and cyanosis may be present because of poor blood return to the tamponaded heart.

First aid procedures. Transportation of these patients to the hospital should be undertaken immediately. The head should be elevated to partially relieve any venous congestion. If shock is present, the legs should also be elevated. If a weapon is still in the chest, it should not be removed.

Follow-up care. The patient who has had a cardiac contusion must rest and avoid physical exertion. His regimen would be similar to that of a post–myocardial infarction patient. Occasionally needle aspiration of the pericardial sac may be all that is necessary to relieve cardiac tamponade after penetrating wounds. Larger stab wounds and gunshot wounds to the heart require immediate suturing of

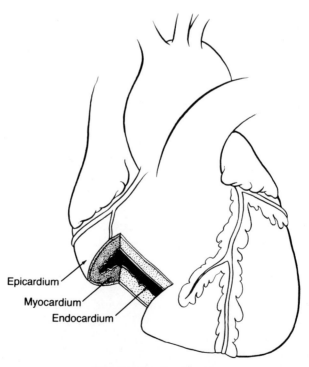

Epicardium
Myocardium
Endocardium

Fig. 5-3. Layers of heart.

the wound in the heart muscle itself. Nearly all patients with large wounds to the heart or rupture of the ventricle after blunt chest trauma die before reaching a hospital.

SUMMARY

The heart functions as a pump to circulate blood throughout the body. Cardiac emergencies occur when the heart is unable to effectively carry out this function. The potential seriousness and the complexity of causative factors make cardiac emergencies one of the most difficult situations for the first aider to deal with. In most cases, cardiac emergencies require prompt medical intervention and treatment. However, it is often the first few minutes of action that make the difference between life and death. The first aider plays an important role by recognizing the seriousness of the emergency, maintaining vital functions, and obtaining medical care.

Cardiopulmonary resuscitation is an essential first aid procedure when the heart fails to sufficiently circulate blood. However, not all cardiac emergencies require CPR. When a patient presents with signs and symptoms of cardiac arrhythmias, heart attack, hypertensive crisis, or cardiac injuries, the first aider must carefully assess the need for CPR. Vital life signs, breathing, pulse, and pupil constriction should be continuously monitored to evaluate the effectiveness of circulation (see Chapter 3 for a more detailed discussion). Do not subject an already damaged heart to the trauma of CPR unless it is necessary to maintain circulation.

FIRST AIDER COMPETENCIES

After studying the material and practicing the techniques presented in this chapter, the student should be able to:

- Define bradycardia and tachycardia, describe signs and symptoms, and explain the first aid procedures for each type of arrhythmia.

- Describe signs and symptoms of angina pectoris and acute myocardial infarction and outline the appropriate first aid procedures.

- Demonstrate the proper position to place a heart attack victim.

- Describe some of the complications that can result from acute myocardial infarction.

- Describe signs and symptoms and outline appropriate first aid procedures for hypertensive crises.

- Identify important factors the first aider should attempt to determine when caring for a patient with a suspected cardiac emergency.

- Describe the types of accidents that might lead to cardiac injuries.

- Describe signs and symptoms and outline appropriate first aid procedures for cardiac injuries.

- Explain under what circumstances it is appropriate to administer CPR for cardiac emergencies.

**REFERENCES AND
RECOMMENDED READINGS**

1. Burch, C. E.: A primer on cardiology, Philadelphia, 1971, Lea & Febiger.
2. Chung, E. K.: Cardiac emergency care, Philadelphia, 1975, Lea & Febiger.
3. Elliot, R. S.: The acute cardiac emergency, diagnosis and management, Mount Kisco, N.Y., 1972, Futura Publishing Co., Inc.
4. Koch-Weser, J.: Hypertensive emergencies, New England Journal of Medicine 290:211-214, 1974.
5. Nixon, P. G.: Coronary heart disease and its emergencies, Practitioner 211:5-16, July, 1973.
6. Phibbs, B.: The human heart: a guide to heart disease, ed. 3, St. Louis, 1975, The C. V. Mosby Co.
7. Renner, W. F.: Emergency medical service: the concept and coronary care, Journal of the American Medical Association 230:251-254, 1974.
8. Selzer, A.: Principles of clinical cardiology, Philadelphia, 1975, W. B. Saunders Co.
9. Services for cardiovascular emergencies, Report of a WHO committee, WHO Technical Reprint Series 562:1-129, 1975.

Trauma emergencies

6

‸‸

PREVENTION AND CARE OF SHOCK

Sally Abston

Shock may result from failure of the cardiovascular system or loss of blood or fluid from the circulation. Shock is a life-threatening situation and requires immediate recognition and early care by the first aider.

STRUCTURE AND FUNCTION OF THE CARDIOVASCULAR SYSTEM

The cardiovascular system consists of the heart and blood vessels and provides for the delivery of oxygen and nutrients to—and the removal of carbon dioxide and waste products from—the cells of all organ systems of the body. Function of the cardiovascular system depends on an efficient pump, the heart, moving a proper volume of fluid, blood, against appropriate resistance, vascular tone. As discussed in Chapter 5, the heart is a four-chambered organ, each side divided into two chambers with a valve between them. The right side of the heart receives blood from the venae cava draining the body and pumps the blood to the lungs. In the lungs, the red cells are saturated by oxygen, and a small amount of oxygen is dissolved in the blood.

Vessels

The left side of the heart receives the oxygenated blood from the lungs and pumps it to the body by way of the aorta. The aorta divides into smaller vessels, arteries, which further divide into arterioles, which divide into a network of capillaries. Capillaries have walls of one cell thickness with microscopic spaces between the cells, providing for exchange of oxygen and nutrients with the cells of the organs. The capillaries drain into venules, which coalesce to form veins, which further unite to form the superior and inferior venae cava, which return the blood to the right side of the heart.

The heart and major vessels are shown in Fig. 6-1.

Blood volume

Blood is composed of formed elements, red and white blood cells, and fluid, plasma. In the normal, healthy individual the total blood volume is constant and is approximately 8.5% of the total body weight. This volume is maintained by the exchange of the fluid portion with the fluids of the extravascular tissue at the capillary level. This exchange and the maintenance of a normal circulating volume

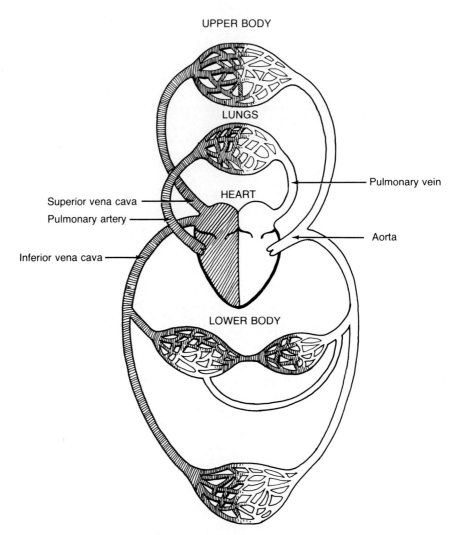

Fig. 6-1. Circulation of blood showing relationship of heart and major vessels.

is dependent on the intake of fluids by the individual equal to the normal physio-logical loss of fluids in respiration, evaporation, urine, and feces. The formed elements of the blood are produced at a rate commensurate with their natural expiration to maintain a fairly constant proportion in the normal healthy state. Red blood cells usually comprise 35% to 40% of the circulating blood volume in the adult woman and 40% to 45% in the adult man.

Blood pressure

The blood is pumped by the heart into the aorta against resistance. This re-sistance maintains constant pressure within the vascular system. The resistance is a result of the elasticity of the aorta, arteries, and arterioles, and the constriction of sphincters in the arterioles. The elasticity of these vessels allows them to distend with each ejection of blood by the heart. At completion of ejection, the vessel walls then recoil to conform to the volume of blood within them. This distention and recoil of the vessels provides the pulses, which may be felt by gentle pressure over arteries at the wrist or in the neck.

The strength of the pulse is dependent on the difference between the size of the artery at the point of maximum distention and the size of the artery at the point of greatest recoil and provides an approximation of the volume of blood. The pulse rate, that is, the number of pulsations a minute, reflects the rate at which the heart is pumping. The pressure within the arteries is determined by inflating a pneumatic cuff about the upper arm with a stethoscope just distal to the cuff. The pressure in the cuff is increased until the artery is totally occluded and then slowly released. When the pressure in the cuff is reduced enough to allow blood to flow through the artery, the sound is transmitted by the stethoscope. This pressure is at the point of maximum distention of the vessel at the end of the heart's ejection and is known as the systolic pressure. As pressure in the cuff is further reduced, the audible pulse will cease as the pressure in the cuff falls below the maximum pressure within the artery. The pulse is no longer audible, and this pressure is the diastolic pressure. The normal blood pressure in the adult is 110 to 140 mm Hg systolic pressure and 70 to 90 mm Hg diastolic pressure and is recorded as, for example, 120/80.

As the arteriole divides to form capillaries, there is a sphincter that is controlled by nervous impulses as well as chemical components within the circulating blood. If this sphincter is relaxed, it allows a more rapid flow of blood into the capillaries. A similar sphincter is located at the venule end of the capillaries. If this sphincter contracts coincident with relaxation of the arteriolar sphincter, the capillaries may hold a large quantity of blood. Such pooling leads to decreased return of blood to the heart as well as decreased resistance and lowered blood pressure.

Cardiac output

Cardiac output is the product of the heart rate and the volume of blood ejected with each contraction. The heart rate is controlled by nervous impulses originating from regulatory centers in the brain. These centers are influenced by changes in the oxygen and carbon dioxide content of the blood, pressure receptors in the arteries and veins, and respiration. The volume of blood ejected is dependent on the heart rate and the contractibility of the cardiac muscle. A slow rate allows enough blood to fill the heart for maximum ejection; a rapid rate, by providing less time for filling, results in a decrease of volume ejected with each contraction. Since cardiac output is a product of the rate and ejection volume, it may remain constant with increase in rate until the rate becomes so rapid that filling becomes greatly diminished.

Shock essentially results from insufficient cardiac output. However, the exact cause of shock is not always the same for every patient. Thus there are several types of shock that can occur as a result of a series of events involved in the interrelationship of blood volume, blood pressure, and heart rate.

TYPES OF SHOCK

Shock results when the cardiovascular system is inadequate in the delivery of oxygen and nutrients to the cells. Shock may result from failure of the heart to function as a pump, loss of resistance or vascular tone, or a decrease of blood volume.

Shock caused by pump failure

Cardiogenic shock, that is, shock caused by inefficiency of the pump, may be due to disease of the muscle of the heart such as myocardial infarction (heart attack) or an infection of the muscle (myocarditis). The injured or diseased muscle is incapable of a forceful contraction, and there is diminished output with each ejection.

Cardiogenic shock may result from arrhythmia (loss of the heart's regular rhythm). An arrhythmia may be an alteration in rate (an abnormally rapid or slow rate) or a change in rhythm with an irregular rhythm (varying times between each beat). Too rapid a rate may result in inadequate filling of the heart before ejection with a diminished volume ejected. A varying time between ejections similarly results in a diminished cardiac output. Changes in rhythm and rate may reflect an increased or diminished sensitivity to the nervous impulses that usually control the heart rate. Arrhythmia may also be the result of cardiac injury with inability to transmit the impulse within the heart.

A third cause of cardiogenic shock is the inability of the heart to distend and fill before ejection. The heart is enclosed within a tissue sac known as the pericardium. In the normal state this sac is empty and allows the heart to distend and contract. In some disease states the sac may be filled with fluid or blood and constrict the heart, preventing its normal filling. This is known as *tamponade* and is encountered most frequently when there has been direct penetrating trauma such as a gunshot or stab wound of the heart with filling of the pericardium with blood.

Shock caused by decreased blood volume

Hypovolemic shock, that is, shock caused by loss of circulating blood volume, may occur with the loss of whole blood or the loss of plasma. Hemorrhage may be the result of trauma with laceration of a blood vessel or injury to an organ. If the injured vessel is in an extremity, the hemorrhage may be obvious as swelling or external bleeding. However, if the injured organ is in the abdomen or chest, the source of bleeding is hidden, and the severity of the injury may be unrecognized until the victim develops shock.

Fractures result in hemorrhage of the vessels in adjacent muscle that are torn coincident with the fracture. The broken bones bleed as the marrow is opened at the site of the fracture. Careless moving of the fractured extremity may lead to the injury of other vessels or dislodge clots, causing further hemorrhage.

Hemorrhage may result from disease rather than trauma. Ulcers of the stomach and duodenum may be complicated by rapid and massive hemorrhage with the patient presenting in shock. Some disease states are characterized by an inability of the blood to clot normally, resulting in major hemorrhage from minor injuries.

Loss of fluids and electrolytes with resultant decrease in circulating volume may occur as a result of vomiting or diarrhea. The absorption of fluids and electrolytes by the mucosal lining of the gastrointestinal tract maintains the normal fluid balance. When the gastrointestinal tract is diseased, this source of fluids is lost. If vomiting and diarrhea occur, there is a loss of fluids that are secreted by the mucosa and normally reabsorbed. The loss of the gastrointestinal tract as the source of fluids, as well as the abnormal loss of fluids, results in a diminished circulating volume.

Plasma loss may occur with serious burn injuries as well as crush injuries. Both of these injuries are characterized by cellular injury and release of cellular metabolic products into the tissues. These products cause changes within the capillaries resulting in a loss of plasma from the capillaries into the surrounding tissue. The total circulating volume decreases, and there is an increase in the percentage of red cell mass.

The quantity of blood or plasma loss necessary to cause hypovolemic shock varies between 10% and 20% of the normal circulating volume. The individual's tolerance to the loss of volume is related to the time span during which the loss is sustained as well as the general condition of the individual before injury. The normal physiological response to hypovolemia is increased heart rate and arteriolar constriction. These two responses maintain the blood pressure, particularly if the patient is supine. Marginal hypovolemia may be recognized in such patients by putting them into a sitting position and recording the pulse and blood pressure. An increase in pulse or fall in pressure greater than 10% should warn the examiner of impending hypovolemia and possibly shock.

Shock caused by lowered blood pressure

Shock caused by loss of vascular tone or peripheral resistance occurs when the arteriolar constrictors do not function and dilatation occurs, allowing pooling of the blood in the capillary bed. This may occur as a result of the loss of nervous control, or it may be the result of circulating toxic substances.

Severe infections may result in the loss of vascular tone, that is, peripheral resistance, as toxic metabolic products of the bacteria or of injured cells enter the circulation. These substances render the arteriolar sphincters unresponsive to nervous impulses, resulting in vasodilation. These toxic substances may also affect the vasomotor centers in the brain, disrupting the nervous control of the sphincters.

A loss in peripheral resistance leads to increased blood in the capillaries, diminished venous return to the heart, and eventually to decreased cardiac output. The loss of resistance and diminished output results in shock.

Fainting. Sudden loss of vascular tone may occur as a result of severe emotional distress or pain. The common faint represents the loss of vascular tone, sudden fall in blood pressure, and transient loss of consciousness. When the patient assumes a reclining position as a result of the faint, cardiac return improves, the blood supply to the brain is improved, those brain centers responsible for vascular tone become active, and vasoconstriction returns.

Correct care for fainting. The victim of a faint should be placed in a reclining position on his or her back. An open airway must be assured by preventing the tongue from obstructing the pharynx (airway) until full consciousness returns. If the faint occurs in a warm or hot environment, the patient should be placed in the shade, and any outer clothing such as a coat should be removed.

On the other hand, if the faint occurs in cold surroundings, the patient should be covered to prevent undue exposure to the cold. Crowding about the victim should be avoided.

What not to do for fainting. An individual who has fainted should not be subjected to a traumatic stimulus such as cold water or a slap in the face.

RECOGNITION OF SHOCK

The recognition of early shock requires a knowledge of those injuries or illnesses that may lead to cardiovascular failure as well as the signs and symptoms of such failure.

Contributing factors

Blood loss. The injuries most frequently associated with shock are those which lead to blood loss. Penetrating wounds of the extremities that injure major vessels are usually recognized by obvious bleeding. The first aider should attempt to determine the amount of blood loss. Two cups is equivalent to 10% of the blood volume of the average adult. Evidence of this quantity of blood loss should warn the first aider of the possibility of shock. The injury resulting from a penetrating wound of the chest or abdomen is more difficult to evaluate, since blood loss is rarely obvious, that is, external. The first aider is dependent on frequent review of the patient with such a wound to constantly assess the likelihood of shock.

Blunt trauma. This most often leads to serious injuries, the consequences of which may be shock. A fracture of a femur, the bone of the thigh, will result in the loss of approximately a pint of blood, which approaches 10% of the blood volume of the average adult. Blunt trauma to the abdomen may result in the tear of blood vessels or injury to intraabdominal organs with resultant loss of blood or plasma. It is apparent that a patient in an auto accident with a fractured femur and blunt trauma to the abdomen may rapidly develop hypovolemic shock.

Fluid loss. Other injuries frequently leading to cardiovascular failure are serious burn injuries and crush injuries. The fluid loss in these injuries is plasma lost through the capillaries. The lost fluid becomes evident as there is rapid swelling of the injured part. A burn involving one entire leg can lead to the loss of 20% to 25% of the circulating blood volume into the leg.

Pain. The sudden onset of severe, unrelenting pain may disrupt the normal nervous balance between vessel contriction and dilation. There may be a sudden loss of vascular tone with an increase in the volume of blood contained in the vessels. The blood pressure fall caused by pain may not be accompanied by an increased heart rate, and this finding may serve to differentiate such shock from hypovolemic shock for the first aider.

Traumatic cardiac failure. Occasionally trauma is associated with shock due to cardiac failure, that is, cardiogenic shock. Such shock may result from a blow to the chest with myocardial injury. The most frequent cause of such an injury is the thrust of a steering wheel or its post in an auto accident. Penetrating wounds of the chest may enter the pericardium, the sac surrounding the heart, and resultant hemorrhage will fill the sac, limit the heart's filling, and diminish its output.

Nontraumatic illnesses. Conditions associated with shock are usually characterized by rapid fluid loss, hemorrhage, or cardiac failure. Gastrointestinal diseases with vomiting and/or diarrhea and the attendant loss of fluids can lead to hypovolemia. Hemorrhage from gastric or duodenal ulcers may result in the rapid loss of large volumes of blood and shock.

The most frequent cause of cardiogenic shock is myocardial infarction, commonly known as heart attack. There is decreased blood supply to a portion of the heart muscle and injury to the muscle results. This is usually accompanied by severe pain and anxiety. There may be a rapid decrease in the cardiac output with shock.

Shock due to loss of vasomotor tone may occur acutely, as mentioned earlier, as a result of severe emotional stress or pain. It may also occur as a result of prolonged standing, particularly in a stressful situation. The frequency of this syndrome occurring at military inspections has led to the name of "parade-ground faint."

Central nervous system injuries may be complicated by the loss of vasomotor tone and shock. Such injuries are unique in that a severe fall in the blood pressure may occur without a concomitant increase in the pulse. Such symptoms should always alert the first aider to the likelihood of a severe head injury or spinal cord injury.

Signs and symptoms of shock

The early signs and symptoms of shock are the signs of compensatory mechanisms, that is, the body's own attempts to maintain an efficient circulation. As the circulation begins to fail, regardless of whether the failure is due to diminished cardiac output or decreased volume, constriction occurs in the arterioles to maintain the pressure to provide perfusion. The constriction initially occurs in the skin, muscles, and intraabdominal organs to provide maximum blood supply to the brain and heart. As this constriction occurs, the patient becomes pale and cool to touch, since there is diminished blood flow through the skin. The skin may be moist, and beads of perspiration appear on the forehead. This sweating occurs because the sweat glands are stimulated by the same nerves that cause constriction of the vessels in the skin. The patient will complain of muscular weakness, since there is diminished flow through the muscles. With similar vasoconstriction occurring to the mucous membranes of the mouth, the patient notes a dryness and thirst.

Coincident with the vasoconstriction, the nervous receptors previously mentioned will lead to an increased heart rate, and the pulse is noted by the examiner to be *more rapid* and *less forceful*. This is often described as a rapid, weak pulse.

Respiration becomes rapid as the nervous centers respond to the decreased delivery of oxygen and the patient may become apprehensive. If shock progresses, the patient may become apathetic.

During the early development of shock, the blood pressure may remain normal, and as shock progresses the pressure may slowly fall. A reclining patient in early to moderate shock may have a normal blood pressure, but when asked to sit up there will be a fall of more than 10% of the blood pressure. The pulse may increase, likewise, when moving from reclining to sitting. Such a test may

Table 1. Summary of signs and symptoms of shock

	Early	Late
Blood pressure	Normal	Less than 90 mm Hg systolic
Pulse	Increase in rate	Increase in rate; weak
Skin color	Normal	Pale
Skin temperature	Cool, moist	Cold
Sensorium	Anxious	Coma
Respiration	Increase in rate and depth	Increase in rate, shallow

be an aid to the first aider in the initial evaluation of a patient to determine the threat of shock.

The first aider should develop the habit of rapidly evaluating the patient's appearance relative to pallor, skin relative to temperature and moisture, the mucous membranes of the mouth relative to moisture, the pulse relative to rate, and strength and the mental status relative to awareness and reaction. The first aider should be fully aware of those injuries and illnesses which may predispose to shock and maintain a constant high level of suspicion and awareness of the early signs of cardiovascular failure.

Signs and symptoms of shock are summarized in Table 1.

CARE FOR SHOCK

Although the definitive care for shock usually requires a hospital and professional personnel, its early recognition and appropriate first aid may be life saving. The first aider's response must be to *diminish the stress* of the injury or illness and prevent progression from early to deep shock.

Physical stress. A brief questioning of the patient or witnesses should be conducted together with a rapid examination of the patient. The patient should be placed at rest and protected from any additional stress on the circulatory system. The head and trunk should be level with the extremities elevated slightly to assist return of blood to the heart. This may be achieved by placing rolled linens or clothing under the feet with the knees extended. The victim should *not* be placed on a litter and the entire litter lifted to elevate the legs above the heart, since this places the head in a dependent position and may decrease blood return from the brain and lead to swelling of the brain. Such a position also restricts respiration as the intraabdominal contents fall against the diaphragm, limiting its movement.

Proper position for a patient in shock is shown in Fig. 6-2.

Any external hemorrhage should be rapidly controlled, and any apparent fractures should be immobilized. The unconscious patient in shock must constantly be observed for respiratory distress. The tongue falling against the back of the throat may obstruct the airway. An open airway should be maintained by keeping the neck in an extended position. The patient in shock often complains of nausea and may vomit. Such a patient should be placed on his side to prevent aspiration of the vomitus and choking on inspiration. If the patient cannot be turned, his head should be turned. If an oxygen mask is in place, it must be removed to permit clearing of the mouth.

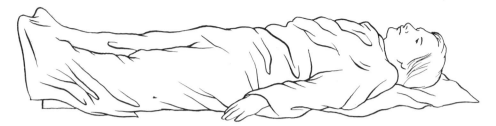

Fig. 6-2. Shock position.

Movement of the patient in shock must be done carefully, particularly if there are fractures. The first aider must have adequate assistance to lift a patient. If the patient has skeletal injuries, he should be placed on a board or stretcher to allow transport without movement of extremities or head.

The victim of major trauma such as auto accidents or falls may have unrecognized intrathoracic injuries that may interfere with oxygenation. Such patients should be given oxygen by mask until the respiratory function can be evaluated. Similarly, serious illnesses may have respiratory dysfunction and benefit from oxygen therapy. Although oxygen may not be necessary for all patients with early shock, its routine use is advisable to assure its benefit to those patients whose condition could deteriorate without oxygen. In other words, the use of oxygen to severely injured or ill patients will not do harm, and the first aider should not hesitate to provide it if available.

Environmental stress. The victim of shock or impending shock should be protected from additional stress of environmental temperature extremes. In a cold environment, that is, less than 13° to 16° C (55° to 60° F), the victim should be covered with blankets to prevent the added stress and energy expenditure of shivering. In extreme cold, the peripheral vasoconstriction due to the cold, particularly of the hands and feet, imposed on an inefficient vascular system may lead to injury of those parts. An environment warmer than 32° C (90° F) may cause increased fluid loss through sweating and an increased oxygen demand due to increased metabolic needs. This increased stress may cause rapid progression to shock.

Psychological stress. The patient in early shock is anxious and should constantly be reassured to allay the anxiety. The first aider should always advise the patient of the procedures being done and explain why they are being done. The victim's questions should be rapidly answered. The student should refer to Chapter 15 for specific procedures to provide psychological care.

Immediate transportation. The definitive treatment of shock requires a hospital setting and professional personnel. The first aider must decide quickly if shock is a realistic expectation for the victim of an injury or illness. If so, plans for transportation as well as care en route should be effected. The successful reversal of shock depends often on how long the shock has existed as well as how severe the shock is.

At the hospital, diagnostic procedures such as electrocardiograms, radiographs, and laboratory work are performed. Therapy is begun with fluid administered intravenously, respiratory support with ventilators, and definitive treatment such as fixation of fractures, surgical exploration of the abdomen, or other operations. Arrhythmias or other complications of myocardial infarctions are treated with specific drugs. Often the patient's recovery is dependent on someone's having recognized the early signs of impending shock, diminished the stresses, and transported the patient to a treatment facility.

PREVENTION OF SHOCK

It is apparent that the prevention of shock requires careful observation of the injuries or illness and the early initiation of first aid before the obvious signs of shock intervene. The first aider must always evaluate the possibility of shock as a routine procedure in rendering emergency first aid.

SUMMARY

Shock, or cardiovascular failure, may result from serious injury or illness. It must be recognized early and progression prevented. When examining a patient for shock, one should consider:
1. What is the injury or illness?
2. What is the appearance of skin color?
3. Is the skin warm and dry or cool and clammy?
4. What is the rate and character of the pulse?
5. Does the patient complain of
    a. Weakness?
    b. Thirst?
6. What is the patient's mental attitude?
7. How is the patient breathing?

FIRST AIDER COMPETENCIES

After studying the material and practicing the techniques presented in this chapter, the student should be able to:
*   Define *shock*.
*   Explain the early signs and symptoms of shock.
*   Define *normal pulse rate* and *blood pressure*.
*   Describe first aid procedures for the patient in shock.
*   Demonstate the correct position for the patient in shock.
*   Explain the need for early transportation of the shock patient.

REFERENCES AND RECOMMENDED READINGS
1. Guyton, A. C.: Textbook of medical physiology, ed. 5, Philadelphia, 1976, W. B. Saunders Co.
2. Shires, G. T., Carrico, C. J., and Canizaro, P. C.: Shock, Philadelphia, 1973, W. B. Saunders Co.
3. Sproul, C. W., and Mullanney, P. J.: Emergency care: assessment and intervention, St. Louis, 1974, The C. V. Mosby Co.

7

▲▼

MANAGEMENT OF WOUNDS AND HEMORRHAGING

Charles Edwin Rinear and Guy S. Parcel

Wounds are injuries to body tissues, either external or internal. External wounds involve injury to the skin or mucous membranes. Internal wounds involve injury to deeper tissues, not associated with the skin or mucous membranes. Often both types of wounds are encountered after traumatic injury.

DANGERS OF WOUNDS

Wounds that are characterized by severe bleeding are life threatening and should be considered second in importance only to cardiopulmonary arrest cases in terms of their medical urgency. If a major artery has been severed, blood loss may be sufficient within 3 minutes or less to cause death. Wounds of the head, chest, back, and abdomen are of particular significance, since injury to these parts may cause serious organic damage or uncontrollable internal bleeding, severe shock, and rapid death.

The dangers of infection must not be overlooked. This is particularly true in cases involving penetrating wounds or in wounds involving diabetics or individuals with various forms of peripheral vascular disease. In such instances, even small wounds can become seriously infected, leading to gangrene and limb amputations. Finally, the dangers of rabies from animal bites or licks on abraded skin should be considered along with the dangers of tetanus, which exist with *all* wounds, including burns.

The major objectives in the management of wounds are to (1) maintain vital functions, (2) control hemorrhaging, (3) care for shock, and (4) prevent wound contamination and further injury while providing for professional medical treatment.

TYPES OF WOUNDS

There are five major types of wounds frequently encountered in emergencies (Fig. 7-1). These include abrasions, punctures, avulsions, incisions, and lacerations. Each type has its particular dangers relative to bleeding, infection, and organic damage.

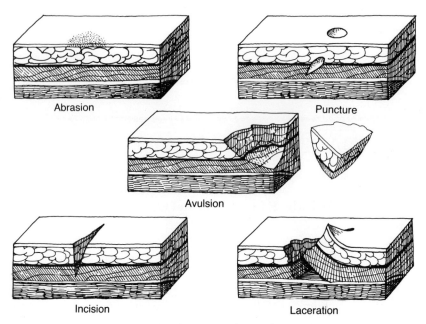

Fig. 7-1. Types of wounds.

Abrasions

Abrasions are wounds in which the outer layers of skin are scraped away. These wounds are usually associated with minimal bleeding but are likely to become contaminated by foreign objects, which may become ground into the wound site. If these wounds are not properly cleansed and cared for, serious infection and a permanent tatoo-like scar may remain.

Punctures

Puncture wounds result from foreign objects that penetrate the skin. Such objects as nails, tacks, knives, or bullets penetrating the body cause puncture wounds of varying severity. Often puncture wounds are associated with minimal bleeding. However, the dangers of internal bleeding, organic damage, and infection are great due to the presence of the foreign object. Animal bites and stings such as those from snakes or bees are also included in this category.

Avulsions

Avulsive wounds result when tissues are torn from the body. These wounds are frequently associated with serious bleeding. If body parts such as fingers, toes, or parts of the ear or nose, have been avulsed, such parts should be brought to the hospital with the patient for possible reattachment.

Incisions

Incised wounds are sharp cuts that often bleed severely. If the wound extends below the skin surface, there is danger of nerve, muscle, or tendon damage. As in all wounds, the dangers of infection must be considered and cared for with respect to these wounds.

Lacerations

Lacerated wounds are jagged, irregular wounds that are associated with much tissue damage. Bleeding and tissue damage with subsequent deep infection are common with these wounds.

TYPES OF BLEEDING

Bleeding from wounds may be of three varieties. *Arterial* bleeding involves blood loss from arteries, which carry blood away from the heart. Arterial bleeding is characterized by bright red blood spurting from a wound. It is the most serious type of bleeding, since it will require medical intervention after initial control to prevent severe shock or death. Venous bleeding, which involves blood loss from veins, which conduct blood back to the heart, is characterized by dark red blood that flows from a wound site. This type of bleeding may also be life threatening, especially when several veins are involved. However, it is generally more readily controlled than arterial bleeding because blood flow in the veins is under less pressure than in the arteries. Venous bleeding should be controlled quickly because of potential blood loss.

The third type of bleeding is capillary. Capillary bleeding results from superficial wounds and is readily controlled by first aid procedures and the body's normal clotting mechanisms. This type of bleeding may be recognized by blood oozing from a wound.

CONTROL OF BLEEDING

When presented with a wound that is associated with significant bleeding, it is imperative that the bleeding be controlled at once. Infection should *not* be a consideration under such circumstances. It is better to have an infected wound than a dead person. Any available material should be used. In the absence of such, a bare hand can be used to save a life. There are essentially three methods for controlling bleeding, which should be followed in order.

Direct pressure

Hard, firm, direct pressure (Fig. 7-2) applied over the wound site will generally prove effective in controlling hemorrhage from most wounds. Pressure should be maintained until a *pressure dressing* is applied to hold pressure over the bleeding site until the services of medical personnel can be obtained. When bleeding starts again after pressure is released, get the patient to medical care at once.

Pressure points

The use of a number of pressure points (Fig. 7-3) in *combination* with direct pressure will control bleeding in virtually all but a few cases. Pressure points can be applied in conjunction with direct pressure. In such cases, the blood vessel supplying blood to the wound is compressed against an underlying bone or muscle tissue in an effort to close it off and decrease the amount of blood flowing through the vessel. The importance of knowing the exact location of

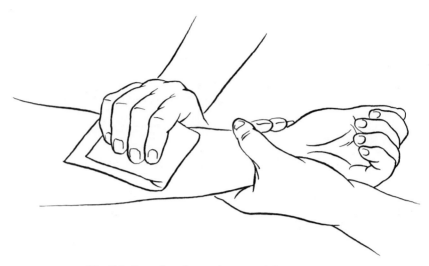

Fig. 7-2. Procedure for application of direct pressure.

such pressure points cannot be overemphasized. Unless the correct pressure point is quickly found, significant blood loss will result. Thus the use of pressure points should be practiced frequently and on a number of different individuals, noting anatomical differences that make a particular pressure point easy to find on one person and difficult to find on another.

Temporal artery. Compression of the temporal artery, which is located about 2.5 cm (1 inch) posterior (in back of) the corner of the eye and slightly above the angle may prove useful in controlling superficial wounds of the frontal part of the scalp or forehead. Because of the extensive circulation to the scalp, pressure may have to be applied to both sides of the head. This should be avoided whenever possible, however. In finding this pressure point, look for the temporal pulse and slight indentation of this area in the location specified.

Facial artery. The facial artery, which supplies blood to the face and lower jaw, can be found by finding the two little notches about 2.5 cm (1 inch) anterior to (in front of) the angle of the jaw. If pressure is applied upward and outward in this area, the facial arteries become occluded, causing a numbness of the facial region and controlling bleeding in this area. The facial artery should be pressed against the jawbone. Two or more fingers may be used effectively for this purpose.

Carotid artery. Located on each side of the neck, slightly away from the trachea (windpipe), are the two common carotid arteries, which supply blood to the head and neck regions. Compression of the carotid artery against the mass of muscle beneath it is useful in controlling the serious hemorrhage from blood vessels in the head. Care must be taken not to obstruct the patient's airway when this pressure point is used. Pressure dressings should not be applied around the person's neck. The pressure point can be located in practice sessions by locating the carotid pulse on each side of the throat, just outward from the trachea.

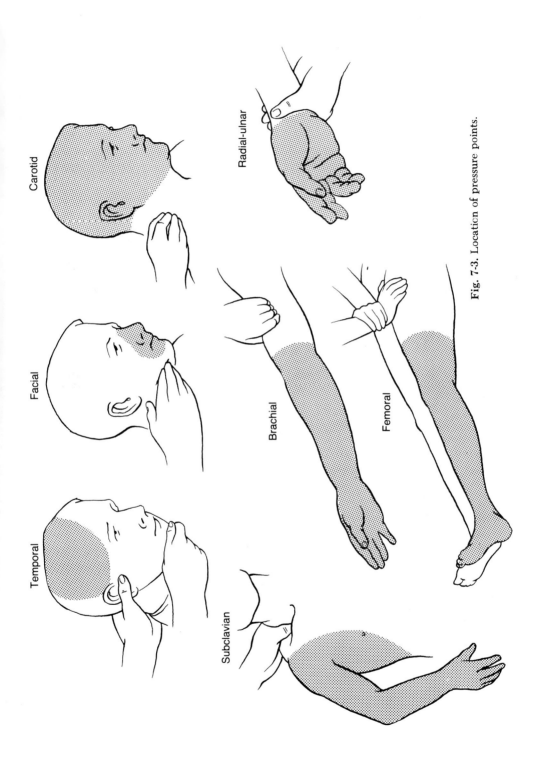

Carotid

Facial

Temporal

Radial-ulnar

Brachial

Femoral

Subclavian

Fig. 7-3. Location of pressure points.

Subclavian artery. The subclavian arteries, one on each side, just under the collar bones, supply the arm and upper shoulder regions with blood flow. Pressure applied with fingers downward just *behind* the collar bone will control bleeding in this region. This pressure point requires considerable practice to locate. It is essential that first aiders know this particular pressure point because of the large volume of blood that passes through this artery from the aorta. When this pressure point is successfully found, the patient will be unable to feel a wrist pulse and will notice a numbness in the arm and hand region.

Brachial artery. This major artery, located on the inner side of the upper arm between the biceps and triceps muscles, supplies the arm, hand, and fingers. Pressure should be applied halfway between the shoulder and the elbow. When the correct pressure point is found, a pulse will be felt in the arm, and the radial pulse should disappear. A numbness will also be felt in hand and arm areas.

Femoral artery. The femoral artery is located near the groin where the leg joins the trunk. When the correct place is found, a femoral pulse will be noted. Bleeding from this artery is profuse and life threatening. Practice this pressure point extensively. It is particularly difficult to find on muscular individuals.

Radial artery. The radial artery, at the anterior surface of the wrist on the thumb side, can be useful in controlling severe bleeding to the hand or fingers. A pulse should be felt and a numbness experienced in the hand areas. It is useful to compress the ulnar artery as well until pressure dressings have been applied.

Ulnar artery. Just across from the radial artery on the small finger side is the ulnar artery, which also supplies the hand with blood. This should be used in conjunction with the radial artery to control profuse hemorrhaging in the hand areas. If there is difficulty stopping bleeding with the use of the ulnar and radial pressure points, move up to the brachial point to control bleeding.

Tourniquet

The use of a tourniquet (Fig. 7-4) is rarely necessary to control bleeding. When direct pressure, elevation of a limb, pressure points, and pressure dressings are used in combination, all but a few cases will respond. However, there are cases in which bleeding will continue and a life could be lost without the use of a tourniquet. Tourniquets should be avoided whenever possible because of the danger of nerve and blood vessel damage. The decision to apply a tourniquet is a decision to risk the person's limb to save a life. When the use of a tourniquet is warranted, the following principles must be observed:

1. Use appropriate materials—stocking or cloth, *not* wire or rope.
2. Apply the tourniquet just above the wound site.
3. Note the time of application.
4. *Never* release a tourniquet.
5. Make the tourniquet tight enough to stop bleeding.
6. Never cover a tourniquet.
7. Elevate the limb slightly if it will not cause further injury.
8. Transport the patient immediately to medical care. Give care for shock while awaiting emergency transportation.
9. Mark on the patient or tag to indicate the time of application of the tourniquet.

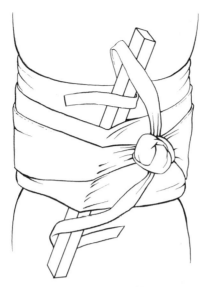

Fig. 7-4. Procedure for application of tourniquet.

Two principles need additional mention. Years ago, first aiders were advised to release a tourniquet periodically. Studies now prove that once a tourniquet is applied it should be released only by a physician who can give supportive treatment for shock.

Tourniquets must be applied tightly enough to stop bleeding. If they are applied too loosely, the bleeding will be *increased* through a shutdown of the venous circulation taking blood back to the heart while allowing the arterial circulation carrying blood into the extremity to continue. If a tourniquet is applied too tightly, injury to underlying nerves and blood vessels may be the result.

In applying a tourniquet, the appropriate material should be wrapped around the limb twice and a secure knot tied. A suitable strong object should be inserted between the two loops and the object turned until bleeding has been controlled. The tails of the cloth should then be wrapped around the object and tied in place. It is important that a strong stick or other strong object be used to tighten the tourniquet. Pens and pencils can be used in practice sessions. However, in real situations they would easily break, making the tourniquet ineffective and further endangering the life of the person injured.

Supportive measures for controlling bleeding

Ice is useful in controlling capillary bleeding, internal bleeding of a limb, and nosebleeds. It is not effective in controlling severe bleeding. Pressure dressings represent a dressing and a bandage applied to a wound to sustain pressure on the wound during transportation or while first aid is being given to other injured persons. Pressure dressings can be used on virtually any part of the body with a few exceptions such as the neck area.

Elevation of a limb in conjunction with other methods of bleeding control is effective in controlling hemorrhage. Elevation of a limb is immediately indicated unless injuries to the limb make this procedure inadvisable. The elevation of a bleeding limb can be performed in a second and reduces the hydrostatic pressure of blood within the limb, thus making the use of direct pressure and pressure point methods more effective.

CARE FOR MINOR WOUNDS

Wounds that involve only the superficial layers of the skin and are not associated with severe bleeding should be properly cleansed, dressed, and bandaged. Wounds in which bleeding has been of significance should not be cleansed. In such cases, bleeding should be controlled, a pressure dressing and bandage applied, and a physician consulted as soon as feasible. The following steps are taken when caring for minor wounds:

1. Wash hands two times using soap and water.
2. Allow the wound to bleed slightly.
3. Using a sterile gauze pad saturated with soap and water, gently wash dirt away from the wound edges. A cleansing agent may be used for this purpose, providing that all of it is removed. Unless a specific cleansing agent is recommended by a physician, use only nonirritating soap plus water.
4. Flush the wound liberally with large quantities of water. Remove all cleansing agents. *Do not apply an antiseptic* or any other ointment cream or spray.
5. Cover the wound with a sterile gauze dressing and bandage.
6. Refer the patient to a physician for follow-up care.

Application of dressings

1. Use commercial sterile materials whenever possible.
2. In the absence of the above, use sterile cloths by boiling the fabric and allowing it to dry, by ironing it, or through other means.
3. Open the package, touching only the corner of the dressing. Be sure the dressing extends well beyond the wound edges.
4. Apply a clean bandage over the dressing. Do not allow the bandage to retard circulation. Allow for swelling in burn cases.
5. Refer the person to a physician. In the meantime keep the part rested and elevated.

SPECIAL WOUNDS
Infected wounds

Infected wounds should receive the immediate attention of a physician, particularly in diabetic persons or individuals with circulatory diseases. Interim care may be given by a first aider until professional medical attention can be obtained.

Symptoms of wound infection. The following symptoms are given so that wound infections may be recognized. Such cases should be promptly referred to a physician for medical treatment when they are recognized. Typical symptoms of wound infections include the following, which may be remembered by the key word SHARP.

Swelling: The area progressively swells as the infection becomes worse. This may include swelling of adjacent lymph nodes, such as those in the neck, under the arms, or in the groin. In addition, the systemic symptoms of headache, fever, and weakness may appear.

*H*eat: The wound area feels warm.

*A*che: There is local pain around the wound site.

*R*edness: There is redness around the wound or red streaks extending from it.

*P*us: Dead white blood cells are often extruded from the wound.

First aid. Care consists of the following:

1. Keep the infected part immobile. Activity helps infection to spread.
2. Elevate the infected part unless this is contraindicated by injuries.
3. Apply warm wet cloths to the infected area followed by the application of sterile dressings and a bandage. Repeat this process four times a day.
4. Give care for shock and obtain medical assistance as early as possible.

Abdominal evisceration

In this emergency, the abdominal organs protrude through the abdomen and are exposed and visible to the first aider (Fig. 7-5). In such instances, the abdominal organs should not be touched nor pushed back into the abdomen. A sterile moist dressing saturated with saline solution or water should be applied and kept

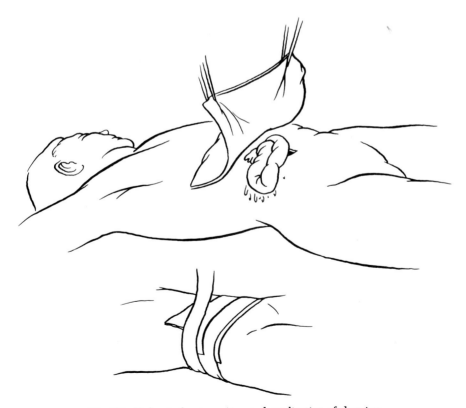

Fig. 7-5. Abdominal evisceration and application of dressing.

moist while awaiting medical treatment. The intestines should be stabilized by dressings and bandages to reduce movement and possibilities of further injury. The patient should be given care for shock, fluids should *not* be administered, and help should be obtained at the earliest time possible. Pulmonary and cardiac resuscitation should be administered if indicated.

Human bites

Human bites are common and represent a potentially serious source of infection if not properly cared for. The wound should be immediately washed with soap and water or a cleansing agent, thoroughly flushed with water, dressed and bandaged, and the patient referred to a physician for immediate follow-up care.

Animal bites

The principal danger of animal bites is rabies. Warm-blooded animals such as dogs, cats, bats, rats, raccoons, and rabbits can transmit the rabies virus through their saliva by means of biting the victim or by licking the individual on abraded skin. Contrary to popular belief, the animal need not be drooling, irritable, or dangerous. In some cases, the animal will appear partially paralyzed, stuporous, quiet, or even affectionate. The most common sites involved are limbs. Bites around the head, facial, or neck areas should be considered more serious because of a shorter incubation period.

An animal in the final stages of rabies infection will usually develop symptoms of the disease and die within a few days of symptomatic infection. The human incubation period for rabies varies considerably but averages around 2 months. The diagnosis of rabies by a physician is based on the history of contact with the animal, laboratory studies of the animal, and the presence of clinical symptoms in the animal. The disease is virtually always fatal in man once the symptoms appear. The total course of symptomatic disease is only 7 days. However, since the total course of survival is long (a range of 24 to 155 days from the time of the bite until the time of death), time is available to treat the person and prevent the symptomatic onset of the disease and death.

The following procedures should be carried out in cases of human-animal contact if rabies infection is suspected:
1. Wash the wound with large quantities of soap and water. Apply a dressing and bandage. Seek prompt medical attention, keeping the part immobile.
2. Call the police, veterinarian, and a physician as soon as possible. Try to restrain the animal if at all possible.
3. If the animal must be killed, avoid injury to the brain, which must be studied to determine viral rabies infection.
4. If the animal cannot be caught, immediately arrange for care with a physician while providing initial care as previously mentioned.

Tetanus infection

The danger of tetanus must be considered in *all* wounds. This is true even in the case of minor wounds, burns, or in drug injection cases. Thus all wounds must be given proper initial care and then referred to a physician for treatment. Booster shots are generally recommended every 10 years, although some physicians recommend a yearly tetanus booster for athletes or other individuals in high-risk activities.

Internal wounds

Internal wounds are generally characterized by pain, tenderness, swelling, and discoloration that takes some time to develop. In cases of severe internal wounds, especially those involving internal organs, progressive shock signs and symptoms may be apparent due to internal bleeding. Care may be provided for internal bleeding of a limb by using the same procedures as for external bleeding. Internal bleeding of the head, chest, abdomen, or internal organs cannot be controlled except by surgical intervention and must be considered a surgical emergency. For minor internal wounds, the following steps are recommended:

1. Keep the part immobile.
2. Apply cold wet cloths or ice to prevent swelling and retard internal bleeding and discoloration.
3. For contusions (bruises), apply ice and compression bandages, and elevate the extremity to reduce bleeding and swelling.
4. In severe wounds, give nothing by mouth and arrange for immediate medical treatment while providing symptomatic care for shock and vital signs.

Poisonous and nonpoisonous snake bites

The emergency care for nonpoisonous snake bites is that for minor wounds. Most snakes found throughout the world are nonpoisonous. Only about 400 of the 2000 kinds of snakes are of a poisonous variety.

In the United States, essentially four kinds of poisonous snakes exist. These include rattlesnakes, copperheads, cottonmouth moccasins, and coral snakes. A description of each of these snakes and where they are to be found follows.

Pit vipers. Each has a pit between the eye and the nostril on each side of the head, two well-developed fangs, elliptical pupils, and one row of plates beneath its tail. Pit vipers include the following snakes:

Rattlesnakes. Diamondback rattlesnakes are found from the central coast region of North Carolina along the lower coastal plain through Florida and westward to eastern Louisiana. Banded rattlers, mountain rattlers, and black rattlers are found in uplands and mountains from southern Maine to northern Florida and westward to central Texas. Pacific rattlesnakes are found in British Columbia to southern California and lower California east to Idaho, Nevada, and Arizona. The Massasauga or pygmy rattlesnake is found in western New York and northwestern Pennsylvania, westward to northeastern Kansas on the south and southeastern Minnesota on the north. Some subspecies extend into Colorado, Arizona, and Texas.

Copperheads. Copperheads are found in Massachusetts to northern Florida, westward to the Mississippi River in Illinois and across to Texas. They are found usually in hilly, rocky country and lowlands in walls, slab sawdust piles, hedges, haystacks, barns, and even in villages and towns.

Water or cottonmouth moccasins. Moccasins are found from southeastern Virginia along coastal plains through Florida, westward to Texas, and up the Mississippi Valley to Indiana.

Pit viper snakes, which are hemotoxic (toxic to blood cells), may be found essentially in all states except Maine.

Coral snake. This neurotoxic snake (poisonous to the nervous system of the body) is found in the midsouthern, southwestern, and western states. Its tubular fang marks are often inconspicuous but produce intense pain. It has a double row of plates beneath its tail and round pupils, which are also features of nonpoisonous snakes.

Contrary to popular belief, there is no need to panic over even poisonous snake bites. Most patients who have been bitten show up at a hospital within a half hour of being bitten. Recent studies show that approximately two thirds of all people bitten by poisonous snakes would survive even if nothing were done. The signs and symptoms of poisonous snake bites are as follows:

1. Burning pain and progressive swelling at the bite site
2. Shock and respiratory depression
3. Swelling of the tongue or about the neck
4. Nausea, dizziness, vomiting, general weakness, convulsions, coma, or paralysis.

The difference between poisonous and nonpoisonous snake bites is shown in Fig. 7-6. In cases of poisonous snake bites, fang marks *may* be visible. When the symptoms just mentioned present themselves, fang marks are visible, or the snake is suspected to be of a poisonous nature, the following steps should be taken as emergency care.

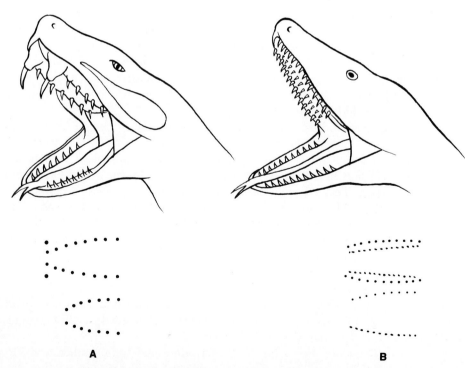

Fig. 7-6. Snake bite. **A,** Pit viper snakes. **B,** Nonpoisonous snakes.

1. Apply a constricting band 2 inches above and below the bite site. (The band should not cut off the arterial flow of blood. This can be determined by checking for a pulse or by seeing if a finger can be wedged under the band.)
2. Keep the part immobile and level.
3. Apply ice or cold applications to retard spread of the venom and swelling. Remove any jewelry such as rings or watches.
4. Care for shock and vital signs.
5. If the snake has been killed, save it for identification.
6. Provide emergency transportation.
7. Do *not* make incisions except under the following circumstances.
   a. The bite is from a poisonous snake and a hospital cannot be reached within an hour, and local signs and symptoms, including pain and swelling, are present; or
   b. The bite is *not* on an extremity, and therefore a constriction band cannot be applied.
8. In such cases, proceed as follows:
   a. Proceed as above, steps 1 through 6.
   b. Make longitudinal incisions, which should be no deeper than the skin, ⅛ to ¼ inch long through the fang marks. Suck on the wound for an hour. Although snake venom is not a stomach poison, it is best not to swallow it. Rinse your mouth after suction has been applied.
   c. Cleanse the wound and apply a sterile dressing and bandage.
   d. If the person must walk, he or she should avoid rapid movement.
   e. Notify the hospital and have them prepare antivenom serum.

General care for idiopathic bites and stings

When an individual has sustained a bite from a spider, jellyfish, or other insect or sea creature of unknown origin, the following steps should be instituted:
1. Remove the stinger if it can be seen.
2. Give supportive care for vital signs and shock. Maintain an open airway. Give pulmonary or cardiac resuscitation if indicated.
3. Apply a constricting band 2 inches above and below the wound site. Check the band to be sure that arterial circulation has not been cut off by taking a pulse below the band or by inserting a finger under the band. Remove the band after a half hour if medical treatment has not been obtained within that time period.
4. Keep the part immobile and below the level of the heart.
5. Apply ice or cold applications to prevent spread of the poison and to prevent and reduce the severity of swelling.
6. Refer all cases to medical treatment at once.

SUMMARY

In caring for individuals with wounds or hemorrhaging, one must institute both specific and generalized care procedures. First and foremost is the control of life-threatening bleeding by direct pressure, pressure points, or a tourniquet, in that order, in conjunction with appropriate supportive measures such as ice, compression dressings, and elevation of affected extremities. Prompt attention must be given to wounds where there is danger of air embolism, gangrene (as in eviscerations), and pneumothorax (sucking chest wounds). Considerations about the reduction of wound contamination should be given priority only in cases of minor wounds not associated with a life-threatening hazard. One must consider the danger of internal bleeding, which tends to be insidious yet often life threatening in many cases.

Generalized emergency care for patients showing evidence of wounds or hemorrhaging includes the important measures of airway establishment and maintenance, supportive care for shock and vital body functions, and emotional support.

As in all other aspects of emergency care, one must use caution in not overlooking a potentially serious condition; thus appropriate referrals are recommended in all cases.

FIRST AIDER COMPETENCIES

After studying the material in this chapter, the student should be able to:
- Demonstrate procedures for airway establishment for neck injury and non-neck injury cases.
- Demonstrate bleeding control skills for direct pressure, pressure points, tourniquet, and supportive measures, including use of ice, compression dressing, and elevation; know when elevation is contraindicated.
- Demonstrate application of constricting bands.
- List signs and symptoms and describe first aid for infected wounds.
- Describe first aid for serious wounds, minor wounds, and special wounds.
- Describe ways of recognizing poisonous snake bites.

REFERENCES AND
RECOMMENDED READINGS

1. Advanced first aid and emergency care, The American National Red Cross, Garden City, N.Y., 1973, Doubleday & Co., Inc.
2. Emergency care and transportation of the sick and injured, Chicago, 1971, The American Academy of Orthopaedic Surgeons.
3. Rinear, C., and Rinear, E.: Emergency bandaging: a wrap-up of better techniques, Nursing '75 **5**:29-35, Jan., 1975.
4. Sproul, C. W., and Mullanney, P. J.: Emergency care: assessment and intervention, St. Louis, 1974, The C. V. Mosby Co.
5. Stephenson, H. E., editor: Immediate care of the acutely ill and injured, St. Louis, 1974, The C. V. Mosby Co.

8

POISONING AND TOXIC REACTIONS

Richard F. McConnell, Jr., Elton Dupree, and Guy S. Parcel

Accidental or intentional poisoning can constitute a serious threat to life. Depending on the amount and type of toxic substance, immediate first aid intervention may be the critical factor in the outcome of a poisoning incident.

Accidental and self-administered poisonings constitute a serious health problem. Poisonings from ingestion of toxic agents and drugs account for nearly 10,000 deaths each year. In addition there occur incidents of nonfatal ingestions of chemicals and drugs. In 1973, the National Clearinghouse for Poison Control Centers processed 163,500 ingestion reports. This number is conservative, since it represents only reports obtained from 517 centers and does not account for numerous cases treated and not reported by private physicians or those receiving no professional attention at all. More realistic figures may range as high as 800,000 cases per year.

CLASSIFICATIONS AND GENERAL EFFECTS OF POISONING

A poison may be defined as any substance, gas, liquid, or drug that damages tissue or adversely alters organ function. This may be accomplished through destruction or irritation of tissues or through physiological alteration of the cardiorespiratory or central nervous systems.

The commonest route of administration is by *ingestion* of solids or liquids, including such things as pills, plants, and cleaning agents. Another common method of exposure is *inhalation* of gases, such as carbon monoxide, gasoline, hair spray, and glue vapors. With the increase in drug abuse over the last several years, *injection* of drugs and chemicals has become another method of exposure to toxic agents. Injection may also occur from natural sources, such as bee stings and pit-viper bites.

Stimulants, such as amphetamines and strychnine (often used to cut street narcotics) increase the heart rate, respiratory rate, and level of excitability of the central nervous system (CNS), which leads to convulsions and usually elevates blood pressure. Depressants include those agents which act on the CNS and cardiorespiratory centers to decrease the level of consciousness, often leading to various stages of sleepiness or actual coma. Many of these agents depress respiration, leading to lack of oxygen, which causes nervous system damage. Lack of oxygen may also cause a drop in blood pressure. Depressants include the narcotics, such as morphine and heroin, the tranquilizers, and barbiturates.

Corrosive compounds containing strong acid or alkali are those agents which combine with tissue and cause rapid and deep destruction of tissue. Included in this category are many household cleaning products that contain lye, forms of sodium hydroxide, chlorinated compounds (such as bleach), or ammonia. Noncorrosive liquids are those which are not associated with significant contact-type tissue damage. This category includes most of the aromatic hydrocarbons, gasoline, kerosene, naphtha, and furniture polishes. Much of the damage done by these agents is delayed and involves drowsiness and damage to organs such as lung, liver, and kidney.

FACTORS RELATING TO INTERNAL POISONING

The frequency with which an agent is involved in poisoning varies with age and to some extent socioeconomic status. The majority of poisoning incidents involve young children. The large number of cases of poisoning found in early childhood parallels the peak of the child's natural inquisitiveness, at about 18 to 24 months. Of all accidents in childhood, 51% involve poisoning. Annually, 250 children under the age of 5 years die from poisoning in the United States. The real tragedy is that the majority of these poisonings are preventable. Agents responsible for most childhood poisonings are readily found in the average household. About 25% of childhood ingestions involve aspirin, most frequently candy-flavored baby aspirin. This is the single most frequently encountered agent responsible for childhood poisoning. The actual percentage of poisoning incidents involving aspirin has dropped from 26% of all poisonings in 1965 to 6.5% in 1973. Contributing factors to this decline include increased awareness of the problem among the public, safety packaging of aspirin, and laws limiting the amount of baby aspirin that can be packaged per bottle. Nevertheless, aspirin still leads the list of substances ingested by children under 5 years of age. Other frequently ingested agents involved in childhood poisoning incidents include tranquilizers and antidepressants, household cleaners, insecticides, antihistamines, bleach, birth control pills, vitamins, and cologne. Aspirin and tranquilizers are by far the leading cause of death from poisoning in childhood. Household cleaners, such as drain cleaners or oven cleaners, and other alkali-containing compounds are particularly devastating because of prolonged and recurrent hospitalizations for reconstructive surgery. Agents frequently involved in adult poisonings include medication for mental disturbances, tranquilizers, and depressant drugs.

Any poisoning incident involves a complex interaction between victim, agent, and environment. The sociocultural influence in a poisoning episode can be appreciated by noting the frequency of lye, kerosene, and lead poisoning in low-income housing areas. The environment also plays an obvious role when gasoline, lye, and furniture polishes are stored in open containers or pop bottles, as is often the case.

Regardless of family economic status, the impact of family stress is often evident in the poisoning incidents. When a child ingests a poison, the physician and health worker should enquire into the home situation for possible underlying turmoil. Frequently one finds that family routine has been broken; the father may be away, a new sibling recently arrived, or the family recently moved. Instances of poisoning tend to increase around 5 to 6 PM, when normal family routine is most rushed.

Self-induced poisoning in teenagers and adults is most often a direct response to pressures and accumulative stresses. A large number of these are accidental and involve instances of overdose from street drugs that have been improperly cut. Often overdoses from narcotics and other illicit drugs are accidental and are the result of acquisition of an unusually strong grade of heroin or barbiturate, or they involve agents added to street narcotics to either enhance their effect or mask the fact that they have been cut (a process known as *lacing*). Often these agents are even more toxic than the drug to which they are added (for example, strychnine).

PREVENTION

Poison prevention in adults centers around education. However, the child is particularly vulnerable to household agents, especially those in colorful or palatable bases, such as ant poison, roach powders, and furniture polish. Boric acid, camphorated oils, merbromin (Mercurochrome), and oil of Wintergreen are potentially toxic and practically ineffective for their purported uses. Objective consumer product testing has shown that lye-containing cleaners are generally ineffective for cleaning sink pipes. The extreme, irreversible damage done to a child's esophagus and stomach after ingestion of even small amounts of these products is reason enough to ban them from the home.

Federally regulated packaging methods have done much within the last few years to decrease the number of poisonings from medication. All drugs and poisons should be totally inaccessible to children. They should be out of normal reach and *locked up* in a cabinet. Drugs should never be left on dressers or in unlocked bathroom cabinets. There are increasing numbers of poisonings from drugs in mothers' purses. The homes of relatives visited by children should be checked for harmful agents. Cabinets beneath the kitchen sink are often a warehouse of injurious agents for children. Several items found in the average household that can be harmful if ingested are the following:

Alcohols/liniments	Furniture polish
Antidepressant drugs	Insecticides
Antihistamines (cold pills)	Kerosene
Aspirin	Lighter fluid
Bleach	Lye°
Cardiac medication (digitalis)	Paints/turpentines
Cough medicines	Paregoric
Detergents	Plants (oleander, elephant ears, toadstools)
Dishwashing detergents°	Tranquilizers/sedatives
Drycleaning fluid	

The best prevention is to make these agents unavailable to young children. It is also suggested that adults should never coax a child into taking medication by referring to it as candy and should be cautious about taking drugs of any sort in front of a child, who may mimic such adult behavior.

°These agents are corrosive and can result in extensive tissue destruction.

EMERGENCY CARE FOR POISONING

Often one can determine the nature, if not the amount, of the ingested substance. Nevertheless, there remain many instances in which ingestion is not suspected until the patient begins to exhibit overt signs of drug or chemical action or begins to behave in an unusual manner. The majority of these symptoms are nonspecific but may give useful clues to medical personnel. Careful observation of vital life signs (respiration, pulse rate, level of consciousness, pupil size) may provide a clue to the pharmacological action of the ingredients, allowing for more rapid and specific treatment.

Indicators of poisoning

The symptoms of poisoning will depend on the type and amount of ingested agent. It is difficult to present specific symptoms because of the wide variation of physiological effects of different agents. However, there are typical indicators that can serve as clues to lead you to suspect poisoning. In addition, there are other important factors that should be taken into consideration in an attempt to determine the nature and severity of a suspected poisoning emergency.

First, look for any physical changes. Poisoning should be suspected when a child in the at-risk age group of 1 to 5 years of age presents with the abrupt onset of an atypical illness, history of previous ingestions, or multiple system involvement, such as depressed consciousness with an irregular heartbeat. There may also be burns or stains around the face and in the mouth indicating poisoning with a caustic substance. The victim might complain of abdominal pain or actually vomit. The breath odor may indicate the type of poison, such as gasoline or perfume.

Second, make a rapid investigation of the surrounding environment. An important clue is the tell-tale container. An empty pill box, a spilled bottle of fluid, or a close-by box of a toxic agent can be a tip-off to what has been ingested. The location of the incident may be important. The bedroom, garage, bathroom, and kitchen, for example, all have characteristic substances that might be toxic.

Third, collect a history to find out the chain of events that led to the incident. This may be obtained directly from the victim; however, if the victim is a small child or is unconscious, the history may have to come from an observer if one was present. It is important to determine if multiple agents are involved. In the case of sedatives, otherwise nonlethal doses may result in death if taken in combination with other agents such as alcohol. In many cases it will not be possible to collect a history, and action will have to be taken on the basis of any observable physical or environmental clues that are present.

First aid

First aid for poisoning is dependent on the nature of the ingested substance. There exists such a great variety of toxic substances that it would be impossible for the first aider to be prepared to know what specific first aid procedure would be necessary for every type of product. Therefore, it is necessary to establish a general framework for approaching all poisoning emergencies. The following steps are included in this general framework.

1. Determine what and how much was taken.
2. Determine *specific* first aid procedures.

3. Administer *specific* first aid.
4. If specific first aid cannot be determined, administer nonspecific first aid.
5. Transport the patient to medical care.

Determine what and how much. Every effort should be made to determine the exact product that was ingested. If possible, identify the specific brand name. This information will be extremely helpful in determining the specific first aid. In cases that involve an unknown substance, determine as much as possible all physical signs, symptoms, breath odor, and circumstances surrounding the incident. By way of an empty container or by questioning, attempt to estimate the amount of the ingested agent. Take into account any spilled product and your knowledge of the original amount in a container.

Determine specific first aid procedures. There are three possible sources to obtain specific first aid procedures: the container of the ingested substance, the poison control center, and a physician. If an obvious container can be identified, look for first aid instructions. Many products will include on the label first aid procedures to follow in case of poisoning. If there are no first aid instructions, do not assume that the product is not toxic. Quickly proceed to one of the other two sources for specific first aid procedures.

Within the last 20 years an intense nationwide effort has been made to establish poison control information centers in the major cities throughout the United States. Since the establishment of the first of these centers in Chicago, several hundred such centers have been established in most major cities of the United States. Most states now have a central poison control center in operation 24 hours a day, serving as a reference library and providing information on the ingredients of several thousand commercially available products and the toxicological potential of their ingredients. Such centers are best contacted either through one's private physician or by calling a local emergency room and obtaining the information or the number of the nearest poison control center. Contact the nearest poison control center for specific instructions, since such centers maintain an up-to-date file of toxic materials and treatment. Information the caller should provide includes:

- Type and amount of poison or drug taken
- Age of the victim
- Care given previously
- Condition of the patient (conscious, blue, convulsive)
- Whether vomiting occurred
- Location (distance from medical assistance)

These centers will provide specific first aid information for the patient and more detailed information to the physician.

If the patient has a physician who can be contacted quickly, it may be possible to obtain the specific first aid from the physician. The major advantage of contacting the patient's physician is that the physician may have important knowledge about the patient that can be taken into consideration when determining the first aid procedures. This alternative is useful only if the physician can be contacted right away. If there is delay, call the poison control center or the hospital.

Administer specific first aid. Once the specific first aid is known, the first aider can proceed to follow instructions. Following these procedures will avoid inappropriate measures and in some cases dangerous practices. In some cases the best first aid is immediate transportation with no additional measures. In cases in which the poison, such as a drug, is already in the bloodstream, there is little that can be done except transportation. In all cases monitor vital life signs, keep an open airway, and if necessary administer CPR.

Nonspecific first aid. There are cases for which specific first aid cannot be determined. There may also be a delay in contacting the poison control center or a physician. If a specific first aid is not known or readily available, treatment may be initiated using several nonspecific measures. Dilution of the poison is often effective; milk is a useful agent for both acid and alkali because of the action of the amino acids and proteins. If milk or a specific antidote is not available, water should be used. Several ounces should be given, but caution should be exercised not to induce vomiting in those cases in which it is not advised. Milk of magnesia is a good agent, available in many homes, for neutralization of acids and induction of catharsis.

Corrosive agents, such as lye, are an absolute contraindication to induction of vomiting because of the danger of rupture of the esophagus or further tissue damage, since tissue will be bathed in regurgitated caustic fluid. Likewise, with rare exception, induction of vomiting after ingestion of petroleum distillates is not advised because of the danger of aspiration of material into the lungs with resultant pneumonia.

Contraindications to the induction of vomiting are as follows:
- *Corrosive compounds*
- *Petroleum products*
- *Unconsciousness or depressed gag reflex*
- *Strychnine (found in some rodent and varmint poisons)*

With the majority of poisons, it is desirable to remove the unabsorbed portion of the offending compound from the stomach. This is most effectively achieved by the induction of vomiting. The patient should be given several ounces of warm water and gagging induced with a finger. Preferably, the patient should be given syrup of ipecac, followed by a couple of glasses of warm water. Procedures should cause vomiting within 15 to 20 minutes. If vomiting fails to occur, the dose can be repeated a second time only (adults may be given 1½ tablespoons, children 1 tablespoon). If the patient is unconscious or poorly responsive, it is best to wait until he or she is transported to a medical facility before attempting removal of the poison.

Syrup of ipecac is a highly effective inducer of vomiting; it is safe and fast acting, and it is available in many states in amounts of an ounce or less without a prescription. It is advisable to keep some in the house where small children may be exposed to toxic material (which is any home). If ipecac is not available, mild soapy water may encourage vomiting. Salt water should not be used, especially in children, since such solutions are unusually high in salt content relative to the concentration found in blood. Recently deaths from the resultant increase in serum sodium have been reported after the use of this mixture.

Activated charcoal (USP) is a highly effective inactivator of many poisons. It should be administered mixed with water in a slurry consistency after vomiting has ceased. It is much more effective than any of the universal antidotes recommended in some older first aid manuals. (The universal antidote usually consisted of burnt toast as a source of charcoal, tannic acid in the form of strong tea, and milk of magnesia. The respective components neutralize each other and absorb what little charcoal results from burning the toast, thus rendering the mixture useless. Preparation and administration of this compound is fruitless and a waste of valuable time.)

Transportation to medical care. Medical care should be obtained for all emergencies involving internal poisoning. Aftereffects or complications may not show up for some time, even if first aid intervention appears to be successful. Arrange for transportation as soon as possible. If there is someone to assist, have them call for an ambulance while first aid is being administered. Transportation is urgent if the poison is a corrosive or a petroleum distillate or if there are indications that the poison has been absorbed into the circulatory system. Effects on the various systems of the body will depend on the drug, but the major symptoms to watch for include abnormal pulse, abnormal breathing, unconsciousness, convulsions, dizziness, or drowsiness.

The patient should be attended by someone who can monitor respiration, pulse rate, and level of consciousness. If vomiting continues, the victim should be bent over or rolled to one side to avoid aspiration of vomited material. Reassurance that treatment has been instituted and that medical help is imminent will help calm the patient. If transportation is available, much of the initial treatment may be better carried out en route for most efficient use of time. In every case the medical facility should be notified of the type of poison involved so that preparation for treatment may be made before arrival. Finally, vomitus should be saved in any available container for analysis of unknown components.

EXAMPLES OF SPECIFIC FIRST AID
Corrosives

As mentioned in the introduction, corrosives are an absolute contraindication to the induction of vomiting. Such agents as lye, drain cleaners, and dishwashing detergent can cause extensive damage to the mouth, throat, and esophagus. Dishwashing detergent is caustic and similar to lye in its action. Although bleach is in this group, it is generally much less damaging than the other chemicals listed. Depending on their concentration, ammonia-containing compounds are also destructive to tissue.

Signs and symptoms. Burns from these compounds to the mouth, lips, and digestive tract result in severe pain. Often the patient drools because of inability to swallow. The absence of burns to the mouth, however, does not exclude the possibility of damage to the esophagus. Pulse rate may be elevated and, if several hours have elapsed since ingestion, fever may develop.

First aid procedures. By the time ingestion of caustic agents is discovered, most of the damage has usually occurred, particularly with alkaloid compounds such as lye. If the patient can swallow, a glass of milk with egg white should be given to neutralize and dilute the offending agent. In addition, skin that has come in contact with the compound should be washed freely with water or any other available liquid to attenuate surface burns. Since extensive injury to the esophagus often occurs after ingestion of these agents, the patient must be placed under a physician's care as soon as possible. Ordinary laundry detergents, taken in modest quantity, usually result only in vomiting and diarrhea accompanied by cramping abdominal pain. Usually supportive therapy with fluid replacement is sufficient.

Noncorrosive cleaning agents

Most noncorrosive cleaning agents found around the house are petroleum distillates (consisting of a hydrocarbon base), as are many other agents, such as floor waxes and furniture polishes. These compounds effect their harmful action through primary depression of the central nervous system. Many are similar structurally to general anesthetic liquids and gases. In addition, persons ingesting these hydrocarbons often vomit spontaneously, and in most of these instances at least some of the material is aspirated into the lungs. Depending on the agent and amount, this may lead to serious tissue damage and a chemical pneumonia.

Signs and symptoms. Drowsiness occurs shortly after ingestion of a significant quantity of these hydrocarbon-based compounds. If the patient should vomit, symptoms of respiratory distress may develop when aspiration has occurred. There is often an increase in pulse rate. In addition, fever may develop several hours after aspiration.

First aid procedures. As in the treatment of ingestion of corrosive compounds, dilution with milk or water is the primary first aid concern. Mineral oil may also be given and will help reduce the irritation of these compounds to the stomach and delay absorption from the gastrointestinal tract. It is important to be careful not to overfill the stomach and predispose to vomiting.

Colognes and perfumes

For practical purposes these may be placed in the same category as hydrocarbons. Most of the colognes manufactured in this country are of relatively low toxicity, but the exact ingredients are carefully guarded commercial secrets. Most poison control centers, however, have specific information regarding the ingredients, or this may be obtained by a physician from the various manufacturers. The first aid procedures are the same as for hydrocarbon ingestions.

Aspirin

Aspirin (salicylates) is such a common household drug that parents often do not realize its danger to small children, especially flavored aspirin preparations. Most often poisoning occurs when children get into medicine bottles in the home. It may also occur chronically when a sick child is given repeated doses over several hours. This is especially dangerous in the presence of decreased fluid intake and dehydration. Salicylate poisoning may also occur from other salicylate-containing compounds, such as oil of Wintergreen, which is a much more concentrated source of salicylates than aspirin tablets.

Signs and symptoms. Early manifestations of aspirin and salicylate intoxication include rapid, deep respirations and rapid pulse. The child may develop a loss of appetite, vomiting, and a high fever (which may lead the unsuspecting parents to give more aspirin). Dehydration results from loss of body water from the respiratory tract because of an increased respiratory rate and from the skin surface at increased body temperature.

First aid procedures. Immediate vomiting should be induced; after vomiting has ceased, activated charcoal should be given. If there is a delay in obtaining medical treatment, fluids known to contain salts and sugar should be given. Soda pop or other soft drinks may be useful. Do not attempt to concoct a home-made solution, since this is usually a gross preparation at best and may harm the patient in the same fashion as home-compounded salt emetics.

Tranquilizers and related drugs

Tranquilizers and related drugs are often involved in poisoning incidents in both children and adults. They are often used in attempted suicides, either alone or in combination with one another or alcohol. Most successful suicide attempts involve barbiturates.

Signs and symptoms. The general symptoms seen after ingestion of this class of compounds include varying degrees of mental depression, drowsiness, stupor, and coma. Depressed respiration follows with a decrease in blood pressure and eventual development of shock. Occasionally restlessness may precede the development of stupor and coma. Symptoms resulting from ingestion of lesser amounts of these drugs may include difficulty in walking, abnormal eye movements, dilation of the pupil, giddiness, and confusion.

First aid procedures. In mild cases of overdoses involving tranquilizers, vomiting should be induced to rid the stomach of unabsorbed drug. In more severe cases involving these agents, the patient may be stuporus or unconscious and have a depressed gag reflex. In such cases, removal of the drugs from the stomach should be carried out by medical personnel because of the high risk of choking on vomited material. Care in these instances revolves around first aid for any complicating problems, such as shock or cessation of respiration. Transport the patient at once to medical care.

Alcohol

Contrary to popular Western myths, alcohol is primarily a central nervous system depressant and effects its acute damage through depression of respiration and induction of stupor or coma. Alcohol is also commonly involved in multiple-agent intoxications. A common problem in this respect involves the ingestion of an ordinarily harmless dose of sleeping medication after a night of heavy drinking. This synergistic* depression induced by the combination of agents can be fatal. Although all alcohols are toxic to varying degrees, ethyl alcohol is the agent most frequently encountered, since it is contained in whiskey and liquors. Other forms of alcohol encountered include methyl (wood) alcohol and isopropyl alcohol (rubbing alcohol). Ethyl alcohol is most often denatured by the addition of compounds that induce nausea and vomiting. Efforts to remove these denaturing substances or to convert wood alcohol into a less harmful compound are futile. Such skid-row maneuvers as filtering wood alcohol through a potato or bread are absolutely worthless. Such myths have been responsible for many cases of intoxication and blindness after consumption of wood alcohol.

Signs and symptoms. The signs and symptoms of mild ethyl alcohol intoxication

---

*Synergy: The combined effect of the two agents is greater than the mere sum of their individual actions.

are widely known and easily recognized. These include initial giddiness and loss of inhibitions with a decrease in the ability to make judgments of time and space. Large doses of ethyl alcohol cause the depression of respiration and drowsiness. Although it usually takes rather large quantities of ethyl alcohol to do serious harm, lesser amounts of wood alcohol can result in such devastating harm as blindness and permanent neurological damage. Consequently, this agent must be removed rapidly from the stomach by induction of vomiting and medical treatment obtained as soon as possible. The most common source of wood alcohol is so-called canned heat and cooking fuels. Isopropyl alcohol, unless taken in rather large quantities, results only in severe gastrointestinal symptoms, such as nausea, vomiting, diarrhea, and dizziness.

First aid procedures. Although all alcohols are absorbed rather quickly from the stomach, rapid induction of vomiting may result in removal of some of the alcohol. If the patient is semiconscious or unconscious, do not induce vomiting, but transport to medical care. Chronic alcohol abuse in recurrent intoxications results in rather extensive damage to the body organs and the nutritional status of the patient. The first aider's role in the treatment of chronic alcohol abusers is referral to the proper medical and social care agencies for assistance.

Common plants

Because of the large variety of common toxic plants, only an overview of first aid for plant ingestions will be presented. Because plants are ubiquitous, they are often involved in accidental ingestions, especially in children. By far, the majority of plants are harmless or, at worst, cause only mild discomfort after ingestion, but severe toxicity or even death may follow consumption of certain household plants and common shrubs. The safest course of action in these cases is to treat all such ingestions as representing a potentially serious situation. Plants are many and varied, and, consequently, few people are familiar with the toxicity of a wide variety of plants. Any substance—plant or otherwise—that is not a known food should be considered a potential toxin. It is best in these cases to contact the nearest poison control center for advice on the proper course of care for plant ingestions.

Probably the most notorious of the poisonous plants are members of the mushroom family, known as *toadstools.* Almost all instances of mushroom poisoning in this country are the result of ingestion of a member of the genus *Amanita,* commonly known as the *death angel.* Many of these mushrooms are extremely toxic, and death may result from ingestion of only a small amount of them. Furthermore, cooking does not denature the toxins contained in all mushrooms. It is sheer folly for the ordinary person to attempt to identify and prepare wild mushrooms. Each year, several amateur experts in this field become severely ill or die from ingesting incorrectly identified mushrooms.

Symptoms of mushroom poisoning may come on rapidly (30 minutes to 2 hours) or develop slowly over a day or longer. Such symptoms as salivation, profuse sweating, abdominal cramps, vomiting, diarrhea, decrease in pupil size, hallucinations, convulsions, and shock may appear. Should the victim recover, liver and kidney damage may occur. First aid for early ingestion is the removal of any remains of the plant from the stomach through vomiting. Giving strong tea as a source of tannic acid may be of some help, and a cathartic should be given. All efforts should then be directed toward getting the patient to a physician as quickly as possible, since aggressive medical treatment will be required.

Several plants found in the home and garden contain toxic substances. Oleander and lily of the valley are similar to foxglove and contain a digitalis-like chemical and may cause severe irregularities of heart rhythm. The death of several members of a family occurred after they had eaten meat smoked over oleander branches. Chinaberries, castor beans, and jimsonweed are toxic and cause gastrointestinal and central nervous system effects of varying degrees.

Common holiday plants are potentially toxic and should be kept away from children, since their bright leaves and berries are coaxing. All parts of the mistletoe plant are toxic and may induce nausea, vomiting and abdominal pain, diarrhea and dehydration, rapid pulse, high blood pressure, seizures, and central nervous system alterations. The colorful red leaves of the poinsettia have been overrated as a source of poison. They are mildly toxic, and consumption results in gastrointestinal symptoms of nausea, vomiting, and diarrhea. The sap may cause irritation of the skin. Initial treatment of the ingestion of these plants should include the induction of vomiting followed by the administration of a demulcent such as milk or milk of magnesia and activated charcoal.

Dieffenbachia and philodendron, known as dumb cane and elephant ears, are popular indoor plants. All parts of these plants contain small, sharp calcium oxalate crystals and enzymes, both of which cause burning and swelling of the mouth and tongue. Pain is often severe, and occasionally occlusion of the airway results from swelling of the tongue. The onset of swelling may be rapid and lasts for 2 to 3 days in severe cases. Injury to the eyes may occur from contact with the sap of these plants. First aid is as for other plant ingestions. Milk and other demulcents may help soothe the pain. Copious irrigation with water of the eyes or skin will help if initiated soon after contact.

Poison ivy

Poison ivy, poison oak, and poison sumac all contain phenol-like substances that are contact irritants. All cause what is often referred to as *Rhus dermatitis.*

Signs and symptoms. Signs of contact with these plants usually appear within several hours, although delays of a day or longer are often seen. Areas of redness and blistering are typical. Intense itching followed by pain often develops. Individual sensitivity to these plants is variable; some persons have only mild redness, others develop severe local reactions, and occasionally systemic illness results.

First aid procedures. If contact with these plants is known to have occurred, the areas involved should be immediately irrigated with large amounts of soapy water, avoiding rubbing the involved area directly. Water dressings with aluminum acetate solution (commercially available as Burow's solution) will help severe topical reactions. Calamine lotion may be useful in attenuating the intense itching. (Caladryl and other topical antihistamines, although proported to decrease itching, are topically sensitizing, and their use on raw skin may induce allergy to these drugs.)

Contact irritants

Contact irritants are found throughout a wide spectrum of chemical classes, including many organic solvents, fuels, cleaning agents, industrial-grade acids, and epoxies.

Signs and symptoms. Contact irritants induce varying degrees of local reaction, usually beginning with redness and progressing occasionally through the equivalent of a second-degree burn with blister formation. Strong acids or alkalis may cause extensive local tissue destruction and result in scar formation. Some of the more volatile agents may be absorbed through the skin and may lead to systemic intoxication, similar to inhalation of the fumes.

First aid procedures. The first procedure is irrigation with copious amounts of water and removal of clothing that may be soaked with solvent. After prolonged irritation, cases that result in blister formation may be initially cared for as second-degree burns. In cases involving contact of these compounds with the eye, again, prolonged irrigation with large amounts of water is the correct procedure. All persons working around these agents should be familiar with the location of showers and eye basins that are required by law in areas where toxic chemicals are used.

Lead and mercury poisoning

Lead intoxication has decreased markedly in the last quarter century due to legislation prohibiting the use of lead-based paints. Chronic lead poisoning still occurs in areas of older housing, principally in children who chew paint flakes from old buildings or lead-containing putty from unrenovated windowsills. Rarely, lead may be ingested as the chemical salt, such as lead acetate (sugar of lead) and result in severe, acute systemic manifestations. Pottery from Mexico has been found on occasion to contain large enough amounts of lead to result in poisoning when these containers were used for cooking.

Chronic lead and heavy metal intoxication is often detected through federally sponsored screening programs for persons living in substandard housing. These cases are best brought to the attention of the public health authorities for further evaluation and medical treatment, as indicated.

Signs and symptoms. Manifestations of lead intoxication include nausea, vomiting, diarrhea, cramping abdominal pain (lead colic), anemia, convulsions, and changes in mental function.

The victim of acute mercury poisoning may present with gastrointestinal upset, bloody diarrhea, and increased salivation with red, tender gums. Often a metallic taste is present. Renal and liver damage may follow, and, in severe cases, cardiovascular and respiratory collapse may result. Ingestion of pure elemental mercury, as from a broken thermometer, is harmless. Mercury fumes, however, are toxic. Consequently, there is some danger associated with working in areas where elemental mercury may be spilled and evaporate slowly from crevices, such as in a chemistry laboratory. Common sources of mercury compounds are fungal and mold retardants.

First aid procedures. Initial management should include induction of vomiting followed by milk and egg white. The albumin in the egg white combines with lead and mercury to form insoluble metal-albuminate. This effectively prevents absorption of much of the ingested metal. A cathartic should then be given (such as milk of magnesia or Epsom salt) and medical care obtained despite lack of symptoms.

Iron poisoning

Iron poisoning occurs almost exclusively after ingestion of medicinal iron, such as ferrous sulfate, used in treatment and prevention of anemia. Because iron is often given for the increased iron requirement during and after pregnancy, these pills are often found in a household where there are young children. Coloring and sugar coating of iron salts make them attractive to the young child. One particular iron preparation closely resembles M&M candy in size and texture. As few as three or four tablets may prove fatal to a child.

Signs and symptoms. Vomiting, diarrhea, lethargy with a fast, weak pulse, and a decreased level of consciousness often occur. The patient may appear blue, and shock may quickly follow. The initial episode may pass rather quickly and be followed by a period of apparent well-being, only to have severe symptoms recur 8 to 24 hours later.

First aid procedures. Early removal of tablets through vomiting is most important. Giving a basic solution, such as bicarbonate of soda in water, before and after vomiting will also increase retrieval of the iron. A cathartic and demulcent should be administered and the patient given care for shock. Prompt medical treatment is mandatory to save the victim's life if relatively large quantities have been taken.

DRUG ABUSE

Drug use and abuse, particularly among teenagers and young adults, has increased dramatically over the last several years. A drug subject to abuse may be defined for purposes of discussion as any chemical or substance that affects one's level of consciousness, mood, or behavior. *Drug abuse* is use of a drug in excess and for recreational or psychological effect, without regard for its usual medical purposes. Drug dependence, on the other hand, is a state in which a person cannot function or suffers extreme discomfort if deprived of the drug. The term *physical dependence* is used when deprivation of the drug results in physiological symptoms that abate when the drug is taken. *Psychological dependency* occurs when the person comes to prefer the state induced by use of a drug and cannot function comfortably without it but suffers no objective physiological symptoms when deprived. With continued and prolonged use of a drug in cases of physiological dependence, *tolerance* may develop, in which case larger doses of the drug are required for the previously desired drug-induced state. Tolerance develops with narcotic and depressant agents but is not seen with hallucinogens or marijuana.

Marijuana and hashish

Marijuana is the dried plant *Cannabis sativa*. The plant grows wild throughout the world and is often cultivated for production of rope fiber. For use as a drug, leaves and flowering tops are dried and small fragments are made into cigarettes, smoked in pipe bowls, and also may be taken as tea, made into brownies, sniffed as powder, and mixed with other foods. When burned, it has a characteristic odor similar to burning alfalfa; consequently, users often attempt to mask the odor by burning incense. Numerous slang terms are used to refer to marijuana cigarettes and to marijuana itself: joints, reefers, roaches, Mary Jane, weed, grass, locoweed, hash, and others.

The potency of marijuana varies greatly with content of the active ingredient, tetrahydrocannabinol (THC). The amount of THC will range from small to large, depending on whether some of the weaker mixes found in the United States are tested or whether the stronger Indian and Asian varieties are checked.

Hashish (hash) is technically the dark resin collected from tops of high quality marijuana plants. It has a much higher content of THC. Although many substances have been sold on the street as THC, the difficulty in isolating it and the expense involved are prohibitive. Consequently, it is extremely unlikely that refined THC is actually available illicitly.

Drug effects. Marijuana quickly enters the bloodstream when smoked and begins to affect the user's feelings and thinking. Circumstances surrounding use of marijuana, the user's previous experiences, and the strength of the drug used all act to yield a given response. Most often time is distorted and may seem much prolonged. Space becomes distorted, and sounds and colors are often intensified. Thought becomes dreamlike, and the idea that one is capable of much more profound thinking than usual is a common feeling in the user. Frank hallucinations, however, are rare with the use of marijuana alone. The user often tends to withdraw into himself, and there may be extreme mood swings. Suspiciousness and frank paranoia may occur, and occasionally fear and anxiety result. Occasionally these symptoms are of such a severe nature that the user may temporarily break with reality. Such effects are uncommon except in the younger user whose personality is still in the stage of rapid evolution.

The long-term physical and psychological effects of marijuana usage are not known; however, it is known that a person under the influence of marijuana may often find it much harder to make decisions and objective judgments. Under the influence of the agent he may feel strongly that his judgment is unimpaired and indeed heightened, when in reality a complex task requiring quick judgment and good reflexes may be markedly impaired. Many of the long-term implications of marijuana usage are still under investigation and are at any rate not the immediate concern of the first aider. Signs of marijuana usage include tachycardia, a slight dilatation of the pupils, reddening of the eyes, dizziness, incoordination, sleepiness, increased appetite, and a rather passive, apathetic attitude in most cases. Occasionally a paranoid reaction will occur, particularly in the younger user.

First aid concerns. Emergency care is usually not necessary unless an adverse paranoid reaction occurs. In these cases, the user is best kept in the company of his friends and calmly talked down in a quiet environment. If an adverse reaction, particularly a paranoid reaction, is persisting, the patient is best treated by a physician.

Sedatives and tranquilizers

Probably the best known and most often abused tranquilizers are the barbiturates and related compounds. Common slang for these agents includes redbirds, yellow jackets, yellow birds, christmas trees, and goofballs. Other tranquilizers frequently abused include methaqualone (Quāālude, Quāās), glutethimide (Doriden), diazepam (Valium), and meprobamate (Miltown). Recently a veterinary tranquilizer, phencyclidine (peace, PCP, crystal), has become a popular street drug. It more closely resembles a hallucinogen than the other agents in this group, although it may also produce a depressive effect.

Drug effects. Barbiturates and tranquilizers are usually taken orally, although they may be given by injection also. Small doses result in relaxation, drowsiness, and good humor. Large doses or a combination of agents may lead to sedation, slurred speech, incoordination, and argumentativeness. The pupils may be dilated or pinpoint, breathing may be shallow and slow, incoordination may be present, and mental activities may be depressed. With large doses or a combination of agents, especially alcohol, coma, hypotension, and cardiovascular collapse may lead to death.

First aid concerns. For cases in which only a small amount of drug has been taken, examination and observation by a physician may be all that is necessary. In cases of frank overdose, symptomatic support should be given, the airway should be secured, and CPR given if needed. Care should be taken to maintain body temperature, and general care for shock should be given. The patient should be transported to a hospital as soon as possible for treatment. (See previous section on sedative overdose.)

Opiates

The opiates commonly available include morphine, meperidine (Demerol), heroin, and paregoric. Slang terms for these agents include the following: for heroin—snow, stuff, H, horse, smack; for codeine—schoolboy; for morphine—M. All are narcotics and can be strongly addicting. They may be sniffed, skin-popped, or mainlined intravenously. Physical dependence and tolerance to rather large doses may develop with repeated use. These drugs are all similar in chemical structure, and cross tolerance develops. Methadone is a narcotic used in attempts to withdraw addicts from other opiate compounds. Abusers of narcotics usually administer them by intravenous injection, and consequently needle tracks can often be found in the folds of the arm, the wrists, top of the hands and feet, and other areas of the body.

Drug effects. Specific symptoms of use include euphoria, a flushed feeling, and blurred vision. Signs may include pinpoint pupils, decreased respirations, and stupor. High doses of narcotics may lead to hypotension, coma, pulmonary edema (fluid on the lungs), and respiratory arrest.

First aid concerns. Maintenance of an airway and support of cardiovascular function are important primary concerns. The patient should be treated for shock and breathing maintained by artificial respiration, if necessary. CPR should be instituted if the patient is in frank shock and no pulse is palpable. The patient should be rushed to a hospital as soon as possible, since specific drug antidotes are available. Street remedies, such as injection of milk, are absolutely ineffective and are dangerous to the victim.

Hallucinogens

LSD-25, psilocybin, mescaline, the tranquilizer PCP, peyote, and STP all produce bizarre mental reactions and striking distortions of perception. Common street names for these agents include acid, beans, cactus, bad seed, and mescal. LSD is taken in microgram quantities and is a colorless, tasteless material. Users typically take it in capsule form or may ingest it on a sugar cube. Other members of this group may be taken in different forms; for instance, peyote cactus buttons can be eaten or made into a thick soup and consumed. All these agents produce approximately the same reactions in recipients with effects lasting approximately 8 to 12 hours after consumption.

Drug effects. Physical effects include flushed face, chills, increase in heart rate, a slight increase in blood pressure, dilated pupils, and changes in affect. The effects of these agents vary considerably according to the amount taken, the circumstances under which the drug is ingested, and the personality of the user. Even in the same subject, the effects may vary from time to time. Vision is markedly altered, and the subject is likely to see unusual and brightly colored patterns. The apparent merging of one sensory experience into another (synesthesia) may occur; for example, the user may think he sees sounds. Hallucinations are common, and the sense of time is markedly altered. Emotional lability is marked and may range from euphoria to frank terror. Simultaneous extremes of emotion are common and may lead to anxiety on the part of the user. A sense of merging with space has been described by several users. In general, serious mental changes always occur during the use of the drug. Psychotic manifestations are possible, and occasional suicidal and homicidal tendencies have been noted. Unfortunately, there is no good way to predict how a user may react to the drug at a given time. Drug users often refer to good or bad trips. A *good trip* is a pleasurable drug experience in which sensation and imagery are pleasant, whereas a *bad trip* or *bummer* is one in which unpleasant sensations and anxiety predominate. Because of impaired time perception a few minutes may seem like several hours or a day, and bad trips can assume the proportions of a near-endless nightmare from which the user cannot escape.

First aid concerns. In general, bad trips are best handled in a quiet, dimly lit area where the patient's friends can attend him. The first aider's role is one of directing the patient's friends to reassure him and protect him from injuring himself until the effects of the drug wear off. Attempts should be made to help the patient realize that the current condition is drug induced and temporary. Repeated attempts to orient the patient are necessary. He should be taken to a physician as soon as possible, accompanied by his friends. In general, a calm, reassuring, humane approach is the most effective method of care for the bad trip.

Stimulants

The central nervous system stimulants include amphetamine-like compounds and cocaine. In street jargon, they are known as speed, crystal, coke, dex, or bennies.

Drug effects. Agitation, euphoria, tachycardia, elevated temperature, visual and auditory hallucinations, dilated pupils, a dry mouth, increased blood pressure, and restlessness are all symptoms of stimulant overdose. Coma and convulsions may occur after large doses of these drugs. The amphetamines may be taken either by mouth or by injection. Cocaine is usually taken by sniffing it after application to the inside of the nose and may lead to ulceration of the nasal passages.

First aid concerns. The patient often demonstrates confusion, suspiciousness, and hallucinations and requires calm reassurance and support. Abusers of cocaine are particularly prone to acts of aggression and violence. The terminal period of a speed run (often referred to as the *crash*) involves such symptoms as extreme faitgue, emotional depression, and hunger. Above all, the user should be protected from harming himself and others. Disturbances of vital signs should be cared for supportively and care provided for convulsions or shock if either occur. Prompt medical help is indicated. Obtain assistance from the police if the abuser becomes violent.

Miscellaneous agents

Alcohol represents a serious drug problem, and, although by itself it does not often represent a threat to life, victims of acute intoxication should be afforded the same careful treatment as abusers of any other drug. Alcohol is the most commonly abused drug. Acute alcoholic intoxication is treated principally as a depressant overdose. Chronic alcoholic abuse requires the evaluation of a physician and long-term assistance from mental health workers and such organizations as Alcoholics Anonymous.

Other agents commonly available and open to abuse include glue, paint thinners, gasoline, hair spray, and nail polish remover. These are often taken by holding a cloth over the nose and mouth with some of the substance on it. Use of these agents results in excitation, rapid heartbeat, and stupor. Liver and central nervous system damage are common complications of the abuse of these agents. Emergency care includes establishment of an airway and removal to fresh air. Asphyxia and convulsions may occur. Respiratory and cardiopulmonary support and care for shock should be given when indicated and medical assistance obtained immediately. Long-term damage to the nervous system and liver may complicate use of these chemicals.

Drug withdrawal

Withdrawal symptoms may occur after the discontinuance of drugs on which the user has become physiologically dependent. Commonly involved drugs include tranquilizers, sedatives, alcohol, and narcotics. Withdrawal symptoms occur after varying periods of abstinence from drug use. In hard-core narcotic users, several hours of abstinence may be all that is required to bring on symptoms of drug withdrawal.

Signs and symptoms. The onset of symptoms may occur as early as 6 hours or as long as 24 to 36 hours after the last dose in an addict. Anxiety and restlessness are early and prominent symptoms. Hot flashes alternating with chills and sweating are also common. Pain in the legs, back, and abdomen occurs frequently, as does vomiting, diarrhea, and increased respiratory and heart rates. As symptoms progress there is an ever increasing craving for the drug, which the patient may freely admit. He will make unreasonable demands and irrational promises in an attempt to obtain the drug. Untreated, these withdrawal symptoms may progress to coma, convulsions, and cardiovascular collapse resulting in death.

First aid concerns. The patient should be reassured in a quiet and supportive manner and normal body temperature maintained. Vital signs should be checked immediately. Should severe symptoms result in shock or convulsions, appropriate supportive first aid care should be given. In every case, the patient should be taken to an emergency medical facility as soon as possible. Attempts at cold-turkey withdrawal are extremely hazardous and may result in death. Since certain drugs mixed with heroin (cocaine, strychnine) may also give symptoms of restlessness and tremors, it is important to obtain a history from the patient in a nonthreatening manner.

SUMMARY

Poisoning represents a significant source of morbidity and death in both adults and children. To a large degree prevention is the only sure method of treatment. Key points to remember are:

1. Always keep harmful chemicals under lock and key.
2. Survey the home and garage for potentially harmful agents.
3. Never refer to medicine as candy to coax children to take it.
4. Syrup of ipecac is the most effective method of inducing vomiting in a conscious poisoning victim. Avoid the use of the so-called universal antidote, which is useless.
5. The poison control center is a valuable source of readily available information concerning the ingestion of toxic compounds.
6. Vomiting should *never* be induced when caustic agents (such as acids and drain cleaner) or hydrocarbon compounds (such as kerosene and furniture polish) have been ingested.
7. Always attempt to obtain the container of the chemical or drug that the victim has ingested to determine specific contents.
8. In the treatment of depressant and narcotic overdoses, check vital signs immediately, and assure the airway as necessary. Institute the usual supportive first aid measures for shock, respiratory arrest, or other symptoms that might be present.
9. Never attempt cold-turkey withdrawal from narcotic agents under any circumstances.
10. When an adverse reaction (bad trip) to a hallucinogen occurs, attempt to establish a near-normal setting for the patient in a quiet, dimly lit room. Work through the patient's friends. Establish a feeling of trust and avoid moralizing or arguing at all costs.
11. In all cases of poisoning, determine what, how much, and when a substance was taken, and make the first aid as specific as possible.

FIRST AIDER COMPETENCIES

After studying the material presented in this chapter, the student should be able to:

- Outline the classifications and general effects of poisoning.
- List the factors that are frequently associated with accidental poisoning.
- List procedures that should be taken to prevent accidental poisoning.
- Describe the typical indicators that can serve as clues to poisoning.

- Outline and explain the five procedures for administering first aid for internal poisoning.
- Indicate under what circumstances and with what types of poisoning vomiting should not be induced.
- Describe specific first aid procedures for the following common types of poisoning: corrosives, noncorrosive cleaning agents, aspirin, tranquilizers, alcohol, and poison ivy.
- Describe the drug effects and important first aid concerns associated with the following drugs: sedatives, opiates, hallucinogens, and stimulants.

REFERENCES AND RECOMMENDED READINGS

1. Done, A. K.: Household poisons, Emergency Medicine **1**:33-37, March, 1969.
2. Dreisbach, R. H.: Handbook of poisoning, Los Altos, Calif., 1969, Lange Medical Publications.
3. Editorial: Childhood poisoning: prevention and first aid management, British Medical Journal **4**:483-484, 1975.
4. Gleason, M. N., et al.: Clinical toxicology of commercial products, Philadelphia, 1969, The Williams & Wilkins Co.
5. Lawrence, F. H., et al.: Activated charcoal: a forgotten antidote, Journal of the Maine Medical Association **63**:311-313, Nov., 1975.
6. Pascoe, D. J.: Drug abuse. In Pascoe, D. J., and Grossman, M., editors: Quick reference to pediatric emergencies, Philadelphia, 1973, J. B. Lippincott Co.
7. Pascoe, D. J.: Poisoning. In Pascoe, D. J., and Grossman, M., editors: Quick reference to pediatric emergencies, Philadelphia, 1973, J. B. Lippincott Co.
8. Smith, D.: The trip, there and back, Emergency Medicine **1**:26-42, Dec., 1969.
9. Soldmann, W. T.: Poisonous reptiles and insects. In Sproul, C. W., and Mullanney, P. J., editors: Emergency care: assessment and intervention, St. Louis, 1974, The C. V. Mosby Co.

9

{{{

BURNS

Sally Abston

Burn injuries vary in severity depending on the amount of the total body surface that is injured. Even the smallest burn causes discomfort that can be relieved by rapid first aid. The severe or major burn involving more than 40% of the body surface may be life threatening. Appropriate early first aid may diminish the later threat to body part or life.

STRUCTURE AND FUNCTION OF THE SKIN

The skin is one of the largest organs of the body, comprising 16% of the total body weight. It is composed of two layers, the dermis and the epidermis (Fig. 9-1). The dermis is composed of dense collagen with many small blood vessels called *capillaries*. The epidermis is the outer layer and is composed of many layers of epithelial cells laid on top of each other like bricks in a wall. The basal layers of cells, that is, those adjacent to the dermis, divide regularly; as these cells reproduce, they push older cells to the surface. As the cell ages, it forms keratin within the cell, and the nucleus diminishes and dies, so that the cells on the surface are primarily keratin.

In addition to providing the surface covering of the body, epithelial cells form specialized structures beneath the dermis, which connect with the surface by small ducts. These are sebaceous glands, which elaborate an oil to coat the skin; the sweat glands, which assist in the body's thermoregulation and fluid control; and the hair follicles, which produce hairs.

The principal functions of the skin are sensory perception, thermoregulation, fluid retention, and protection against bacterial invasion. The skin is supplied with many sensory nerve endings, allowing perception of harmful stimuli, such as temperature extremes, as well as pleasant stimuli.

The skin participates in thermoregulation as an insulator against extremes in environmental temperature as well as by retaining or eliminating heat created by the body. The rich network of capillaries in the dermis, by dilating, allows for the transmission and elimination of a large quantity of heat. Conversely, by constriction and decreasing the flow of blood, this same network of vessels will serve to retain heat. The sweat glands, by the elaboration of the fluid, sweat, its secretion on the surface, and its evaporation, allows for further elimination of heat. The subcutaneous tissue, that is, tissue beneath the dermis, is primarily fat, which

116

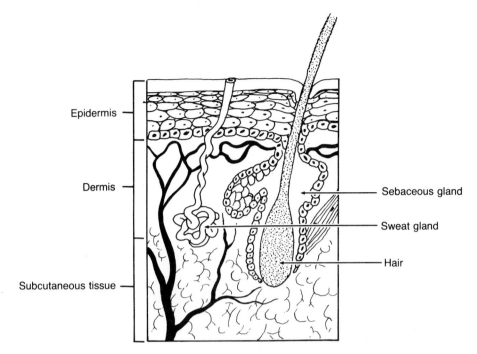

Epidermis

Dermis

Sebaceous gland

Sweat gland

Subcutaneous tissue

Hair

Fig. 9-1. Cross section showing structures of skin.

serves as a poor conductor of heat and assists the skin and the dermis in their function as insulators against environmental heat or cold.

The outer layer of the skin prevents dehydration of the body. This layer provides a cover for the deeper cells, which exist in a fluid environment, and prevents evaporation. A demonstration of this is seen in a superficial abrasion (scrape) wound in which the deeper layer of epithelial cells is intact but moist. Exposure to the air of such a wound leads to painful drying.

Protection against invasion by bacteria in the environment is provided both by the outer layer and by the oily secretion of the sebaceous glands. The intact outer skin is impervious to bacteria, and the secretion elaborated by the sebaceous glands discourages colonization of the skin by harmful bacteria.

CLASSIFICATION OF BURN INJURIES

Thermal burn injuries. Thermal injuries may occur as a result of scald by hot liquids or contact with flames, hot surfaces, or electricity. The injury is classified according to its depth (Fig. 9-2) and to the percentage of the body surface it involves.

First-degree burns. Burns are superficial injuries, involving only the outer layers of epithelium. They are painful, and the wound is red and heals within 2 or 3 days without treatment. The classic example of a first-degree burn is a sunburn that does not peel.

Second-degree burns. Burns involve deeper layers of the epidermis. These wounds characteristically form blisters, are painful, and require 7 to 30 days to

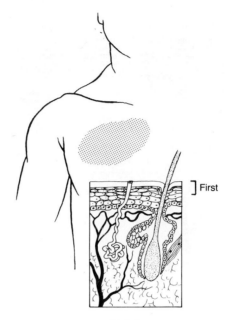

First degree

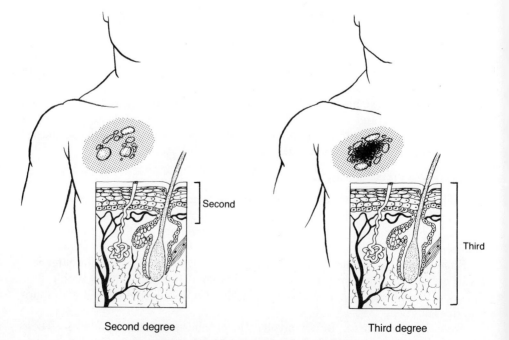

Second degree

Third degree

Fig. 9-2. Classification of burns by degree.

heal. Without appropriate care these wounds may become infected with resultant loss of the full thickness of epidermis and will require skin grafting to heal.

Third-degree burns. Burns involve the full thickness of the epidermis as well as the sebaceous and sweat glands and the hair follicles. The wound is firm and dry, and coagulated blood vessels may be visible. The wounds are painless because of the loss of the sensory receptors. Third-degree burns caused by flame injury may result in charring of the skin.

Body surface. Severity of the burn injury is dependent usually on the percentage of the total body surface involved. The rule of nine divides the body surface into areas approximating 9% or a multiple of 9% (Fig. 9-3). Each arm is 9%, each leg 18%, the front or back of the trunk is 18%, and the head and neck is 9% of the total body surface.

Any second- or third-degree burn involving more than 20% of the body surface is considered a serious injury. Severe burn injury implies greater than 40%

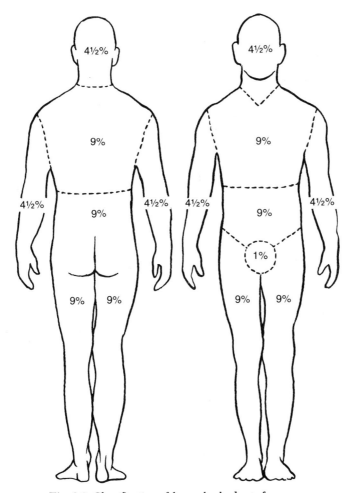

Fig. 9-3. Classification of burns by body surface area.

total body surface involvement. Exceptions to these definitions are third-degree burns involving the face, hands, feet, or genitalia, all of which are considered serious.

Scald injuries are usually first or second degree due to the rapid loss of heat as well as to the short contact time of the hot liquid. If the injury is a result of immersion or if clothing is soaked, holding the hot liquid in contact with the skin, the burn wound may be third degree. Flame burns, if the flame involves the clothing, are most often third degree. The wound may be more superficial if clothing is not involved. Burn wounds due to electric contact may involve deeper tissues than the skin, since the heat of the electricity is transmitted along nerves and vessels.

Chemical burn injuries. The depth of burn wounds due to chemicals is related to the nature of the compound and the length of time it remains on the skin. Generally, alkaline compounds are more rapidly destructive than acid compounds.

PATHOPHYSIOLOGY OF BURN WOUNDS

After a thermal injury there is a rapid loss of fluid into and around the injury site seen as swelling of the tissues or edema. If the wound involves less than 10% of the body surface, then the fluid lost will not be significant. On the other hand, if the wound is greater than 20%, the fluid lost may be enough to cause hypovolemic shock. (See Chapter 6.) As the outer layer is lost as a result of the injury, there will be fluid loss by evaporation.

With the loss of the outer layer and sebaceous glands, the barrier to infection is diminished, and common bacteria may invade the wound and cause infection. If the injury involves greater than 20% of the body surface, thermoregulation may be compromised, and maintaining normal body temperature may be difficult.

EMERGENCY CARE FOR BURNS
Examination of the burned patient

Initial examination should include an assessment of the depth of the injury, the amount of total body surface involved, and assessment of associated injuries.

Depth can be established by the presence or absence of blisters, sensation, pain, and vascularity. Blisters are collections of fluid between epithelial layers and almost always are indicative of second-degree injury. Sensation is usually absent in the third-degree wound because of the loss of the sensory receptors. Vascularity is assessed by gentle pressure on the wound with a finger. If the wound is blanched on removing your finger but rapidly becomes red, then the injury is second degree, and vascularity is intact. If the wound is rigid, firm, and leathery, it is third degree.

Tabulation of the total body surface involved is rapidly done using the rule of nines previously described. Any second- or third-degree burn wound involving more than 20% requires hospitalization and treatment.

Associated injuries should be assessed on the initial examination. The most common injuries occurring with burn wounds are inhalation injuries and injury to the eyes. If the burn injury occurred in a closed space such as a vehicle or closed room, inhalation of smoke and debris may occur. This leads rapidly to hoarseness and respiratory distress. Respirations should be observed for depth and rate as well as signs of upper airway obstruction. Examination of the nose for ashes or burn injury of the external areas may give an early suggestion the victim may have inhaled noxious substances. The eyes should be examined for burned lashes or other debris.

Blood pressure and pulse should be assessed early and repeatedly to recognize impending hypovolemic shock.

First aid for the burned patient

Minor burns. First aid for the patient with a minor burn wound is intended to relieve pain and diminish the risk of infection.

If the agent of injury is a chemical solution, the wound should immediately be washed with large quantities of water. The washing should be done with running water from a hose or faucet to assure removal of the chemical. Simple immersion may provide only dilution. After thorough washing it may be treated as any other burn wound. Flushing chemicals from the eye is shown in Fig. 9-4.

The simplest and most effective way to relieve the pain of a small-area burn wound is to immerse it or cover it with an ice-water solution. This is maintained until the cold causes pain and the injured part is removed from the cold. Within a few minutes, the pain of the burn wound will return. The injured part is again covered with the ice-water solution until the cold causes pain. This procedure is repeated three or four times until the burn wound no longer becomes painful with

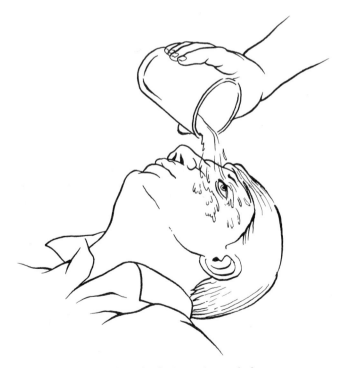

Fig. 9-4. Procedure for flushing chemicals from eye.

removal of the ice water. The wound is then washed in soap and water, and medical attention may be sought for further care.

Serious burns. First aid for the victim of a major injury is intended to diminish pain, the threat of later infection, and the immediate threat of hypovolemic shock.

The injured person should be placed in a reclining position. Any debris such as burned clothing should be removed from the wound. If there is dirt on the wound, it should be washed off before it becomes adherent. The wound should be covered with a clean sheet. If the wounds are second degree, wetting the sheet may diminish the pain. If the wet dressing causes shivering, a light blanket should be placed over the dressing to decrease draft and chilling.

If there is debris in or about the eyes, they should be irrigated if water is available. To irrigate the eye, the lids are held open, and water is placed in the part of the eye next to the nose and allowed to flow out the side of the eye. The head may be turned slightly toward the side so the water flows to the side. If hoarseness or other evidence of respiratory distress is present, oxygen may be given.

The first aider should not apply such things as butter, bacon, oils, or ointments to the burn wound. These substances adhere to the wound and make cleansing more difficult. The victim with a large-surface-area burn should not be packed in ice, since this will cause constriction of the blood vessels to the wound, diminishing the blood supply, which may increase the depth of the injury. The patient with a burn injury greater than 20% should be transported as rapidly as possible to a hospital.

Follow-up

While awaiting transportation of the patient with a severe burn injury, the pulse, respiration, and blood pressure should be frequently checked to assess impending shock. The patient should be kept at rest. Chilling must be avoided, since shivering increases discomfort and energy loss. On the other hand, excessive cover may cause overheating with sweating and increase the fluid loss. The wound should be protected from contamination by dirt and debris. The patient may experience thirst but should not be given fluids, since these may provoke vomiting. The severely burned patient may be anxious and apprehensive and should be reassured constantly and advised before any movement.

FIRST AIDER COMPETENCIES

After studying the material in this chapter, the student should be able to:
- Identify and describe first-degree, second-degree, and third-degree burn wounds.
- Describe how to calculate the total body surface burned.
- Describe first aid for a minor, second- or third-degree burn.

REFERENCES AND RECOMMENDED READINGS

1. Artz, C. P., and Moncrief, J. A.: The treatment of burns, Philadelphia, 1969, W. B. Saunders Co.

2. Curreri, P. W., Asch, M. J., and Pruitt, B.: The treatment of chemical burns: specialized diagnostic, therapeutic, and prog-

nostic conditions, Journal of Trauma **10:** 634-642, 1970.

3. Epstein, M. F., and Crawford, J. D.: Cooling in emergency treatment of burns, Pediatrics **52:**430, 1973.

4. Hartford, C. E.: The early treatment of burns, Nursing Clinics of North America **8:**447-455, 1973.

5. Kravitz, H.: First aid therapy for burns—cool it, Clinical Pediatrics **9:**695, 1970.

6. Polk, H. C., and Stone, H. H.: Contemporary burn management, Boston, 1971, Little, Brown & Co.

7. Sdurim, H. S.: The treatment of electrical injuries, Journal of Trauma **11:**959-965, 1971.

10

COLD INJURY

Edward L. Schor and Charles Edwin Rinear

Excessive loss of heat from the body or from a body part may cause damage or death of tissue. Proper precautions in cold environments may prevent injury. Appropriate emergency care can minimize disability.

SOURCES OF BODY HEAT

The normal body temperature, measured with an oral thermometer, is about 37° C (98.6° F). This temperature is maintained within a wide range of environmental temperatures. Heat may be absorbed by body tissues from outside, external sources, such as direct or indirect sunlight, heating elements, or from eating or drinking warm foods.

Internally the body is able to produce its own heat by burning calories obtained from food. When food has not been recently eaten, body stores of carbohydrates and fat are broken down and metabolized to produce heat and energy.

Elevations of body temperature may result either from abnormal increases in external sources of heat, increases in internally produced heat such as from fever or muscular activity, or from inability to release heat from the body.

LOSS OF BODY HEAT

There are five ways in which the body normally may lose heat. When any of these cause a loss of heat faster than the external and internal sources can replace the heat, a cold injury can result. The five ways of losing body heat are *conduction, convection, evaporation, radiation,* and *respiration.*

When a person's body is touching an object that is colder, the body heat is transferred to that object. This is *conductive* heat loss. For example, immersing an extremity in cold water, touching a cold piece of metal, or lying on cold ground will all allow a loss of body heat to the colder material.

When body heat is transferred to air, it is called heat loss by *convection.* The more rapidly cold air moves past a warmer body, the greater the amount of heat that is lost. This effect is referred to in weather reports as the *windchill index.* As much body heat will be lost on a day when the temperature is −4° C (25° F) and a 15 mph wind is present, as on a day when the temperature is −15° C (5° F) but there is no wind present.

Moisture on the body surface will be warmed by body heat. If the water

124

content of the surrounding air (humidity) is low, the warmed water on the body surface will vaporize. This process of *evaporation* can account for considerable loss of body heat.

The body may lose heat by transferring it to objects with which it is not in direct contact. Heat lost in this way is in the form of infrared waves. The amount of heat lost is directly related to the amount of exposed surface area. Body parts with a large surface-area-to-volume ratio, such as the head, ears, hands, and feet are particularly likely to lose heat by *radiation*.

The fifth way in which body heat is lost is through *respiration*. When a person inhales, the air is warmed to body temperature; when this air is exhaled, body heat is lost with it.

THERMAL REGULATION

Heat produced from deep body tissues such as muscles and the organs (for example, liver, kidney, or lungs) warms the blood circulating through those tissues. The warmed blood then flows through the superficial blood vessels of the skin, allowing heat to be lost by convection to the air. Increasing the amount of blood flow through the skin by dilating the blood vessels in the skin will increase heat loss. This *vasodilatation* produces a reddening of the skin, and the skin feels warm to the touch.

If the body needs to decrease heat loss, the superficial blood vessels will constrict, thereby reducing the blood flow through the skin. This *vasoconstriction* causes the skin to appear pale and to feel cool or cold to the touch. Both vasodilatation and vasoconstriction are automatic, involuntary processes.

Another involuntary mechanism for temperature control is *shivering*. Through many continuous localized muscle contractions, the body is able to generate additional heat.

In summary, maintaining normal body temperature is a complex process involving external and internal sources of heat, five mechanisms by which heat may be lost, and automatic body controls of heat regulation.

Maintaining healthy body tissues depends on continual chemical reactions occurring within body cells. These reactions require an energy source such as sugar, a sufficient supply of oxygen carried to the cells by the circulatory system, and a constant, normal body temperature. A reduction in the temperature of the tissues will slow down the chemical reactions, and the tissue will begin to die. The longer the abnormally low temperatures are present, the greater will be the damage to the tissue.

TYPES OF COLD INJURIES AND THEIR RECOGNITION

Cold injuries may be classified according to whether the entire body or only a body part is involved. They may also be classified by the degree of tissue damage produced—reversible tissue injury or tissue death.

Destruction of tissue by freezing is called *frostbite*. In this condition the involved tissues die, and surrounding tissues are injured. The frozen area is usually small and most commonly occurs on the nose, cheeks, ears, fingers, or toes.

Before the onset of frostbite, the affected area may be slightly flushed, reddened. The skin then changes to a grayish yellow or white color. Pain may be felt initially but later subsides. Occasionally there is no pain, and only a sensation of coldness and numbness is perceived. In many instances, the person is unaware of the condition until it is brought to his attention by others.

Tissue may be damaged by cold exposure short of freezing. In mild cases the injury is characterized by itching and burning sensations. In the case of longer or more severe exposure, the injured tissue will first become reddened, accompanied by pain or itching, followed by swelling and scabbing ulcerations of the affected area. The severity and extent of a cold injury cannot be accurately assessed by initial examination, and repeated examination is necessary.

When the core body temperature is reduced, this generalized condition is called *hypothermia*. Symptoms arise from a reduction in the rate of all of the metabolic processes of the body. Affected individuals may have abnormal behavior, weakness, and incoordination, eventually leading to collapse and loss of consciousness.

FIRST AID PROCEDURES

Care of cold injuries should begin with prevention. Heat loss can best be prevented by wearing dry clothing as insulating garments. Shelter should be sought when necessary. Drugs that affect judgment and/or peripheral vascular function, such as alcohol, should be avoided. Damaged tissue and severely ill persons need to be handled *gently!*

Local tissue injury

1. Remove the individual from the cold environment or to a protective environment while providing immediate additional protection in the form of additional layers of clothing or blankets.
2. Give the person a warm drink if conscious and not in need of early surgery.
3. Rapidly rewarm the frozen part(s) in water 38.9° to 40.6° C (102° to 105° F). A thermometer should be utilized and warm temperature constantly monitored. If thawing is slow, tissue damage increases, whereas tissue injury will occur if the temperature rises over 42.8° C (109° F). Discontinue warming as soon as the part becomes flushed. Once rewarmed, have the person exercise the part.
4. The frostbitten or injured areas should be handled with care. Massage should *not* be applied to frostbitten areas.
5. A blister should *not* be broken. Cleanse the affected area with mild soap and water (*not* laundry or dishwasher detergent), rinse thoroughly, and then blot dry. Apply a dressing only if the person is to be transported to medical aid. Dressings should be placed between the patient's toes and fingers if these areas are involved. Jewelry should be removed in anticipation of swelling.
6. Frostbitten parts should be elevated and protected from contact with bedclothes. Such parts should be splinted during transportation to a medical facility. Parts should be kept elevated during transportation.
7. Additional heat should not be applied. The patient should not be placed near a radiator, stove, or fire.
8. Medical help should be obtained at the earliest possible time with vital

signs monitored and recorded frequently before definitive therapy by a physician.

Hypothermia

1. Remove the patient from the cold environment while providing for immediate emergency transportation to a medical facility.
2. Monitor the patient's vital signs constantly while caring for shock. Additional clothing or blankets should be utilized to increase body temperature. In cases of mild to moderate hypothermia (27° to 35° C [81° to 95° F]) with a conscious patient, increase body temperature by administration of hot drinks unless other medical problems contraindicate this. Wet clothing should be removed. Loosen constrictive clothing and administer oxygen if available.
3. Rapidly rewarm the patient with mild to moderate hypothermia (30° C [86° F]) in a tub of water at 40.6° to 43.3° C (105 to 110° F). Dry the patient thoroughly.
4. Administer calories in the form of sugar, especially glucose tablets or hot sweet drinks. Do not give alcoholic beverages to the individual.
5. As part of generalized shock care, during transporation, the patient should be moved gently, avoiding sudden jolts, and should be transported with his head lower than his feet. The patient must be constantly observed for ventricular fibrillation, which can occur at body temperatures below 27° C (81° F).

FIRST AIDER COMPETENCIES

After studying the material presented in this chapter, the student should be able to:
- Explain the processes of cold injury to local tissue and generalized effects on the body.
- Describe the symptoms and outline the first aid procedures for frostbite.
- Describe the symptoms and outline the first aid procedures for hypothermia.

REFERENCES AND RECOMMENDED READINGS

1. The American National Red Cross: Advanced first aid and emergency care, New York, 1973, Doubleday & Co.
2. Bowman, W., and Bunce, G.: Injuries in the winter environment, Emergency Product News, ed. 34, Oct., 1975.
3. Holvey, D. N., et al.: The Merck manual of diagnosis and therapy, ed. 12, Rahway, N.J., 1972, Merck, Sharp, & Dohme Research Laboratories.

11

▼▼

MUSCULOSKELETAL INJURIES

Guy S. Parcel

Musculoskeletal injuries commonly result from falls, collisions, and overexertions causing damage to bones, joints, and/or muscles. Proper care by the first aider may prevent serious complications and permanent crippling.

Injuries to structures of the muscular or skeletal systems are usually not life threatening. Yet improper care may lead to painful or serious complications and permanent damage. When caring for musculoskeletal injuries, no injury should be thought of as only minor but should be considered potentially dangerous and disabling. Proper care of musculoskeletal injuries depends not only on a knowledge of first aid techniques but also on an understanding of the structure and function of the muscular and skeletal systems.

STRUCTURE AND FUNCTION OF THE MUSCULAR AND SKELETAL SYSTEMS

The muscular and skeletal systems work together to provide movements of the body. In addition, the skeletal system gives support and protection to body structures. As shown in Fig. 11-1, the skeleton consists of numerous bones connected together to form the various segments of the body. A joint is formed at the place where the individual bones articulate (come together). Bones are held in place at the joint by bands of dense connective tissue called ligaments. It is at the joints that movement takes place.

To accomplish movement, a muscle or group of muscles must contract to decrease or increase the angles formed by two or more bones at the joint. As shown in Fig. 11-2, muscles are usually attached to the bone by means of a tendon. The origin of the muscle attaches to one bone, and the other end, the insertion, crosses a joint and by means of a tendon connects to another bone.

Musculoskeletal injuries are classified according to the structures damaged and the nature and extent of the damage. For example, fractures are injuries to the bones; sprains, the ligaments; strains, the muscles and tendons; dislocations and subluxations, the joints; and contusions, the muscles and surrounding soft tissue. In examining an injured person, it would be helpful to know the major structures of the muscular and skeletal systems to make an intelligent supposition as to what structure has been damaged. Knowing what structure has been damaged will make it easier to classify the injury and apply the proper first aid care.

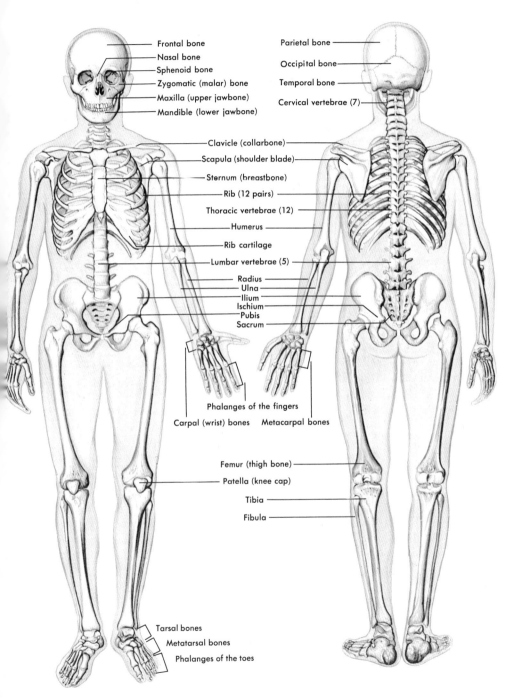

Fig. 11-1. Skeletal system. (From Francis, C. C, and Martin, A.: Introduction to human anatomy, ed. 7, St. Louis, 1975, The C. V. Mosby Co.)

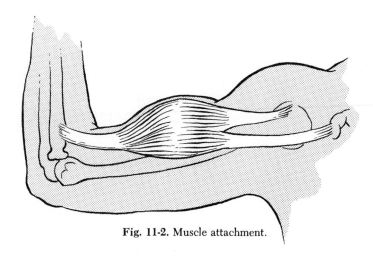

Fig. 11-2. Muscle attachment.

EXAMINATION OF AN INJURED PATIENT

When examining a patient for musculoskeletal injuries, do not move the patient until the nature and extent of the injuries have been determined.

The history of the accident should be the first consideration in making a decision whether musculoskeletal injuries are involved. Histories involving auto accidents, athletic injuries, falls, collisions, overexertions, twisting, or impacts usually lead to musculoskeletal injuries. After you have determined that the patient is breathing effectively and is not bleeding seriously, proceed to examine for musculoskeletal injuries, but *do not* move the patient. In an emergency, people often overreact by moving the patient prematurely. Many of the musculoskeletal injuries will be aggravated by movement and must be properly splinted before any movement takes place.

To guide you through your examination, musculoskeletal injuries can be ranked according to their potential danger. The greatest danger is presented by fractures. Fragments of bone may sever nerves or blood vessels or may puncture organs. Examine first for fractures, especially fractures of the bones in the back and neck. Dislocations are usually painful and may lead to fainting or shock. Therefore dislocations are ranked second in order of examination. Examine for the remainder of the musculoskeletal injuries in the following order: subluxations, sprains, strains, and contusions.

FRACTURES

A fracture is defined as a break in the continuity of a bone. A fracture may result from a direct blow producing a break at the site of the impact, such as the impact of a moving object in a collision. Falls or a twisting of body parts may cause a fracture by applying a force at one part of the bone while the break occurs at some other site in the bone. A forceful muscle contraction will sometimes cause the tendon to pull a piece of bone away from the bone, resulting in what is referred to as an avulsion fracture. Any accident history including any of these mechanisms should be suspected as possibly resulting in a fracture.

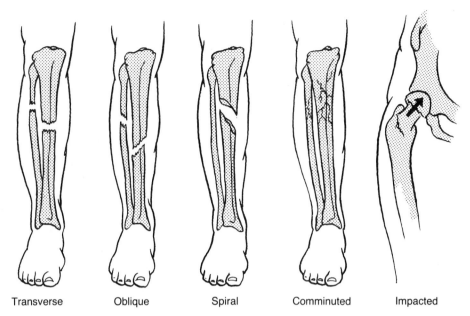

| Transverse | Oblique | Spiral | Comminuted | Impacted |

Fig. 11-3. Types of fractures.

Classifications of fractures

Fractures may be broadly classified into two types: open fractures or closed fractures. An *open fracture* is one that produces an open wound resulting from a piece of the bone penetrating through the skin. If the skin is not penetrated by the fractured bone, it is a *closed fracture*. For many years the terms compound and simple have been used to designate these two classifications. Because simple and compound do not adequately describe the situations, these terms are no longer recommended for use in classifying fractures.

In addition to the two broad classifications, a fracture may be classified according to the nature of the break in the bone. Fractures may be further designated as *complete* (broken parts no longer intact) and *incomplete* (break does not go all the way through the bone) (Fig. 11-3). It is important to be aware of the extensive variety of fracture conditions that may occur.

Signs and symptoms of fractures

The signs and symptoms presented by a fracture will vary greatly from one situation to another. It is important to be aware of all the possibilities to make an accurate decision, and whenever in doubt assume a fracture.

A fractured bone may not prevent the patient from moving the injured part. Movement may cause additional harm or permanent damage. Therefore do not ask the patient to move to determine whether a fracture has occurred. Unnecessary movement is one of the most serious errors made while caring for a patient with a fracture. Asking the patient if he or she can move is not effective in determining whether there is a fracture and can be dangerous. Keeping this concept in mind, proceed to look for the following signs and symptoms:

1. *History:* Ask the question, how did the injury occur? Look for the mechanisms that frequently cause fractures. Ask the patient what happened, *letting him or her provide the information.* Do not ask leading questions, such as, "Did you hear it crack?" "Did you feel it snap?" Leading questions may put false ideas in the mind of a patient in pain or emotional stress.
2. *Open wound:* In the case of an open fracture, the bone may be protruding through the wound, or the bone may have made a wound and withdrawn beneath the skin.
3. *Deformity:* Look for unusual or abnormal angles presented by a body part. It is useful to compare the uninjured part to the injured part to detect a difference.
4. *Point of extreme sensitivity to pain:* Palpate the part, being careful not to move it, and apply slight pressure at the suspected fracture site. If this pressure produces extreme pain, assume a fracture.
5. *Swelling:* If the injury causes internal bleeding, swelling may appear rapidly at the suspected site of the fracture. This sign may not always be present and cannot be depended on to occur in all cases. Whenever swelling persists over several days after an injury, the possibility of a fracture should be considered and the patient referred to medical care.
6. *Discoloration:* Bleeding into the tissue produces discoloration. Because it is rarely present until several hours after an injury, discoloration is not an effective means to determine a fracture.
7. *Radiograph:* Many fractures can only be determined by radiographic examination; therefore it is important to refer *all* suspicious cases to medical care.

First aid care for fractures

Immobilize the injured part before moving or transporting a patient with a suspected fracture. The old first aid saying, "Splint them where they lie," is an important concept to keep in mind. Immobilization reduces pain to help prevent or control shock and prevents additional damage to soft tissue, blood vessels, and nerves. Proper immobilization will also keep a closed fracture from becoming an open fracture.

If the fracture is open, the first procedure is to control any serious bleeding from the wound. Direct pressure may be applied if the bone is not protruding through the wound and if the pressure does not cause excessive pain. Digital pressure to the main artery supplying blood to the wound should be applied if direct pressure cannot be used or is not effective. Be careful not to further contaminate the wound of an open fracture. Contamination may result in an infection of the bone, which is a serious complication. Cover the wound with a sterile dressing and bandage in place before applying immobilization procedures.

Immobilization is accomplished by applying splints, slings, and bandages to keep the body part from moving. Specific immobilization techniques will be

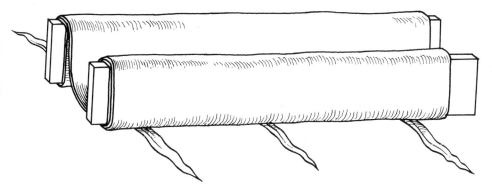

Fig. 11-4. Fixation splint.

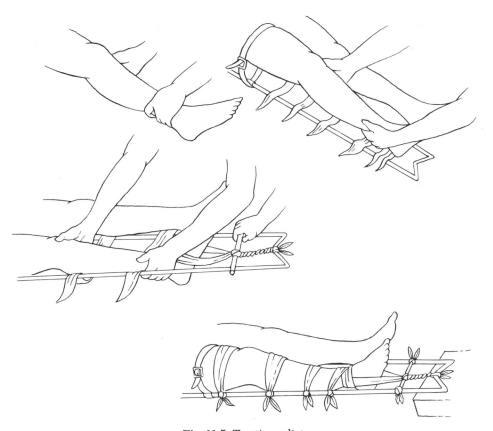

Fig. 11-5. Traction splint.

presented later in the chapter. However, the following general guidelines will apply to all immobilization procedures:

1. Immobilize the joint above and below the fracture site.
2. Make sure splints or bandages do not interfere with normal circulation.
3. Pad the splints where they come in contact with the body to prevent undue pressure and injury.
4. Place the patient on a litter to transport.
5. When possible, use specialized splints and specially trained emergency personnel.
6. Care for shock.
7. Transport the patient to medical care.

Types of splints

Several types of splints are available to be used to immobilize a body part. The type to be selected will depend on the body part injured and the availability of material.

Fixation splints. A fixation splint consists of a firm material and is usually applied on each side of the fractured limb extending beyond the joints above and below the fracture site (Fig. 11-4). Commercial splints are made of light wood, metal, or fiber. Fixation splints may be easily applied with a minimum amount of training. Follow the guidelines in the preceding part of the chapter.

Traction splints. Traction splints are designed for the extremities to prevent muscle contraction from causing the ends of the fractured bones to override (Fig. 11-5). A traction splint is difficult to apply and should only be attempted if the first aider has been specifically trained to use this technique. A traction splint is usually applied if there has been a complete fracture of a large bone and it will be a long period of time before the patient can receive medical attention.

Pneumatic splints. The pneumatic splint, or air splint, consists of a double-walled plastic sheath that can be inflated with air to make it rigid enough to immobilize an extremity (Fig. 11-6). Most pneumatic splints on the market today are transparent and have a zipper to make application easier. Six sizes are available to meet the needs of various fracture sites. The pneumatic splints present many advantages over other types of splints. When deflated, they can be folded and occupy a small space. They are simple and easy to apply, requiring little movement. The transparency of the splints allows observation of skin

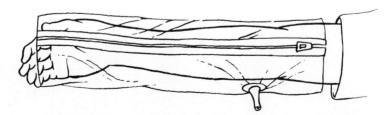

Fig. 11-6. Pneumatic splint.

color and other conditions of the limb. The pressure provided by the splint may also assist in controlling bleeding from an open wound.

Despite the many advantages, the pneumatic splint is potentially dangerous. If the splint is overinflated or remains on a limb too long, normal circulation may be disrupted, causing tissue death in the limb. Pneumatic splints should only be used as a temporary measure while transporting the patient to medical care. To avoid complications, follow the procedures listed below for applying pneumatic splints.

1. Place sterile dressings on any open wounds.
2. Place the splint over the extremity, avoiding unnecessary movement, and close the zipper.
3. Inflate the splint using lung pressure, being careful not to overinflate. Do not use a pump or other means of artificial inflation.
4. Check skin color to determine whether circulation is cut off. If the skin turns blue or the patient feels a throbbing, release some of the pressure.
5. If transportation is long or medical care will be delayed, release most of the pressure until movement of the part is again necessary.

When properly used, the pneumatic splint is an excellent and effective means of immobilizing fractures of bones in the extremities. First aid stations, emergency rooms, emergency vehicles, and rescue squads should be equipped with a set of pneumatic splints. Because of the potential danger, all personnel should be trained in the proper application before using the splints.

Improvised splints. In time of an emergency, specialized splints may not be available. Efforts should be made to obtain specialized splints before turning to improvising splints. If they cannot be obtained in a short period of time, it will then be necessary to make use of what material is available. Ingenuity and imagination are the only limits to making improvised splints. Examples of material that may be used include boards, poles, sticks, tree limbs, rolled magazines or newspapers, cardboard, pillows, and blankets. When material is not available for a splint, the fractured part may be secured to another part of the body. For example, a fracture of the upper arm may be immobilized by bandaging to the side of the chest, or a fracture of the lower leg may be immobilized by bandaging to the uninjured leg. Be sure to follow the guidelines for splinting outlined earlier in the chapter whenever improvising splints. Improvised splints are only a substitute for specifically designed splints and should only be used when necessary.

Specific fractures

In addition to the general guidelines for administering first aid care for fractures, certain fractures will require special attention and care.

Skull fractures. If a patient has received a blow to the head or has hit his head during a fall, examine for the possibility of a skull fracture. Keep the patient quiet, keep the head elevated, and look for any abnormal depressions in the skull. A fractured skull will sometimes cause fluid or blood to drain through the ears or nose. If fluid or blood is draining from the ears or nose, assume the possibility of a skull fracture. *Do not* apply pressure to the fracture site. Pressure may force fragments of bone into the brain tissue.

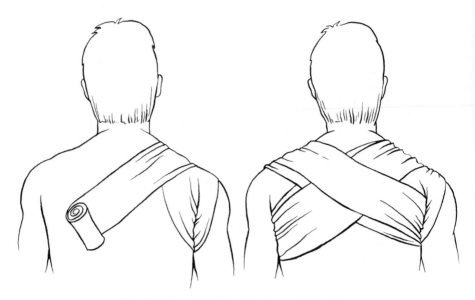

Fig. 11-7. Immobilization for fractured clavicle.

Proper first aid consists of keeping the head elevated, immobilizing the head by placing clothing or other material on each side so that the head cannot move, and transporting the patient on a litter to the hospital. If there is bleeding, apply a dressing and bandage lightly in place without applying pressure to the fracture site. (Additional information is presented in Chapter 12.)

Clavicle. The clavicle (collarbone) is the small **S**-shaped bone that runs from the scapula to the sternum. A fracture of the clavicle is usually painful and makes it difficult for the patient to support his or her arm. To detect the fracture, compare the injured part to the normal side. You should be able to notice a lump at the site of the fracture if it is complete. If a lump is not present, apply gentle pressure to determine a point of extreme sensitivity to pain. The pain may be reduced and the fracture immobilized by applying a bandage as illustrated in Fig. 11-7. Start by looping the bandage around the affected shoulder and pull gently back, bringing the bandage across the back and looping it around the other shoulder. Bring the bandage back around the affected shoulder, forming a figure eight. Place the arm in a sling and transport the patient to medical care.

Upper extremities. A fracture of the humerus (upper arm bone) should be splinted to immobilize both the shoulder joint and the elbow joint. This can be accomplished by applying splints on both sides of the upper arm, placing the arm in a sling, and securing the arm to the body with bandages as shown in Fig. 11-8. A similar type of procedure can be applied for a fracture of the ulna and/or the radius in the lower arm. Fractures of the carpal bones (eight small bones in the wrist) are most difficult to detect. There may be little or no deformity. Palpate the area, applying pressure at suspected sites, and assume a fracture if there is a point of extreme sensitivity to pressure. Immobilize the wrist so that it will not move in any direction. Refer all doubtful cases to medical care for further examination. Frac-

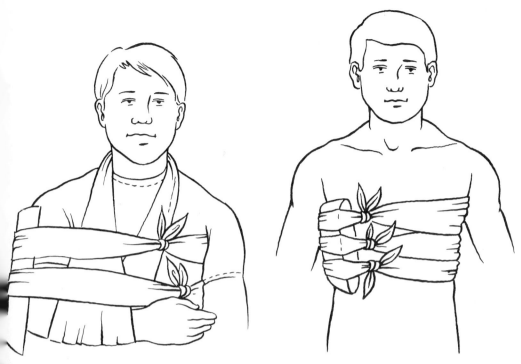

Fig. 11-8. Immobilization for fracture of upper arm.   Fig. 11-9. Immobilization for fractured ribs.

tures of the phalanges (bones in the fingers) can be partially immobilized by securing the injured finger to uninjured fingers.

Ribs. Suspected fractures of the ribs may be immobilized by tying cravat bandages around the chest (Fig. 11-9). Have the patient exhale each time you tighten a bandage around the chest. A patient with fractured ribs must be handled carefully to prevent broken bones from puncturing the lungs.

Pelvis. The pelvic bone is actually made up of three separate bones that connect, forming immovable joints. The pelvis serves to protect many vital organs. Improper handling of a patient with a fractured pelvis may result in serious damage to internal organs. A fractured pelvis is a common injury in auto accidents and falls, especially in accidents involving elderly people. Any time there is severe pain in the pelvic area after an injury, assume the possibility of a fractured pelvis and apply the proper first aid care. With wide bandages, tie the patient's legs together and place a bandage around the hip area. Carefully place the patient on a flat board or firm stretcher, secure the patient so that he or she cannot move, and transport the patient to medical care.

Lower extremities. Fractures of the femur (upper leg bone) can usually be identified by deformity and severe pain. Immobilize the leg by applying splints from the hip to the lower leg as shown in Fig. 11-10.

Fractures to the lower leg may be to either or both the tibia and fibula. The tibia is the large shinbone that runs from the ankle to the knee. A fracture of the tibia will be more disabling than a fracture of the fibula. The fibula is on the

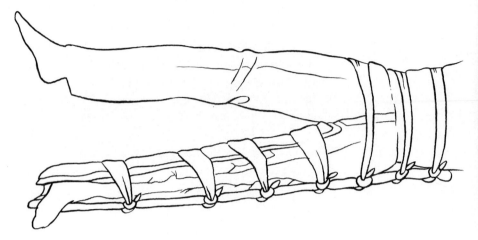

Fig. 11-10. Immobilization for fractured upper leg.

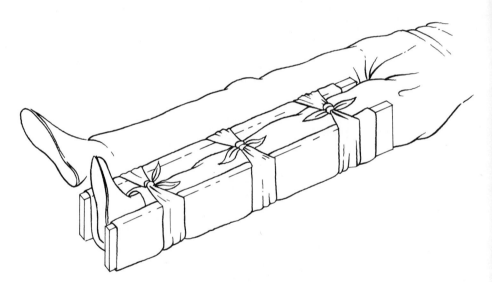

Fig. 11-11. Immobilization for fractured lower leg.

outside of the lower leg and runs from the ankle to the outer portion of the tibia near the knee joint, but the fibula is not part of the knee joint. A fractured fibula is less disabling than a fractured tibia and, in fact, may go undetected. Careful examination should be made by palpating the lower leg looking for any deformity and a point of extreme sensitivity to pain. Immobilization may be accomplished by applying splints as shown in Fig. 11-11.

Fractures of the tarsals (bones in the ankle) are common, especially in recreational and athletic events. It is often difficult to distinguish a fractured ankle from a sprained ankle. Both may be disabling. The key symptom to look for is a

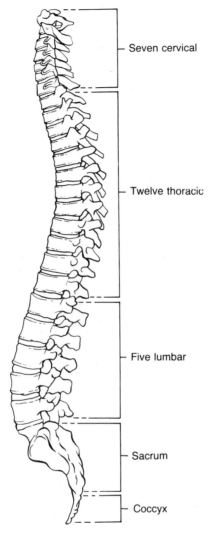

Seven cervical

Twelve thoracic

Five lumbar

Sacrum

Coccyx

Fig. 11-12. Bones of spinal column.

point of extreme sensitivity to pain. Whenever in doubt, assume a fracture, and immobilize the joint with splints.

Vertebral column. The vertebral column (backbone) is made up of twenty-four or more separate small bones called *vertebrae* (Fig. 11-12). The vertebral column functions to support the erect body and to protect the spinal cord, which passes through the vertebral foramen (opening in the vertebrae). Nerves controlling body functions pass through the spinal cord to parts of the body. Fractures of the vertebral column are extremely dangerous because bone fragments may damage or sever nerves controlling vital body processes. When a person receives a fracture to the vertebral column, the result—life or death, normal functioning or permanent paralysis—is often dependent on the immediate care. Improper care may be disastrous.

Most lay people, including many trained first aiders, picture all patients with a fractured back or neck as being completely paralyzed from the waist down or the neck down. They often erroneously assume that if paralysis is absent, the back or neck has not been broken. Bones of the vertebral column can be fractured in many ways. The majority of fractures do not involve spinal cord damage and will not show symptoms of paralysis. But all suspected vertebral column fractures must be handled to protect the spinal cord because it must be assumed that there exists a potential for spinal cord damage.

To determine a suspected fracture of the vertebral column, first consider the history of the accident. Falls, direct blows, forceful extension or flexion of the spine, and collisions are common mechanisms that produce fractures. *Do not move the patient.* Examine the patient in the exact position you find him or her. Check for feeling in all four extremities by pinching the skin and muscles hard enough to produce pain. Ask the patient to move his or her fingers and toes. If the patient does not feel the pain when you pinch and cannot move fingers or toes, assume a vertebra fracture involving the spinal cord.

If the patient does have feeling and movement in the extremities, do not rule out a fracture but continue examination. Ask the patient where he or she feels the pain. Determine whether the pain is located in the area of the vertebral column.

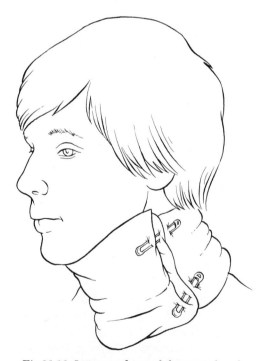

Fig.11-13. Improvised immobilization of neck.

Palpate the area, being careful not to move the patient, and look for a point of extreme sensitivity to pain. If you locate the pain in the area of the vertebral column, assume a fracture and apply the proper first aid.

The first aid for fractures of the vertebral column must be carefully planned and administered. There is little room for error. Keep in mind that in most cases there is no need to hurry, and proper technique is more important than time. The first principle of first aid is not to cause further harm. If you lack the confidence to cope with a situation presenting a fractured vertebra, keep the patient still and send for specifically trained emergency medical personnel.

When possible, obtain specific emergency equipment designed to immobilize the neck and back. If the injury is to the neck, first apply a neck collar to keep the head from moving (Fig. 11-13). Additional specific procedures are presented in Chapter 12. Regardless of whether the injury is to the neck or back, immobilize the vertebral column by applying an orthopedic stretcher as shown in Fig. 11-14. The orthopedic stretcher is the preferred method of immobilization because it can be applied without moving the patient. It comes apart in two pieces and can be put under the patient in any position and is then put back together for transportation. Request this type of apparatus whenever there is a suspected vertebral column fracture.

A substitute for the orthopedic stretcher can be made out of ½-inch plywood 2 feet wide and 7 feet in length. Apply the back board by having helpers support the vertebral column and lift the patient an inch off the ground while the board is slid under the patient. Carefully place the patient on the board and tie to the back board so that he or she cannot move. The neck board, a smaller version of the back board, can be applied to a patient in a car to immobilize the neck to get the patient out of the car.

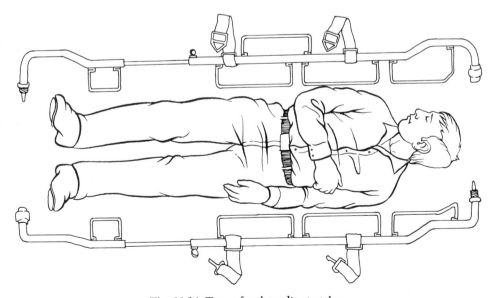

Fig. 11-14. Type of orthopedic stretcher.

When transporting a patient with a suspected fracture to the vertebral column, *do not* use a litter or stretcher that is not firm. Rule out the use of the typical soft ambulance stretcher, the canvas stretcher, and improvised blanket stretchers. Unless life is in danger, do not move the patient with a suspected vertebral column fracture until the proper equipment has been obtained.

DISLOCATIONS

A dislocation is defined as a displacement or separation of a bone from its normal place of articulation. A dislocation may result from a blow, fall, or violent muscular contraction. Signs and symptoms to look for to detect a dislocation include the following:

1. *Pain:* There is extreme pain located in and around a joint.
2. *Immobility:* It will be too painful for the patient to move the part at the joint that is dislocated.
3. *Deformity:* When compared to the uninjured side, the joint will appear deformed (lump, ridge, or excavation present).
4. *Swelling:* If internal bleeding takes place, swelling will occur at the time of injury, but it may take several hours for swelling to develop.

Suspect a dislocation when these signs and symptoms appear after an accident.

First aid for dislocations

Do not attempt to put a dislocated joint back into place. Complications may be associated with a dislocated joint that may be aggravated by the attempts of unqualified persons to reduce the dislocation. The proper first aid is to:

1. Immobilize the joint so that further movement doesn't contribute to pain.
2. Apply ice or cold packs to assist in controlling internal bleeding.
3. Care for shock, since pain is usually severe and shock will frequently occur.
4. Transport to medical care; in most cases a litter is recommended.

Specific dislocations

Information concerning common sites of dislocated joints will be helpful in making decisions and applying the proper first aid.

Lower jaw. The lower jaw may be dislocated by a direct blow or sometimes by exaggerated opening of the mouth. The patient will be unable to completely close his or her mouth so that the upper and lower teeth meet in a normal position. Use a bandage to immobilize the jaw similar to immobilization for a fracture.

Shoulder. Dislocation of the humerus (upper arm bone) from its socket at the shoulder is one of the most frequent. As shown in Fig. 11-15, the head of the humerus usually displaces downward and forward, making the shoulder appear pointed rather than rounded. This deformity will usually be apparent when compared to the uninjured shoulder. The patient will tend to hold the extremity at the side and will be unable to lift his or her arm sideward. The recommended technique for immobilization is to bend the arm at the elbow, place in a sling, and secure the upper arm to the body with bandages. If it will be an extended period of time before medical attention can be obtained, the patient may be placed lying face down at the edge of a table with the arm extending down. Traction may be applied by fastening a weight of 10 to 15 pounds to the wrist as

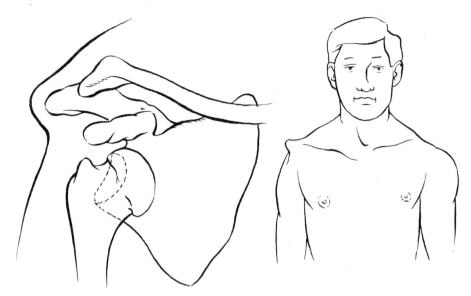

Fig. 11-15. Dislocated shoulder showing position of head of humerus and typical disfiguration.

shown in Fig. 11-16. Sometimes this procedure will result in a reduction of the dislocation. If it does, remove the weight and allow the patient to put his or her arm at the side. Always refer to medical care.

A-C joint. The joint where the clavicle and scapula come together is called the *A-C joint*. The bones are held in place by ligaments. The joint becomes dislocated when these ligaments are torn (Fig. 11-17). A point or lump will appear at the top of the shoulder. The patient will be unable to move his or her arm across the chest toward the other shoulder. Place the arm in a sling and transport the patient to medical care.

Elbow. The elbow is a well-protected joint and does not easily dislocate. A dislocated elbow usually results from the patient trying to break a fall with an outstretched arm. As shown in Fig. 11-18, *A*, the deformity looks like a bump at the end of the elbow. A radiograph (Fig. 11-18, *B*) shows that the upper arm bone has been displaced forward, causing the end of the lower arm bone to protrude outward. Splint the elbow in the position it is found, and transport the patient to medical care.

Fingers and toes. A dislocation of the fingers or toes will usually cause one phalange to override the adjacent phalange. The deformity will look like a lump at the joint. Secure the finger or toe to uninjured fingers or toes, and take the patient to medical personnel for reduction.

Hip. A dislocated hip will display signs and symptoms similar to a fractured pelvis. Apply the same first aid care as you would for a fractured pelvis.

Patella. The patella (kneecap) will usually dislocate to the outside of the knee, leaving an excavation on top of the knee joint and a lump appearing at the side of the knee joint. Splint the leg so that it cannot bend at the knee, and transport the patient to medical care.

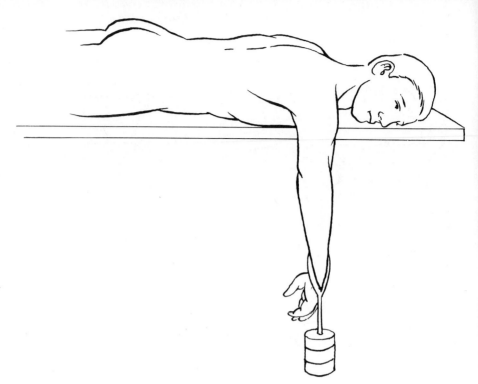

Fig. 11-16. Position for placing patient with dislocated shoulder.

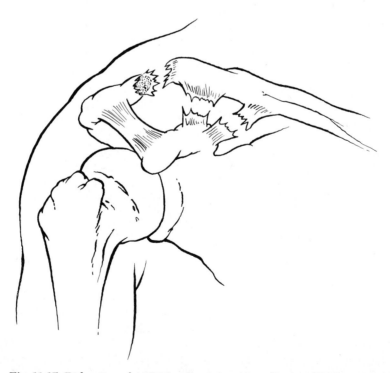

Fig. 11-17. Dislocation of A-C joint showing tearing of supporting ligaments.

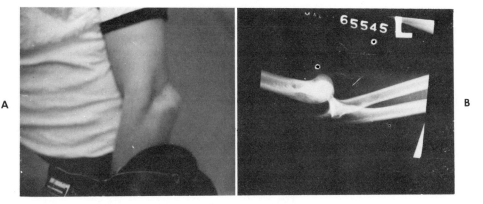

Fig. 11-18. A, Dislocated elbow showing typical disfiguration. **B,** Radiograph of dislocation showing displacement of distal end of humerus.

SUBLUXATIONS

A subluxation is similar to a dislocation and results from the same type of mechanism. The bone displaces from its normal place of articulation, but it returns spontaneously to its normal position. It is a difficult injury to determine because almost all signs and symptoms will be absent when the bone goes back into place. The history reported by the patient may be the only clue to a subluxation. Ask the patient to describe what happened. If he or she reports the bone sliding out of the joint and back in again accompanied by pain, assume the possibility of a subluxation.

A suspected subluxation should be cared for in the same manner as a dislocation. Immobilize the joint and refer to medical care. There is often a tendency to slough off such an injury as nothing serious because of the lack of signs and symptoms, but serious damage may have been done to the structures of the joint. All subluxations should be evaluated by qualified medical personnel to determine the extent of the damage. Repeated injury and permanent damage may result from inadequate and improper care.

SPRAINS

A sprain is defined as a stretching and/or tearing of ligament and soft tissue surrounding a joint. A sprain results from a blow or movement that forces a joint to go beyond its normal range of motion. Sprains may be classified according to the degree of damage to the ligaments. A *mild* sprain is one in which the ligaments are stretched and not torn. A *moderate* sprain is characterized by stretching and some tearing of the ligament fibers. A *severe* sprain is one in which the ligament is completely torn.

When examining a patient for a sprained joint, first look carefully for the possibility of a fracture. The mechanisms that cause a sprain may also cause a fracture. This possibility should not be overlooked. Look for a point of extreme sensitivity to pain by applying pressure at the site of the injury. If there is doubt, immobilize the part as you would a fracture. If you think you can rule out the possibility of a fracture, proceed with the examination, looking for the following signs and symptoms:

1. *Pain:* The pain will be located in the joint area and will usually be increased by moving the joint through its range of motion.
2. *Swelling:* The amount of swelling will depend on the damage to the vessels around the joint and will usually appear shortly after the injury has occurred.
3. *Discoloration:* It will probably take several hours for discoloration, which indicates internal bleeding.

First aid for sprains

Do not allow the patient to move or put weight on the moving part. Apply a compression bandage to help control the swelling. An elastic bandage serves as an excellent compression bandage. Be careful to avoid cutting off normal circulation by applying the bandage too tightly. Apply ice or cold packs to assist in controlling internal bleeding. Elevate the limb to keep gravity from pooling excess fluid into the injured joint. Transport the patient to medical care for further examination and treatment.

The first aid care for sprains can be summarized by using the three letters of the word ICE:

I : ice or cold pack
C: compression
E: elevation

STRAINS

A strain is defined as a stretching and/or tearing of muscle and tendon fibers. Overexertion, such as lifting something too heavy or working a muscle beyond the point of fatigue, may result in a strain. An uncoordinated movement may also cause a strain. The hamstrings (muscles in the back of the upper leg) are frequently strained while running because they contract when they should be relaxed.

Strains may be distinguished from other musculoskeletal injuries by the history and location of the pain. The history will indicate an injury caused by overexertion or movement and will not include a fall or a direct blow. The pain will be located in a muscle or its tendon and not in a joint or bone. Pain can be elicited by having the patient contract the suspected injured muscle against a fixed object. Swelling may occur, but it will not be as apparent as it is in the case of a sprain.

First aid for strains

Essentially, the same physiological reactions occur with a strain as in the case of a sprain, only in different parts of the body. Tissue has been torn, capillaries have been ruptured, and internal bleeding occurs in both strains and sprains. Therefore, as with sprains, think of the three letters in ICE for the first aid care for strains.

I : ice or cold pack
C: compression
E: elevation

First aid care and follow-up medical treatment should be provided for even those strains thought to be minor. Minor strains are often neglected at the time of injury. This sometimes results in reinjury, which may lead to chronic injuries and more serious complications. Many sources suggest that the first aid care for strains include the application of heat or warm compresses. The application of heat is contraindicated (not recommended) because heat will increase any internal bleeding and thereby increase the severity of the injury.

CONTUSIONS

A contusion is commonly referred to as a bruise. It occurs as a result of a direct blow causing tissue damage. Signs and symptoms may include local pain, stiffness, and some disability of the part. The pain is more dispersed than that of a fracture, and a contusion will usually not display a single point of extreme sensitivity to pain. Swelling may occur but may not be noticeable, depending on the depth of the tissue injury. Discoloration will usually not appear until several hours after the injury has occurred.

First aid for contusions

The first aid should be easy to remember because, again, the three letters of the word ICE apply to contusions. Contusions are perhaps the most neglected and poorly cared for injuries. Often it is said, "Oh well, it's just a bruise. Don't worry about it." Contusions through neglect or repeated injury may develop into more serious conditions such as myositis ossificans (calcification of the damaged tissue mass). What started out to be a simple bruise may result in disability over a prolonged period of time. Therefore provide the proper first aid for even minor contusions and refer patients with contusions for follow-up medical treatment.

SUMMARY

Musculoskeletal injuries most often are not an immediate threat to life, but the prevention of serious complication and permanent damage frequently depends on the application of proper first aid care. When examining an injured patient for musculoskeletal injuries, it may be helpful to consider the following questions:

1. What happened?
2. How did it happen?
3. Where is the pain located?
   a. At the location of a bone
   b. Joint
   c. Muscle or tendon
4. What is the nature of the pain?
   a. Point of extreme sensitivity
   b. Dispersed
   c. Intense
   d. Mild
5. How does the injured side compare to the normal side?
   a. Deformity present
   b. Deformity absent
6. Is there any loss of function?

After determining the nature and severity of the injury, proceed to administer the appropriate first aid.

FIRST AIDER COMPETENCIES

After studying the material and practicing the techniques presented in this chapter, the student should be able to:

- Define *fracture* and describe the different types of fractures.
- Explain the signs and symptoms that may indicate a possible fracture.
- Outline the first aid procedures for fractures.
- Explain what special measures need to be taken for suspected fractures of the vertebral column.
- Explain how a first aider should examine a patient with a back or neck injury.
- Describe the different types of splints and indicate under what conditions each one would be utilized for immobilization.
- Define *dislocation* and indicate what joints are most often dislocated.
- Outline first aid procedures for a dislocation.
- Define *subluxation* and indicate the first aid care.
- Define *sprain* and describe the three classifications of sprains.
- Outline first aid procedures for a sprain.
- Define *strain* and describe how the injury usually occurs.
- Outline the first aid procedures for a strain.
- Define *contusion* and explain the signs and symptoms of a contusion.
- Outline the first aid procedures for a contusion.
- Explain how a first aider could determine whether an injury is a fracture, a dislocation, a subluxation, a sprain, a strain, or a contusion.
- Indicate what first aid procedures are common to most musculoskeletal injuries.
- Apply compression bandages, support bandages, slings, and splints to various parts of the body.
- Demonstrate procedures for transporting a patient with a suspected fractured vertebra.

REFERENCES AND RECOMMENDED READINGS

1. Artz, C.: Trauma can be conquered, Emergency Medicine Today, pp. 1-6, July, 1974.
2. Blaisdell, F. W.: Multiple trauma. In Pascoe, D. J., and Grossman, M., editors: Quick reference to pediatric emergencies, Philadelphia, 1973, J. B. Lippincott Co.
3. Bovill, E. G., and Chapman, M.: Skeletal injuries. In Pascoe, D. J., and Grossman, M., editors: Quick reference to pediatric emergencies, Philadelphia, 1973, J. B. Lippincott Co.
4. Brodeur, A. E.: Fracture or suspicious trauma? Emergency Medicine **1**:26-28, Feb., 1969.
5. Cantrell, J. R.: Injuries of the musculoskeletal system. In Miller, R. H., and Cantrell, J. R., editors: Textbook of basic emergency medicine, St. Louis, 1975, The C. V. Mosby Co.
6. Diving injuries, Emergency Medicine **1**: 13-16, July, 1969.
7. Earle, A. S., et al.: Inflatable splints, Journal of the American Medical Association **192**:152-154, 1965.
8. Ralston, E. L.: Handbook of fractures, St. Louis, 1967, The C. V. Mosby Co.
9. Wolff, G. T.: The scene of an accident, Emergency Medicine Today, pp. 1-4, Feb., 1974.

12

▰▰▰

HEAD, NECK, AND FACIAL INJURIES

Byron J. Bailey

Injuries that involve the head and cervical spine must be considered to be life threatening. These are commonly the result of vehicular accidents, personal assaults, and falls. Injuries to the soft tissue and bony skeleton of the face may be life threatening if there is compromise of the upper airway. Injuries to the eyes or ears may produce serious functional disabilities in terms of posttraumatic sensory deficits of these important organs. Prompt and effective emergency treatment is vital in the avoidance of fatalities and serious sensory deficits.

Serious injury that involves the head or cervical spine may be fatal or may produce permanent paralysis that may totally incapacitate the victim. Careful surveys have shown that when individuals sustain significant injuries as a result of vehicular accidents (autos and cycles), two thirds of these victims have injuries involving the head and neck.[2] Proper treatment must begin at the scene of the injury with the use of accepted techniques for extrication of and moving the injured person. Eye injuries (including burns and foreign bodies) must be evaluated and treated properly if impairment of vision is to be prevented. Ear injuries similarly must be appreciated to avoid defects of hearing. Facial bone fractures and soft tissue lacerations of the face must be evaluated in relation to their potential for upper airway obstruction and the resulting fatality. The initial evaluation is a pivotal point in management if long-term disability is to be avoided.

STRUCTURE AND FUNCTION

This section will present a review of the basic anatomy and physiology of the organs under consideration in this chapter. We shall consider these organs in the following sequence: brain (cerebrum, cerebellum, and brainstem), spinal cord, covering tissues, skull, spine, facial bones, eye, and ear.

A brief discussion of these organ systems will be presented. For more exhaustive or detailed descriptions of each of these structures, the reader is referred to anatomy texts. Additional review of these organs is strongly recommended.

The brain

The brain (Fig. 12-1) is a unique organ that is the seat of consciousness, the organ that permits a person to be aware of his or her environment and to interact

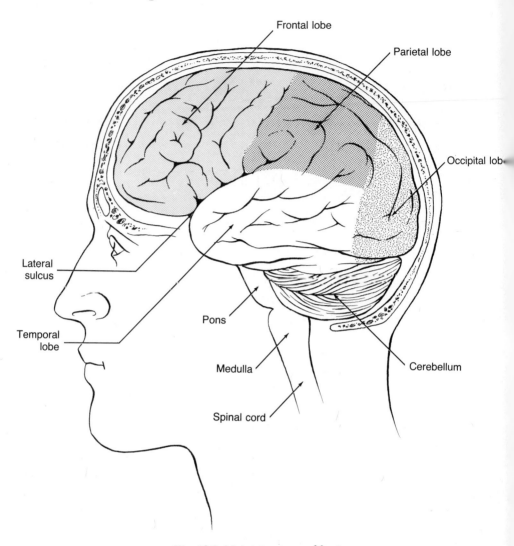

Fig. 12-1. Major structures of brain.

with it, and that senses and moves the body. Within the brain resides the capacity for learning, memory, and the regulation of many body functions that are not under voluntary control.

The brain occupies almost all of the cranial (skull) cavity and is divided into three major parts: the cerebrum, the cerebellum, and the brain stem. The *cerebrum* is the largest portion and houses the segments of the brain that deal with judgment, memory, emotion, and all of the higher functions that characterize us as human beings and separate us from other forms of animal life. It is also the site for all sensation and its interpretation and for all voluntary motor (movement) activities. Vision, hearing, speech, balance, perception of temperature and pressure, all have their ultimate termination in the cerebrum, which functions as a compact and intricate computer.

The *cerebellum* is a segment of the brain that deals primarily with coordination of all motor functions. It houses the connections that reflexly provide for adjustments that the body must make to each intended motion. For example, if a person decides to raise one foot off the floor while standing, there are many delicate adjustments that must be made in the opposite leg and foot, and it is within the cerebellum that these bits of learned behavior are all coordinated without giving careful thought to them.

The *brain stem* is the most primitive portion of the brain and houses the center for vital functions, such as respiration, cardiac activity, blood vessel tone, intestinal tract regulation, and other involuntary body function regulation that is not under direct and conscious control.

In terms of injury, several general concepts are important. First, brain tissue is sensitive to injury. A fall from a horse in which a person strikes his or her head on the ground results in a sudden shock wave being sent through the brain tissue, which may not produce lasting injury. It may, however, result in temporary loss of consciousness by disrupting the normal neural activity of the brain. This temporary loss of consciousness from a direct blow without bleeding into the brain tissue or tearing of the brain tissue is referred to as a *concussion*. The second characteristic of the brain that is unique to nervous tissue is its marked sensitivity to pressure. Increased pressure on the brain tissue or spinal cord will result in a loss of function of that tissue. This is the mechanism responsible for motor or sensory deficits that are seen after injuries in which there is no evidence of skull fracture or spinal fracture. If proper treatment is instituted early, this process can be reversed by measures that relieve the pressure, and no permanent deficits are left. However, if the pressure persists for a sufficient length of time (usually several days) or if the pressure is great enough, the loss of nervous tissue function may be permanent.

The third unique feature of nervous tissue is its limited ability to withstand mechanical injury and to repair itself. If a muscle is cut or if a bone is broken, the tissue has an inherent biological capability for repair. After the repair is completed, bone or muscle may function as well as it did before the injury. This is not the case with nervous tissue. If it is cut or torn, it is usually permanently damaged. This factor must be borne in mind constantly by those who provide emergency care to accident victims. Improper lifting, moving, or handling of persons with nervous system trauma may result in injuries that will be fatal or that will leave the victim permanently disabled.

The spinal cord

The spinal cord (Fig. 12-2) is made up of nerve fibers that run through the cord from sensory end organs to the brain, where the sensations are perceived, and fibers that carry impulses from the brain to muscles, where messages are translated into muscle contraction. In an oversimplified sense, the spinal cord can be compared to a telephone cable that contains thousands of tiny wires capable of carrying messages. These nerve fibers enter and leave the spinal cord through small openings between each of the vertebrae that make up the spine.

The same precautions mentioned in terms of avoiding injury to brain tissue apply to the spinal cord. The cord itself occupies a safe position within the normal spine by virtue of its tough covering and the liquid that surrounds it (cerebrospinal fluid). When the spine has sustained fracture, it becomes unstable, and it is possible for one vertebra to move abnormally forward and backward or laterally (sideward) on the one adjacent to it. This abnormal motion puts the spinal cord at risk of injury by permitting the normally protective vertebral arch to compress or actually tear the spinal cord. This damage to the spinal cord may result at the time of injury or could possibly be the result of careless extrication of the victim from a wrecked automobile or unsafe lifting and moving of the victim between the scene of the accident and the emergency room. Proper techniques in this regard will be stressed later in the chapter.

The covering tissues

The brain and spinal cord are covered by three layers of connective tissue—the dura, the arachnoid, and the pia mater (Fig. 12-3). The dura is a tough and tense protective covering that completely encircles the brain and the spinal cord. The arachnoid and pia mater are thin, delicate layers that afford no protection but that carry the blood vessels that nourish the brain and the spinal cord substance. Between the tough dura and the other two layers, there is a space filled with a watery liquid, the cerebrospinal fluid. This fluid also affords an element of protection by allowing the brain and spinal cord to float freely.

As a result of severe head injuries, with or without skull fracture, bleeding

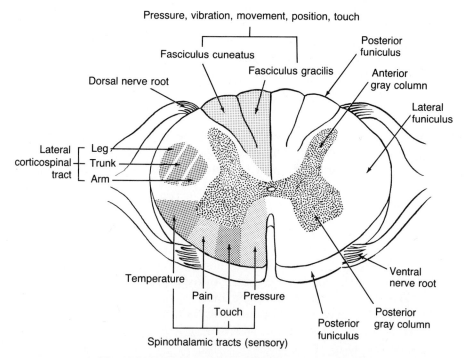

Fig. 12-2. Major structures and functions of spinal cord.

may occur superficial to the dura (extradural hematoma) or between the dura and the arachnoid (subdural hematoma). This collection of blood produces pressure on the nervous tissue and may interfere with the blood supply to and from the brain or spinal cord. This bleeding may occur slowly and may be responsible for the slow deterioration of the vital signs and consciousness of a patient who initially is thought to be free of serious injury and who later develops signs of life-threatening complications.

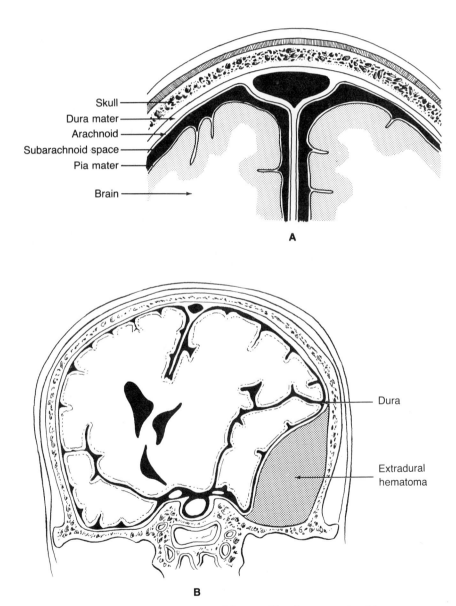

Fig. 12-3. **A,** Relationship of structural layers of head. **B,** Extradural hematoma.

Continued.

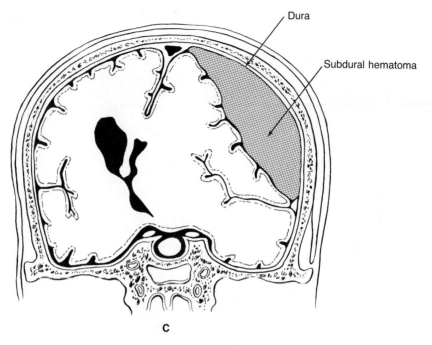

Fig. 12-3, cont'd. C, Subdural hematoma.

The skull (cranium)

The cranium or skull (Fig. 12-4) is the bony case that completely surrounds the brain. It is comprised of dense bone throughout most of its surface but includes some rather delicate areas in the roof of the nose and around the portion of bone that houses the deeper ear structures.

The skull is resistant to fracture from minor blows but may sustain linear (in a straight or broken line), stellate (star-shaped fracture lines coming from a central point), or depressed (fragments of bone pushed into the cranial cavity) fractures when exposed to high-impact levels of energy. Fractures that involve the base of the skull (the area where the cranial bones join the facial bones) may be difficult to detect but are of great importance. These may be suspected when an injured victim with a decreased level of consciousness develops discoloration around the eyes or over the mastoid tip behind either ear. Another sign of basal skull fracture is the presence of bleeding or clear fluid from either the nose or from the ear canal. If you observe either of these two phenomena, it is important to appreciate that this means that the space surrounding the brain is now in open continuity with the outside environment and that every precaution possible must be taken to avoid contaminating this wound. It is also important to remember that no effort should be made to control bleeding from the ear by packing a dressing tightly into the ear. This could result in the accumulation of blood around the brain, which would cause life-threatening pressure within the cranial cavity.

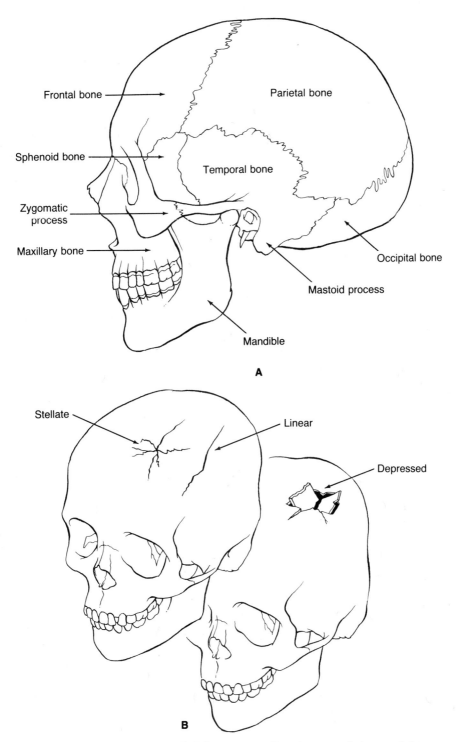

Fig. 12-4. A, Lateral view showing skull bones. **B,** Stellate, linear, and depressed fractures of skull.

The spine

The spine (Fig. 12-5) is usually comprised of twenty-four individual bony vertebrae, which articulate with each other at several points, which permits flexible motion of the back and neck. There are usually seven cervical vertebrae, twelve thoracic vertebrae, and five lumbar vertebrae. Each vertebra is comprised of a large vertebral body, located anterior to the spinal cord, which articulates with the vertebral body above and below it by means of an intervertebral disc. This disc is made up of a dense fibrous ring called the *anulus fibrosus,* which encircles and contains a looser substance called the *nucleus pulposus.* When there is a weakness of the anulus, the nucleus pulposus may be pushed through this weak spot in such a way that it compresses the spinal cord or the spinal nerves

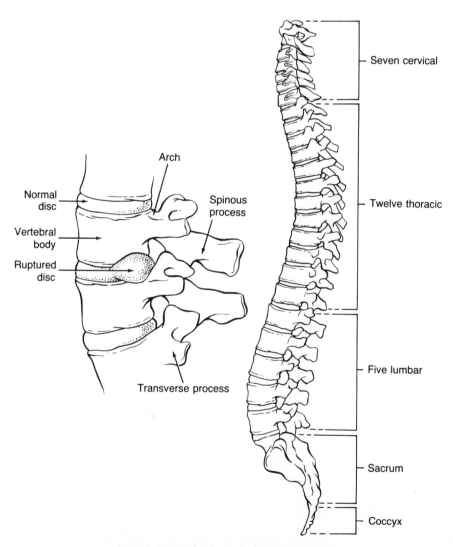

Fig. 12-5. Spinal column and herniated disc.

as they exit from the spinal cord. Such a condition is commonly called a *ruptured disc*, which may produce sensory defects, pain, or motor weakness involving the back and legs by virtue of pressure on the nearby nervous tissue. The vertebral arch is a portion of each vertebra that surrounds the spinal cord. Coming off from the lateral aspect of each arch are the two transverse processes, which have joints with the transverse processes above and below each vertebra. Directly posteriorly (in back of) and arising from the arch is the spinous process, which is a bony extension of the vertebrae onto which the paraspinous muscles attach.

In the intact spine, the vertebral arch surrounds and protects the spinal cord, and the motion of one vertebra on the next is of no danger to the spinal cord. When there are fractures of the transverse processes or of the vertebral arch itself, this series of bony elements becomes unstable, and the stage is set for abnormal motion of one vertebra on the next, which will permit serious damage to the spinal cord.

The facial bones

The major facial bones (Fig. 12-6) are the mandible (lower jaw), the maxilla (upper jaw), the zygomas (cheekbones), and the nasal bones. In regard to emergency treatment, the mandible is the most important of the facial bones because it is essential for chewing and serves as the anchoring point for the tongue. If the mandible is fractured in two areas, it can be unstable, and this permits the

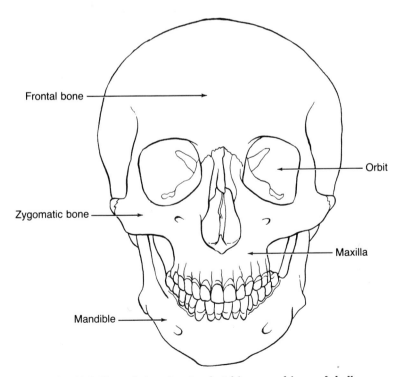

Frontal bone

Zygomatic bone

Mandible

Orbit

Maxilla

Fig. 12-6. Frontal view showing facial bones and bone of skull.

tongue to be displaced posteriorly, where it may occlude the upper airway. In this situation, it is essential that the mandible be grasped securely and pulled forward so that the airway may be opened.

It is also important to check for loosened or absent teeth. Fractures of the mandible or maxilla may result in the avulsion (violent pulling out; traumatic loss) of teeth and their displacement into the airway passages. It is also important to check for dentures, which may have been dislodged and which may be obstructing the airway in the same anatomical locations. Fractures involving any of the facial bones are usually associated with bleeding into the nose or mouth. This blood may then clot and obstruct the airway.

Fractures of the nasal bones are especially common. This pair of bones is rather delicate and occupies a prominent and exposed position on the face. Fractures of the nasal bones are usually associated with nasal bleeding and nasal obstruction. Examination often reveals tenderness, crepitus (a crunching sensation on attempted movement), deformity, and false motion of the nasal bones. If none of these situations are present, the fractures of the nasal bones are not otherwise significant in regard to emergency care.

In many instances, trauma victims have sustained multiple injuries, and because of this factor, these patients are usually treated most effectively by a team of specialists who are experienced in trauma management. Such a team usually consists of a general surgeon, a thoracic (chest) surgeon, a neurosurgeon, an otolaryngologist (ear, nose, and throat specialist), an ophthalmologist (eye specialist), and a general plastic surgeon. Dentists may serve an important consultative role when there are dental injuries.

The eye

Injuries involving the eye (Fig. 12-7) may cause damage to one or more elements of a group of related anatomical structures, and it is important to clarify

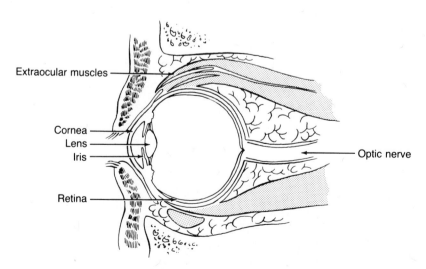

Fig. 12-7. Structures of eye.

the anatomy and physiology of each of these component segments. These segments include the lids, conjunctiva, globe, periorbital muscles and fat, lacrimal glands, and bony orbital cavity.

The eyelids form a protective covering for the globe and close by reflex when any threatening injury is perceived. The act of blinking enables them to moisten the conjunctiva (the protective covering on the undersurface of the lids and the outer surface of the eye itself), which dries rather quickly when exposed to the air. The lower lid is passive and serves as a pad for the upper lid to meet as it moves downward. Both the upper and lower lids consist of a layer of skin, then a layer of muscle, a layer of cartilage or dense connective tissue, and then the inner layer of conjunctiva. The eye is moistened by tears produced in the lacrimal gland, which is located in the upper and outer quadrant of the eye. The tears then collect at the medial angle of the eye, where they drain through the lacrimal canaliculi into the lacrimal sac and then into the lower portion of the nose.

The globe (commonly called the eye) is made up of several significant parts. On the outer surface is the conjunctiva, which is a thin, moist membrane and covers all of the exposed portion of the eyeball except for the cornea. The cornea is a thin, tough layer of tissue with few blood vessels that serves to protect the next portion of the eye which is the anterior chamber. This chamber is between the cornea and the lens and iris and is filled with a fluid called *aqueous humor.* This fluid serves to maintain a normal state of pressure within the eye and gives the cornea the shape it must have for the eye to function properly in terms of vision. The iris is the colored portion of the eye that surrounds the dark, central, circular portion called the *pupil.* The pupil size is determined by the degree of muscle contraction on the iris to enlarge it or to constrict it. The next structure toward the back of the eye is the lens, which is normally clear and tends to focus the light rays on the retina. Between the lens and the retina is a large spherical space filled with a jelly-like material called the *vitreous humor.* The retina is located on the posterior surface of the eyeball and is the site of the rods and cones, which are the nerve cells that perceive light and color. These nerve cells then pass toward the brain through the optic nerve, which leaves the bony eye socket through a foramen (opening) located posteriorly and medially (toward the center).

The ear

A variety of injuries may involve the ear (Fig. 12-8). The external ear (auricle) is susceptible to lacerations, blunt trauma, and thermal injury (burns and frostbite). These problems seldom present major difficulties in detection. First aid care consists of applying a moist, sterile dressing and securing this with a turban-like bandage.

Foreign bodies in the ear canal are especially common in children. Because of the probability of damaging the ear canal skin or tympanic membrane (ear drumhead), get this patient to an ear specialist without making any effort to remove the object yourself.

Bleeding from the ear after a blow presents several diagnostic possibilities. If the blow was not characterized by extreme force but was inflicted over the

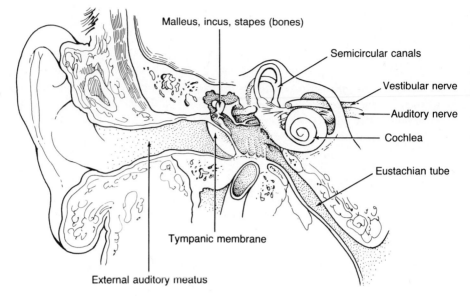

Fig. 12-8. Structures of ear.

opening of the ear canal, one suspects a traumatic tympanic membrane perforation. If the force was severe, the bleeding may be associated with a fracture of the base of the skull. Hearing loss, dizziness, and ringing noise in the ear may be seen with either of the problems just mentioned. More exact diagnosis and treatment will follow referral to the ear specialist. Do *not* make any effort to prevent the blood from coming from the ear in any event.

EVALUATION OF THE INJURED VICTIM

As previously stated, over half the patients who have been involved in a serious vehicular accident, personal assault, or fall will have sustained injuries to the head and neck area. Usually these injuries will be obvious in terms of skin bruises, abrasions, or lacerations with bleeding, but in other instances, the injuries will be more subtle.

Remember that life-threatening injuries may be present without evidence of any significant external injury. Also, it is essential to remember the following points:

1. An accident victim with a serious head injury may also have an associated, equally serious injury of the spine.
2. An injured person may have survived without serious disability the initial trauma of the accident but may become disabled as the result of attempts to move him or her in an inappropriate manner.
3. Accident victims who have sustained serious head injury may be alert and neurologically intact when they are first seen but may deteriorate rapidly if there is bleeding inside the skull or swelling of the brain tissue.
4. Victims of serious head and neck injuries may have or may develop respiratory obstruction from a variety of causes, and the airway must be

kept open and vital signs monitored frequently to detect and treat any deterioration of respiration or cardiac function.

History and physical examination

Information crucial to the management of these patients can be obtained by means of a careful history and physical examination.

History. One of the key steps in the effective management of trauma victims is the obtaining of an adequate history from the injured person or from others who have observed the accident. In some instances, immediate examination and treatment must be done at the same time the history is being obtained. The significance of historical information is that it provides important clues relating to the possible severity of the injury, the possible presence of associated injuries that are not obvious, and the probability of later complications. This information is not only of importance to those who are stabilizing the patient at the scene of the accident but may be also crucial to the further medical management on arrival at the hospital. It is essential in many cases and must be conveyed accurately to the attending physician.

With any given injury, the history should include certain *general* information and information that is *specific* to the patient's status after the injury. In dealing with the general information first, it is important to record the following observations:

1. *The nature of the accident.* For example, in an automobile accident, where was the patient sitting, what was the approximate speed of the vehicle, what was the approximate angle of impact, and was the patient thrown from the car?
2. *Status of the patient immediately after the injury.* For example, in an assault, was the patient unconscious for a period of time after the injury, were there signs of irrational behavior, were there complaints of pain or visual impairment, and has there been any change in the patient's status since the time of the injury?
3. *Other factors that may alter the emergency care of the victim.* For example, has the patient been drinking or taking drugs of any kind, does the patient have a history of cardiac or respiratory disease, is the patient allergic to any medication, such as penicillin, and has the patient been immunized for tetanus?

On arriving at the scene of the accident, your information gathering should begin with at least the following ten items:

1. Check the patient quickly for signs of an obstructed airway, check the patient's vital signs, and examine the patient for any evidence of serious bleeding. Although this is not strictly historical information, it is where your evaluation must begin, and with the passage of time, it will become valuable historical information.
2. Determine the state of the patient's consciousness. Note specific general observations such as agitated, alert, depressed, confused, semiconscious, or unconscious. Ask the patient (or other observers if the patient is unconscious) whether the state of consciousness has changed in the time period since the accident.

3. Determine the degree of orientation. Find out whether the patient is able to tell you who he is, where he is, the approximate date and time, and any recollections of the accident itself.
4. Determine whether the patient's status in general is stable or unstable. Is there evidence that the patient is improving or deteriorating?
5. Determine the presence or absence of pain. Is there headache, neck pain, back pain, or pain in any other part of the body or its extremities?
6. Has movement been painful?
7. Is the patient aware of numbness or decreased sensation in any area of the scalp, face, body, or extremities?
8. Is the patient aware of weakness or paralysis in any part of the body?
9. Is the patient aware of any deformity of the skull, facial bones, teeth, or spine?
10. Is the patient aware of significant blood loss?

Evaluating the unconscious patient may be a great deal more difficult. If there are observers, ask the same questions of them. It is essential to remember that any injury serious enough to have caused unconsciousness may be associated with a serious injury to the neck or back. Ask observers whether the patient appears to have had any uncontrolled movements while unconscious (seizures).

Physical examination. The examination of the accident victim must include the entire body. The following ten points are provided in reference to the examination of the patient who may have sustained serious head or neck injuries. Begin by reevaluating the airway, the vital signs, and looking for any evidence of significant bleeding. Then proceed with the following ten essential steps:

1. Inspect the scalp, face, and neck for any lacerations, bruises, or visual evidence of deformity.
2. Check the eyes for any evidence of serious head injury. Determine whether the pupils are equal in size, and remember that a dilated pupil in one eye suggests the presence of increasing intracranial pressure (usually as the result of brain swelling from trauma or bleeding within the skull) on that side. Determine whether the eyes move in a coordinated way. Have the patient follow your finger as you move it from side to side and up and down. The patient who cannot follow your finger movements evenly with both eyes may have either a local injury around the eye or central brain damage.
3. Check for signs of tenderness by palpating (pushing lightly on) the skull, around the eyes, the facial bones, the throat, and the neck spine.
4. Check the patient carefully for evidence of painful movement. Pain on opening and closing the mouth suggests the possibility of a fracture of the mandible. Pain on slight movements of the neck suggests a possible fracture of the neck spine.
5. Check the patient for evidence of local areas of numbness. Fractures or other significant injuries should be suspected when there is decreased sensation to touch above or below either eye, on either side of the chin, or in any other localized areas of the neck, the body, or the extremities.
6. Check for signs of bony deformity. This may be felt over the skull when

there is a depressed skull fracture, over the facial bones when they are fractured, or along the bony elements of the spine.

7. Check for evidence of significant bleeding, especially as it might involve the upper airway.
8. Look for blood or watery fluid (cerebrospinal fluid) that might be oozing from the nose or from either ear. The presence of this finding would strongly suggest a skull fracture.
9. Check for evidence of hoarseness or breathing difficulties, which might suggest an injury to the upper airway in the region of the larynx (voice box).
10. Determine whether the patient's condition is stable or whether it is changing in any way.

One of the common errors in evaluating the patient with head and neck injuries is for the examiner to be distracted by serious lacerations on the face. These are seldom life threatening, and attention to them should not prevent your carefully examining all of the areas just mentioned.

EMERGENCY MANAGEMENT OF SPECIFIC INJURIES
Head injuries

Injuries to the brain may vary considerably in regard to their seriousness. The three terms most commonly used to describe the severity are as follows:

1. A *concussion* is a temporary loss of consciousness resulting from the force of an impact that produces a transient interruption of the brain's normal neurological activity and loss of awareness of the victim's surroundings without producing permanent brain damage.
2. A *contusion* is a brain injury in which there is actual loss of blood into the brain tissue substance (bruising). This may produce a longer period of unconsciousness but is usually not fatal and not associated with permanent brain dysfunction.
3. *Brain tissue laceration* usually results from a depressed skull fracture in which there is actual tearing of the brain coverings and the brain substance itself. This may be associated with permanent loss of function and with the development of episodes of seizures for long periods of time after the injury.

The two keys to the effective management of brain injury are to maintain adequate respiration and to avoid any action that could conceivably make the patient's condition worse. The patient's respiratory efforts may be hampered by associated injuries that produce airway obstruction, by paralysis of the chest muscles of respiration or the diaphragm, or by direct damage to the brain's centers that control respiration. The vital signs must be monitored carefully, and one must be prepared to assist the patient's respiration should problems arise.

The most serious injuries are usually those in which brain tissue may actually be visible from the outside. Make no effort to clean these wounds or to apply pressure in these areas. Place a sterile dressing over the head wound and moisten it with sterile saline, if this is available. Secure the dressing with a bandage wrapped around the head. If the patient is on a stretcher, elevate the head of the stretcher slightly, but do not place the patient's head on a pillow, since this tends to flex the neck, which may be injured also. If the patient is comatose (unresponsive to verbal commands or painful stimuli), be especially protective of the airway, and be prepared to suction blood or vomited material from the throat during the time that the patient is being transported. Of course, in most first aid situations, suction equipment will not be available. This situation highlights the importance, in each community, of an emergency medical service with well-trained and properly equipped paramedics who can respond promptly to this type of life-threatening emergency situation.

Some serious injuries to the head are subtle. The patient may be alert and oriented when first seen and gradually slip into a decreased level of consciousness. Remember that this may be the result of bleeding inside the skull and that this event may produce compression of the vital brain tissue. In its most serious form, it may result in cardiac arrest and respiratory arrest. Observe the pupils and vital signs frequently for any evidence of intracranial bleeding. If the pupil begins to dilate, the blood pressure begins to rise, or the state of consciousness begins to recede, this is strong evidence that suggests an elevation of intracranial pressure.

Seizure activity may follow as a result of head injury. These seizures are usually observed as violent, uncontrollable convulsive shaking actions of the patient. They may be associated with postseizure loss of consciousness and with nausea and vomiting. The patient should be prevented from injuring himself during the seizure by placing a bite block or series of five or six tongue depressors between the teeth so that the airway can be maintained and the tongue and cheek will not be bitten. The patient must be watched carefully during seizure activity for vomiting, and, should this occur, immediate suction must be instituted (if available).

It is usually considered ideal in terms of safety to position the patient on his side during transportation to the hospital. This will minimize the danger of vomiting and aspiration and will provide maximum protection to the airway.

Injuries to the neck and back spine

These injuries are extremely serious because of the potential for further injury and lifelong disability in the event of improper handling. On arriving at the scene of any serious vehicular accident or fall, it is the safest course of action to assume that the victim may have sustained a spinal injury. Similarly, injury resulting from diving into the shallow end of a pool, or any injury that has produced unconsciousness, is best assumed to have potentially produced a spinal injury. After the airway has been checked carefully and adequate ventilation is secured, attention may be directed to the problem of extricating, lifting, and moving the patient. This is done with the greatest safety by securing the patient to a firm backboard in whatever position he or she is found if this can be done (Fig. 12-9).

If the injured person must be moved before being placed on a backboard, this must be accomplished without producing any bending or twisting of the spine. This requires the cooperative effort of a number of individuals. One must securely hold the head to prevent its being flexed forward, extended backward, or moved laterally. This person should maintain a light traction (pull) of the head away from the body. Two or three other persons must then lift and support

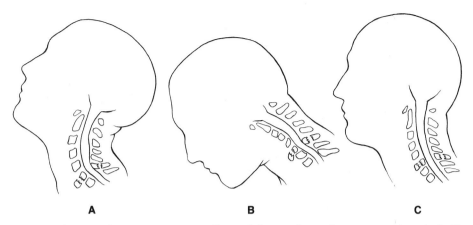

Fig. 12-9. Three head positions showing effects of fractured vertebrae on spinal cord. **A,** Hyperextension. **B,** Hyperflexion. **C,** Neutral.

the body and extremities and move the patient without any twisting or bending actions. The head, neck, and spine must be moved as if they were a delicate, rigid log without any portion being permitted to move in relation to another portion.

The patient is then secured on a firm stretcher or backboard and, if unconscious, must be placed in a lateral position on his or her side. The head is secured with sandbags or cushions, and the head and body are strapped into position (Fig. 12-10). At this point, further evaluation may be performed and other emergency care may be provided. If respiratory assistance is necessary, this must be accomplished without hyperextending the patient's neck by placing your fingers behind the patient's mandible and exerting forward traction. This will displace the mandible forward and secondarily pull the tongue forward and open the airway for forced ventilation. In the event of cardiac arrest, cardiopulmonary resuscitation must be performed in an effective manner, regardless of the possible difficulties that may ensue if a spinal injury is present.

Injuries to the eye

Eye injuries may include penetrating injuries of the eyeball itself, foreign bodies, chemical and thermal burns, and injuries to the structures around the eye.

Begin by obtaining a reasonable estimate of visual function (acuity) by asking the patient to indicate how many fingers you are holding up and testing his ability to read any available printed material. In the case of a chemical injury to the eye, the first step is to begin irrigating immediately with any available source of water such as a hose or faucet, or preferably with sterile saline through intravenous tubing if this is available. Large amounts of irrigating solution are recommended.

In most cases, no effort should be made to remove any foreign body or foreign material from the eye. Care of eye injuries in most cases consists of the application of a light patch to the eye to protect it from further injury. In most cases the eye will be more comfortable if the lids are closed. Prevent the patient from injuring himself further by rubbing his eye in the event of a possible burn or foreign body.

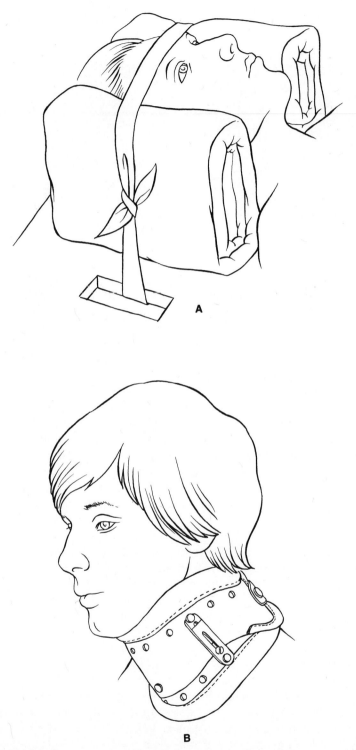

Fig. 12-10. Immobilization for fractured cervical spine. **A,** Sandbag head restraints. **B,** Cervical collar.

In the event of severe lacerations of the lid, there may be profuse bleeding. As long as the eyeball itself has not been injured, it is proper to control this bleeding by direct finger pressure. Avoid any possibility of applying pressure of any sort to an eye in which there is an obvious damage or laceration of the eyeball. Definitive follow-up care for these patients should be provided by an eye specialist. Rapid transportation (in excess of posted speed limits) is seldom, if ever, indicated for these injuries.

Facial bones

Fractures of the facial bones are often associated with rather severe bleeding and may result in obstruction of the upper airway. Therefore the primary principle involved in this instance is protection and maintenance of an open airway. Little definitive action can be taken to control this bleeding in some instances, and suction will be the only mechanism available to prevent the development of clots in the throat or aspiration of blood into the lungs. If suction equipment is not available, you will have to permit the blood to flow freely from the nose and mouth; do *not* have the patient lying on his or her back.

Facial bone fractures may be associated with abnormalities of the bite (the manner in which the lower teeth meet and touch the upper teeth). Palpation may also provide good evidence of facial bone fractures. Tenderness over specific points on the face is generally observed when facial bone fractures exist. In the case of mandibular fractures, there may be pain with swallowing or general movement of the patient. This can be relieved by means of a Barton bandage, which provides good immobilization of the lower jaw during the period before definitive surgical treatment (Fig. 12-11).

Facial bone fractures are usually not life-threatening emergencies, and no specific first aid care is necessary other than close attention to the airway and the detection of any problems causing airway obstruction. Obtain medical attention for all suspected fractures of facial bones.

Nasal bleeding (epistaxis)

Spontaneous nasal bleeding (without nasal fracture or other serious trauma) is a common medical problem. Usually these hemorrhages are minor and stop without any treatment, but occasionally this problem can be fatal.

Most of these episodes of nasal bleeding arise from the anterior-inferior (forward and lower) part of the nasal septum (the partition between the two halves of the nose). Therefore it is frequently possible to control this bleeding by pinching the lower half of the nose between the thumb and index finger for 10 minutes.

Those persons who do not respond to the above will require a further effort for control. Ice packs may be applied to the nasal and facial area. Moisten a gauze pad or cotton tampon with the water and gently insert it into the bleeding nasal cavity. Then pinch the nose between the thumb and index finger for 10 minutes. If this does not control the bleeding, medical attention should be obtained.

Lacerations

Lacerations of the face, neck, and scalp are usually associated with brisk bleeding. The general management of these injuries consists of controlling the

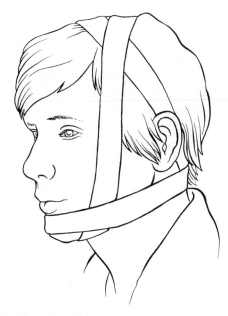

Fig. 12-11. Immobilization for fractured lower jaw.

hemorrhage by finger pressure on a gauze dressing and the avoidance of contamination of the wound.

Pressure is applied to a laceration by placing the fingers on a sterile bandage that has been placed along the edge of the wound. The tissue is then pushed down on the underlying bony structures after it has been determined that there is not a skull or facial bone fracture. This pressure must be held for 5 to 10 minutes to allow a clot to form in the bleeding vessel.

After bleeding has been controlled, the wound should be inspected for the presence of any significant foreign bodies or contamination. Occasionally a sizable piece of glass or other foreign material will be firmly impaled in the depths of the wound, and in this case no effort should be made to remove this foreign body. This will be accomplished by the physician in the emergency room, who will then be prepared to control any heavy bleeding that may result from this technique.

Once you are certain that bleeding has been adequately controlled, the wound should be bandaged to protect it from further contamination. If gross contamination is observed at the scene and if the capability to irrigate the wound with sterile saline water exists, this should be accomplished while the patient is being transported to the emergency room.

Dental injuries

Fractures of the facial bones will often result in avulsion or loosening of one or more teeth. If it is obvious that teeth have been lost from the upper or lower jaw, the mouth and throat should be inspected to rule out the presence of these foreign bodies. In the event of markedly loosened teeth, care must be taken during the emergency care and transportation that these do not become dislodged and become airway foreign bodies.

If the patient is known to have dentures or partial plates, this should be noted, and it is extremely important that these be brought with the patient to the emergency room. They may play an important role in the further management and treatment of fractures involving the upper or lower jaw.

SUMMARY

This chapter has reviewed the major points of evaluation and management of injuries to the head, face, and neck. In discussing all of these injuries, many principles of a universal nature have been expressed. These include the following:

1. Maintenance of an adequate airway and adequate respiration hold the highest priority for these accident victims.
2. The avoidance of injury during the course of rendering emergency care must constantly be kept in mind. Inappropriate handling of patients with skull fractures or spinal injuries may result in death or permanent disability and incapacitation of these victims.
3. Continuous monitoring of the patient's condition and vital signs is essential to chart the progress of the patient from the time of injury until the time of arrival in the emergency room.
4. Patients who have sustained head trauma sufficient to render them unconscious may well have associated spinal injuries.

Remember that trauma is the leading cause of death in the United States for individuals between 1 and 42 years of age. Approximately two thirds of the persons who have sustained serious vehicular trauma or falls will have some degree of injury in the head and neck. You should be aware constantly of the types of injuries that may be present and the general principles for safe and effective management.

FIRST AIDER COMPETENCIES

After studying the material presented in this chapter, the student should be able to:

- Demonstrate procedures for evaluating the patient for skull and/or cervical spine fractures, brain and/or spinal cord injuries, facial bone fractures, eye injuries, ear injuries, and lacerations in these areas.
- Describe the appropriate first aid procedures for the above injuries.
- Demonstrate procedures for transporting a patient with serious head injuries and/or suspected cervical spine fractures.
- Demonstrate procedures for establishing an open airway in a patient with a suspected cervical spine fracture.

REFERENCES AND RECOMMENDED READINGS

1. Emergency care and transportation of the sick and injured, Chicago, 1971, American Academy of Orthopaedic Surgeons.
2. Haller, J. A., Jr., and Talbert, J. L.: Trauma and the child. In Ballinger, W. F., Rutherford, R. B., and Zuidema, G. D., editors: The management of trauma, ed. 2, Philadelphia, 1973, W. B. Saunders Co.
3. National Safety Council: Accident facts, Chicago, 1974.
4. Sproul, C. W., and Mullanney, P. J.: Emergency care: assessment and intervention, St. Louis, 1974, The C. V. Mosby Co.
5. Stephenson, H. E., Jr., editor: Immediate care of the acutely ill and injured, St. Louis, 1974, The C. V. Mosby Co.

SECTION IV

Medical emergencies

13

~~~~~~

SUDDEN ILLNESS

John N. O'Connor and Robert H. Miller

A medical emergency is any nontraumatic illness that may result in death or disability if no care is provided within the first hour. Medical emergencies and related problems are covered in this section, starting with sudden illness.

This chapter will deal with acute sudden illness emergencies, excluding previously discussed cardiorespiratory emergencies, that are not a result of a wound or injury. Central nervous system dysfunction resulting in changes in levels of consciousness or unconsciousness as well as acute abdominal disorders will be the primary emphasis. However, some nonemergency conditions likely to be encountered by the first aider, such as motion sickness, will also be discussed.

ALTERATIONS IN THE STATE OF CONSCIOUSNESS

When the first aider is confronted with a patient who has an altered state of consciousness, certain observations must be made. Specifically, the first aider should (1) assess the state of consciousness, (2) examine for the presence or absence of weakness or paralysis of the extremities, (3) assess the pupilary size and response to light, and (4) observe the pattern of respiration. If you are with the patient for any significant period of time, the observation should be repeated to see if there has been any change in the patient status. All observations should be reported to those who provide continuing medical care. This information may be exceedingly valuable to the physician in terms of both diagnosis and decisions regarding management.

Assessments of the state of consciousness

Alterations in the state of consciousness may range from mild confusion to profound coma in which the patient will respond to neither verbal nor painful stimuli. Many terms are utilized to describe various states of depression of consciousness, such as lethargy, obtundation, or semicoma. Each of these terms has different meanings to different people. In assessing a patient's state of consciousness, if the patient is talking, one first assesses his orientation as to time, place, and person. This is accomplished by asking the patient his or her name, where he or she is, and the date. Other questions concerning the circumstances surrounding the patient may be asked to further assess the degree of confusion. If

173

you must shout at or shake a patient to arouse him or her, then the first aider should describe just that, rather than use a term such as semicomatose, which has little in the way of specific meaning. If shouting at or shaking the patient fails to elicit any response, an extremity may be pinched to see whether the limb is withdrawn. Presence or absence of withdrawal from a painful stimulus should be similarly described.

Determining the presence or absence of weakness or paralysis. The simplest way to determine whether paralysis exists is initially to observe the patient. If the patient is spontaneously noted to move all extremities, one can assume that no paralysis is present. If the patient is conscious enough to follow verbal commands, yet is not moving spontaneously, ask the patient to move each extremity. Check strength in the upper extremities by asking the patient to grab one finger and squeeze, comparing the grasp on the left with the grasp on the right. If there is any difference, it should be noted. The first aider should not be concerned with any more detailed assessment of muscle strength.

Assessment of pupillary size and response to light. The nerve fibers that cause pupils to constrict are carried by a nerve called the *oculomotor nerve,* which travels from the brain to the eyeball. Since the skull is a closed space, bleeding within the skull or swelling of the brain from any cause may result in pressure on one or both of these nerves. One of the early findings of increased pressure within the skull will be dilation of one or both pupils. Because the constricted fibers are damaged, the pupils will be dilated and will not respond to light. In the normal individual, shining a light in either eye will result in constriction of both pupils. Examine both pupils under the existing lighting to determine whether they are equal in size. If they are unequal, note which is larger. Then shine a light into each pupil to determine whether the pupil constricts normally. If either or both pupils fail to constrict to light, this should be noted.

Assessment of respiratory pattern. Again, with bleeding into the skull or brain swelling, regardless of the cause, ultimately the brain stem is damaged. The brain stem is the lowest portion of the brain adjacent to the spinal cord and controls the most primitive functions, such as respiration and heart beat. With progressive damage to the brain stem, respiratory patterns begin to change. The first aider should observe the chest and abdomen, noting the respiratory pattern. The pattern should be described according to observations made, for example, normal depth and regular rate of twelve a minute; periods of gradual increasing depth of respiration followed by cessation of respiration for a period of 10 seconds; deep, regular respirations at approximately thirty a minute; or totally erratic respiratory pattern.

As long as the first aider remains with the patient, these observations should all be repeated at regular intervals. Any change in the status of the level of consciousness, weakness or paralysis, pupillary size and response to light, or respiratory pattern may be extremely significant to those who will later care for the patient.

First aid care for the unconscious patient. The unconscious patient is defined as the individual who is unresponsive to verbal commands and who is making no purposeful or meaningful movements. The patient may or may not withdraw from painful stimuli. In the unconscious state, muscle control of the mandible (lower jaw) is lost. If the patient is lying on his back, the tongue will fall backward, resulting in an anatomical obstruction of the airway. Since unconscious patients lose their gag reflex, vomiting is a serious complication in that they are likely, with vomiting, to aspirate vomitus into the lungs. This may result in immediate airway obstruction and death or later pneumonia, which may be the primary contributing factor to the patient's death.

The first concern in the unconscious patient is to protect the airway. Two methods may be utilized to open the airway. Tilting the head back will force the lower jaw forward and move the tongue from its position of blocking the airway. The jaw may also be pulled forward, which will prevent the tongue from blocking the airway (Figs. 3-4 and 3-6). It should be remembered that many times patients with head injuries also have cervical spine injuries. The patient with a cervical spine injury must be attended carefully to avoid damage to the spinal cord. Since the head should not be moved, it is wise to use the second maneuver (pulling the mandible forward) to establish a patent airway and immobilize the neck as quickly as possible (Chapter 12). The unconscious patient should, whenever possible, be positioned on his or her side so that vomited material will not be aspirated into the lungs. Artificial respiration and external cardiac compression must be provided as needed (Chapter 3). Transport the patient as soon as possible to medical care facilities.

Metabolic coma

When any of the normal physiological processes essential to the maintenance of health are altered, the resultant abnormalities may be generically called metabolic disturbances. Maintenance of normal metabolic status requires autoregulation of a myriad of chemical substances, such as hormones, enzymes, electrolytes, and glucose. Fluid balance must be maintained, and acid base balance (the pH of the body fluids) must be kept within a narrow range to preserve cellular function.

Metabolic disturbances may result from a wide variety of causes. Depression of central nervous system function ultimately resulting in coma is one of the more severe, life-threatening manifestations of metabolic derangements. Metabolic coma may result from ingestion of a drug that depresses central nervous system function, diseases that affect serum calcium levels, abnormalities in serum sodium levels and, commonly, abnormalities in blood glucose (sugar) levels. Metabolic abnormalities generally affect brain function diffusely and, therefore, usually do not produce localized findings such as weakness or paralysis on one side. Metabolic brain disease is frequently reversible if the underlying problem is appropriately and promptly treated. The problem is then functional rather than structural, that is, there is no mechanical damage to brain tissue. In contrast, such events as head trauma and stroke produce abnormalities in brain function as a result of damage to brain tissue.

Diabetic coma. Insulin is a substance secreted by the pancreas into the bloodstream. Insulin acts to permit transportation of glucose from the bloodstream into cells, a process essential for the maintenance of cellular life. Diabetes mellitus is a disease in which the pancreas is unable to produce adequate amounts of insulin. Therefore, in the untreated diabetic, glucose is unable to pass from the bloodstream into cells, resulting in a progressive rise in the blood glucose level (hyperglycemia). Hyperglycemia causes the kidneys to excrete excessive amounts of urine, which ultimately results in a profound loss of body fluid or hypovolemia. Deficiency of glucose within the cells produces further metabolic abnormalities, which result in accumulation of various acid end products within the body with a lowering of the pH of body fluids (metabolic acidosis).

This series of events produces, most importantly, a progressive deterioration in central nervous system function, ranging from early confusion to progressive depression of consciousness and, ultimately, coma. Administration of insulin and intravenous fluids will reverse this process.

Signs and symptoms of hyperglycemia (diabetic coma). Diabetic coma may occur in the diabetic patient who is not taking insulin at all, who is not taking a sufficient amount of insulin in relation to the amount of glucose ingested, or who is well treated but has an infection such as pneumonia. The metabolic abnormalities just described occur gradually, usually over a period of several days. Major signs and symptoms include air hunger manifested by heavy, labored respirations. Loss of body fluid (hypovolemia) produces decreased blood pressure. As hypovolemia becomes increasingly profound, the pulse rate increases, and ultimately the patient will have a weak, rapid pulse. The patient may be noted to have a sweet, fruity odor to the breath. Ultimately the patient becomes comatose, and death will ensue if medical intervention is not provided.

Emergency management. Definitive management of diabetic coma can be provided only at a medical care facility. As with any comatose patient, the first aider must initially attend to the patient's airway, providing respiratory and circulatory support if necessary. Immediate provision should be made to transport the patient to a hospital.

Treated diabetics frequently know a great deal about their disease. If a known diabetic is ill but still responsive enough to answer questions, he or she will often be able to tell you specifically what the problem is and what to do. If a known diabetic is ill, confused, but still able to take oral fluids, it is wise to provide that patient with some oral glucose such as a glass of orange juice. If the problem is low blood sugar (hypoglycemia), the patient will be substantially benefitted.

Hypoglycemia (insulin shock). Hypoglycemia will most frequently be encountered in the diabetic who has taken too much insulin in relation to the amount of glucose ingested. Although all cells require an adequate supply of glucose to function, the brain, in particular, cannot tolerate significant decreases in blood glucose. As the blood glucose level falls, the brain then becomes progressively affected, and death to brain tissue will occur if significant hypoglycemia persists.

Signs and symptoms of hypoglycemia. The signs and symptoms of hypoglycemia are the result both of the fall in blood glucose level and the efforts of the body to increase the blood glucose level. When hypoglycemia occurs, a substance called *epinephrine* is released into the blood. Epinephrine, in addition to other action, serves to increase blood glucose levels and is a part of the normal, everyday regulation of blood glucose. Patients may complain of being weak, fatigued, and tremulous (shaky). The first aider will observe sweating, tremulousness, a rapid heart rate, and, occasionally, nausea and vomiting. As the blood glucose level continues to fall, central nervous system function is affected. The patient first becomes confused, and, if untreated, progressive depression of central nervous function results ultimately in unconsciousness. Seizures may occur.

First aid care for hypoglycemia. As just noted, the first aider must recognize that prolonged hypoglycemia results in death of brain cells, and, therefore, immediate management is essential to prevent irreversible brain damage. In a patient who is conscious and able to swallow, management consists of immediate administration of oral glucose, such as sugar cubes, candy in any form, carbonated beverages, or fruit juices sweetened with additional sugar if available. In the unconscious patient, a cube of sugar or concentrated glucose can be placed under the tongue. Such administrations should be performed with great caution with attention to protection of the airway, and the patient should be transported to a medical facility immediately. Patients should also be searched for a Medic Alert emergency identification symbol, which may be found as a bracelet, necklace, or wallet card. Medic Alert tags may be used to identify any known medical problem (Fig. 13-1).

Cerebrovascular accidents (stroke)

A cerebrovascular accident (CVA), often referred to as a stroke, represents loss of function of a portion of brain as a result of impairment of the blood supply to that portion of brain tissue. Cerebrovascular accidents may result from occlusion of an artery supplying a portion of brain tissue or from rupture of a blood vessel, causing hemorrhage into brain tissue. Occlusion of an artery may be sec-

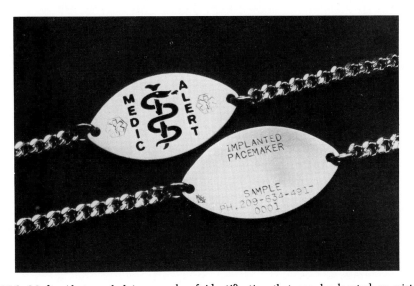

Fig. 13-1. Medic Alert symbol is example of identification that can be located on victim of injury or sudden illness to provide vital information for administering emergency care. Emergency medical identification may be provided in form of necklace, bracelet, or wallet card. Identification can alert first aider to health problems such as diabetes or epilepsy, blood type, allergies, frequently used medications, special conditions, or procedures to follow in case of medical emergency. (Courtesy Medic Alert Foundation International, Turlock, Calif.)

ondary to arteriosclerosis or from a clot arising from a more distant source. Regardless of the cause, the result of any cerebrovascular accident is a loss of brain tissue and, therefore, a loss of function. The specific function or functions lost depend on the area of brain involved.

The majority of cerebrovascular accidents occur in the elderly and are secondary to occlusion of a blood vessel. Hemorrhage may be the result of an aneurysm, which represents a weakened area in the arterial wall that ruptures either into the space surrounding the brain or into brain tissue. With hemorrhage, severe headache may precede the onset of neurological deficits. Hemorrhage from small vessels deep within the brain may occur in patients with long-standing hypertension. Again, the specific neurological deficits depend on the area of brain involved.

Signs and symptoms. The elderly patient who has suddenly lost blood supply to a portion of brain most often presents with the sudden onset of weakness (paresis) or paralysis (plegia) on one side of the body (hemiparesis or hemiplegia). The facial muscles may be involved as well as the arm and the leg on that side. The state of consciousness may vary from awake and alert to comatose. Patients may have difficulty in speaking and in swallowing. Difficulty in speaking may be due to paralysis of the facial muscles and involvement of the tongue, making it impossible for the patient to form various sounds. Difficulty in speaking may also be caused by the effect of the stroke on the portion of the brain that enables an individual to express himself. The patient may be unable to get the appropriate words out but can understand everything the examiner is saying. The area of the brain that receives and interprets messages may also be involved, in which case the patient will hear perfectly well but will be unable to comprehend what the examiner is saying. Keep in mind that with depression of consciousness, the gag reflex may be lost, and the patient may be unable to clear his own airway. Attention to the airway will, therefore, be exceedingly important. Patients not infrequently will lose bladder and bowel control. Convulsions may occur.

First aid care. Emergency management of victims of cerebrovascular accidents is identical to that described for any unconscious patient. In the case of conscious victims, particular attention to airway management is required, as well as continuous monitoring to detect any changes in the level of consciousness. Always keep in mind, as just noted, that although the patient is seemingly unaware of what is going on around him, he may, in fact, hear and comprehend everything. For this reason, be sure that you provide constant reassurance and say nothing that might create anxiety.

Seizures

Seizures or convulsions are the peripheral manifestations of an abnormal stimulus to the brain. Abnormal stimuli can occur as a result of such varied causes as traumatic injury to the brain, tumors, high fever in children, extreme anxiety, and epilepsy. Epilepsy is a chronic seizure disorder, usually of unknown origin. There are two main types of epilepsy. Petit-mal seizures usually present as brief, repetitive, automatic acts of behavior, such as lip smacking or staring. Grand-mal seizures may be focal (involving only a part of the body, such as an extremity) or generalized (involving the entire body). Patients with grand-mal seizures have loss of consciousness during the seizure and frequently will have bladder and/or bowel incontinence during the seizure, followed by a gradual period of awakening. Actual seizure activity usually lasts only for a few minutes.

Signs and symptoms. Epileptics with grand-mal seizures may have a premonition or aura immediately before the onset of the seizure. Some epileptics have learned to recognize this warning and are able to quickly prepare themselves for the imminent seizure. During a generalized, grand-mal seizure, the patient may bite or chew his tongue. There may be evidence of involuntary urination or defecation. During the seizure, the patient is always unresponsive. As the individual regains consciousness, there is a period of gradual recovery during which there may be confusion and lethargy, which gradually resolves.

Petit-mal seizures are usually of short duration. Seizure activity, such as lip smacking, staring into space for brief periods, interrupted speech, or minor convulsive movements of an extremity or the eyes may be observed. The patient seems to be perfectly normal before and after the seizure.

First aid care. Emergency management is primarily directed toward protecting the patient from causing himself injury during the seizure. If a padded bite block is available and can be placed between the teeth for protection against biting the tongue, it is recommended. If force is required to place the bite block, the effort should be abandoned. In most emergency situations, the first aider is not equipped with an appropriate bite block. Rather than risk possible damage from an inappropriate object, it is preferable not to attempt placing something between the teeth. Protect the patient's head at all times; a skull fracture is possible from striking the head on any hard surface. Do not forcibly restrain the seizure activity; movement should be guided and controlled to prevent injury.

Airway management *during* the seizure is difficult if not impossible to manage but is of considerable importance immediately after the seizure. If the patient has bitten his tongue, he may be bleeding into the oropharynx, in which case the patient should be placed on his side to prevent aspiration of blood. The patient should also be protected from curious onlookers.

A single seizure is not considered an emergency, although any person who has had a seizure should be seen by a physician. If seizure activity is continuous or if one attack follows the other in rapid succession, the patient should be taken immediately to the hospital.

Almost as important as the immediate care for seizures is a careful description of the seizure activity to the physician or persons providing continuing emergency care. If possible, the description should include whether the seizure activity was generalized or localized, how it started (in all extremities, simultaneously, or in one portion of the body spreading to involve the entire body), and the number and duration of the seizures.

Fainting (syncope)

Syncope is a sudden loss of consciousness of limited duration. Syncope may occur in certain individuals who have no evidence of any underlying disease. These individuals may, on occasion, react to stressful circumstances by fainting. Although the exact mechanisms are not totally understood, fainting may correlate with sudden wide spread dilatation of veins, which results in pooling of large amounts of blood no longer accessible to the effective circulation. There is an immediate reduction in blood volume and, therefore, a reduction in the amount of blood circulated to the brain, resulting in loss of consciousness.

Some individuals required to stand motionless for long periods of time may experience syncope as a result of pooling of blood in the legs. This is caused by both a loss of vascular tone in the legs and loss of the massaging effect of muscle activity on the veins, which is an important part of augmenting venous return from the lower extremities to the heart. The reduction in effective circulating blood volume will result in decreased perfusion of the brain and may result in syncope.

Signs and symptoms. Syncope in the otherwise healthy individuals may be preceded by dizziness, nausea, pallor, sweating, and pupillary dilatation. During the syncopal episode, the pulse will be noted to be somewhat weak and rapid. With appropriate management, these signs and symptoms will rapidly reverse.

First aid care. As just described, the basic problem in this form of syncope is a decreased circulating blood volume caused by an increase in pooling of blood in dilated peripheral vessels. Care will be directed toward increasing venous return, thereby increasing effective circulating blood volume. Since the lower extremities will contain blood that can be returned to the circulatory compartment, the patient will often treat himself, since almost invariably he or she will assume the recumbent position when syncope occurs. This will automatically augment venous return from the legs to the right heart, and the patient will begin to awaken. Management consists of placing the patient in a lying-down position and raising the legs to further augment venous return. If, for any reason, it is impossible to place the patient in a lying-down position, placing the head between the knees is an acceptable alternative, provided you guard against the patient falling forward.

Other causes of syncope. Syncope may be the result of significant underlying disease, the two most common causes being cardiac disease or cerebrovascular disease. Abnormalities in cardiac rhythm constitute the bulk of cardiac-related syncopal episodes. Patients may develop heart rates that are exceedingly slow or exceedingly fast. Either may result in a sudden dramatic fall in cardiac output, inadequate perfusion of the brain, and loss of consciousness. Since abnormalities in cardiac rhythm may be transient, the first aider can make a significant contribution to the diagnosis by carefully checking the pulse and noting both the rate and rhythm. If an individual who has fainted has a strong pulse, a normal heart rate, and dry warm skin (that is, evidence of adequate circulation), the first aider should suspect the possibility of a cerebrovascular accident. Briefly check the patient to ascertain whether or not one-sided weakness or paralysis is present. If any neurological abnormalities are noted, it is wise to keep the patient in the lying-down position but not to raise the legs.

Syncope may also be seen in patients who have a poorly functioning autonomic nervous system. One of the functions of the autonomic nervous system is to regulate blood pressure when the normal individual changes from the recumbent to the sitting or standing position. With autonomic nervous system disease, the individual who rapidly assumes the upright position may have a syncopal episode or feel like he or she is about to faint. By lying down and then assuming the upright position gradually, the patient can avoid the possibility of having a syncopal episode. When syncope does occur, these individuals rapidly regain consciousness on assuming the recumbent position.

It may be difficult in the individual patient to determine whether syncope is or is not the result of significant underlying disease. For this reason, the first aider should make the observations previously noted, provide immediate management, and always recommend that the individual seek medical attention.

Headache

Headache may result from a variety of causes, including tension, sinus congestion, hypertension, and brain tumors. Since headache may be secondary to a significant underlying disease, any individual with recurrent, severe, or prolonged headache should be evaluated by a physician. Tension is by far the most common cause of headache pain. A first aider might become alarmed at the patient who is having a migraine headache, since migraine may be accompanied by associated signs and symptoms that may lead one to think that something more serious is occurring. Tension headache and migraine headache are the two most common types of headache encountered.

Tension headache. Tension headache is generally linked to emotional stress and is associated with prolonged contraction of the muscles of the head and neck. Tension headache usually begins in the back of the head or the neck, but it may involve the entire head. Most commonly, it occurs toward the end of the day as a result of prolonged stress. The pain is usually constant; however, it may be throbbing. When a headache is severe, there may be some associated nausea. Aside from use of over-the-counter pain relievers such as aspirin, local heat and massage to the neck muscles, as well as rest and quiet in a darkened room, can be of considerable relief.

Migraine headache. The exact cause of migraine headache is unknown. In the majority of patients with migraine, a rather predictable series of events will occur. The initial phase of migraine occurs before the onset of the headache. There is evidence that this initial phase correlates with constriction of arteries supplying the brain. With this arterial constriction, blood flow is diminished to certain portions of the brain, which may produce symptoms such as the individual seeing spots before the eyes, being extremely sensitive to light, and, on occasion, a feeling of fatigue. After this initial phase, within a variable amount of time, the headache phase begins. Now the arteries that were previously constricted dilate, and a severe throbbing headache ensues, which is usually isolated to half of the head. The headache phase may be of variable duration.

There is decreased blood flow to certain portions of the brain. For this reason, in some patients with migraine, neurological deficits such as localized weakness or paralysis may occur. This may lead one to believe that a stroke is occurring. This preheadache phase is followed by the onset of headache, which is commonly associated with nausea and vomiting.

Many patients who have a long history of migraine know their disease well and have medications on hand to attempt to abort development of the headache phase. The first aider may assist the patient with migraine by assuring that he or she has access to a place to lie down where it is quiet and the lights are darkened. The patient may request that his or her medications be provided along with suitable fluid for ingestion of tablets. Since headache may be a symptom of significant underlying disease, the patient with severe, prolonged, or chronic headache should seek medical attention.

ACUTE ABDOMINAL EMERGENCIES

The term *acute abdomen* is used to describe any acute intraabdominal disorder not associated with trauma.

Abdominal organs may be classified into two general categories, hollow organs and solid organs. Hollow organs include the entire digestive tract, beginning with the esophagus as it enters the abdomen, the stomach, small intestine, and large intestine. The gallbladder is a hollow organ, and the great vessels (aorta and inferior vena cava) may also be classified as hollow organs. Solid organs include the liver, spleen, pancreas, kidneys, and adrenals. The peritoneum is a thin sheet of tissue that lines the inside of the abdominal wall and either completely or partially covers all the abdominal organs. The total surface area of the peritoneum is equal to the surface area of the skin, and it is richly supplied with nerves.

Disease processes in the abdomen

Pathological processes within the abdomen can be broken down into five general categories: inflammation, hemorrhage, perforation, obstruction, and ischemia (poor blood supply).

Inflammation. Although, on occasion, an inflammatory process in the abdomen can occur suddenly, more often the process occurs over at least several hours and, not infrequently, several days. Inflammation may involve either solid organs (for example, pyelonephritis, an inflammatory disease of the kidneys) or hollow organs (for example, cholecystitis, an inflammatory disease of the gallbladder). The specific symptoms vary, depending on the organ involved, and, therefore, discussion would be beyond the scope of this section. As a general principle, inflammation of an abdominal organ is accompanied by fever, often associated with chills, and may initially be accompanied by pain located near the area of the organ involved. If the peritoneum becomes involved in the inflammatory process, generalized peritonitis (inflammation of the peritoneum) and, therefore, generalized abdominal pain may result.

Hemorrhage. Hemorrhage within the abdomen may result from a variety of causes, including erosion of an ulcer into an artery or rupture of an abdominal aortic aneurysm (a weak spot in the wall of the aorta). Hemorrhage may be sudden and massive, or it may occur over a longer period of time. If homorrhage occurs into the gastrointestinal (GI) tract, the patient may give a history of vomiting or may be observed to vomit blood, appearing either bright red or like coffee grounds, or the patient may have a history of passing either bright red or black, tarry stools. If blood loss has been significant, signs and symptoms of hypovolemic shock may be noted.

Perforation. Hollow abdominal organs may be perforated. In the absence of trauma, the most common cause of perforation of a hollow abdominal organ would be ulcer disease, usually in the stomach or the first part of the small intestine. Perforation anywhere in the gastrointestinal tract will result in spilling of the contents of the gastrointestinal tract into the peritoneal cavity, leading to peritonitis. Pain may be initially localized, becoming generalized with development of diffuse peritonitis. Although fever and chills may be present, with perforation, pain will precede the onset of signs and symptoms of inflammation.

Obstruction. Hollow abdominal organs may become obstructed for a variety of reasons, ranging from impaction of fecal material to a constricting tumor. Gastrointestinal tract obstruction may be either of slow or rapid onset. Pain is a prominent symptom, which early in the course of obstruction may be intermittent or crampy progressing to a steady, intense pain. Nausea and vomiting may occur. Fever will usually not be present.

Ischemia (poor blood supply). Whenever a blood vessel becomes significantly obstructed, the tissue supplied by that vessel becomes ischemic. Obstruction may be the result of an atherosclerotic plaque, an embolus, or a combination thereof. Blood vessels supplying abdominal organs may become obstructed, resutling in ischemia to the organ or portion of organ involved. Most commonly, in the abdomen, a portion of bowel will become ischemic. When this occurs, the onset of symptoms is usually rapid, and the predominant symptom is pain. Fever may be present later in the stage of the disease process when inflammation complicates the picture.

Signs and symptoms

All the signs and symptoms associated with various disease processes occurring within the abdomen have been discussed in the previous paragraphs. The signs and symptoms of specific disease processes are beyond the scope of this section. In general, pain is a major manifestation of acute intraabdominal disease. This may initially be localized, becoming generalized when the peritoneum becomes involved in the process. With peritonitis, the abdomen may be exquisitely tender to touch. When peritonitis occurs, there is a loss of fluid into the abdominal cavity. This fluid loss may result in hypovolemic shock. The onset of shock is generally over a much longer period of time than would be seen with hypovolemic shock secondary to hemorrhage.

Peritonitis is also associated with paralysis of the normal peristaltic movement of the intestine. This will result in distention of the intestine with gases and markedly distended abdomen. This picture can also be seen in long-standing intestinal obstruction. With peritonitis, the patient, to relieve tension on the peritoneum, may be seen to draw the legs up or may prefer a position lying on his or her side and curled up. Lowering the legs may cause marked intensification of the pain.

In summary, the general symptoms and signs of an acute abdomen may include either singly or in combination any of the following: (1) local or diffuse abdominal pain, which may be crampy or steady; (2) abdominal tenderness; (3) vomiting; (4) hematemesis (vomiting of blood), which may appear as bright red or coffee-ground material; (5) black, tarry stool or bright red blood in the stool; (6) abdominal distention; (7) abdominal rigidity; or (8) signs and symptoms of hypovolemic shock.

Emergency care and first aid

The acute abdomen most often requires surgical therapy, although some acute abdominal processes may be treated medically. In either case, immediate care by a physician is mandatory; this is a medical emergency. Care rendered by the first aider should be generally supportive in nature. Never give the patient with signs and symptoms of an acute abdomen anything to eat or drink, recognize the possibility of vomiting if it has not already occurred, and maintain the patient in a position where the airway can be rapidly cleared.

MOTION SICKNESS

Motion sickness may range from a mild sensation of nausea, encountered in an individual who has been riding for a long time in any standard method of conveyance, to a feeling of extreme ill-being and even impending doom, especially to the individual who is being subjected to an unfamiliar kind of motion, such as an initial bumpy airplane ride or the first time on a roller coaster.

The patient may be somewhat drowsy and is frequently dizzy. If symptoms are more intense, there may be pallor, cool, clammy skin, and a rapid heart rate.

Care consists primarily of isolating the individual from unpleasant stimuli and providing plenty of fresh air and reassurance. Fixing the eyes on a given spot may facilitate relief of dizziness and nausea. Individuals who have knowledge of their susceptibility to motion sickness and who are about to travel should consult their physician, since medication may be provided to prevent these episodes.

FIRST AIDER COMPETENCIES

After studying the material presented in this chapter, the student should be able to:

- Describe the methods of assessing levels of consciousness.
- Describe the methods of determining presence or absence of weakness or paralysis.
- Explain the significance of determining differences in pupillary size and response to light stimulus.
- Describe the general first aid care for an unconscious victim.
- Describe the difference between diabetic coma and hypoglycemia as well as the difference in first aid care.
- Describe the first aid care for grand-mal seizures.
- Define syncope and its first aid care.
- Explain the difference between migraine and tension headache and the first aid care for both.
- Define *acute abdomen.*
- List the five general categories of pathological disease processes in the abdomen.
- Define *peritonitis.*
- List the eight general symptoms and signs of the acute abdomen.
- Describe the emergency care and first aid for a victim with a suspected acute abdomen.
- Describe the first aid care for motion sickness.

REFERENCES AND RECOMMENDED READINGS

1. Cole, W. H., and Puestow, C. B.: First aid: diagnosis and management, ed. 6, New York, 1965, Appleton-Century-Crofts.
2. Emergency care and transportation of the sick and injured, Chicago, 1971, American Academy of Orthopaedic Surgeons.
3. Henderson, J.: Emergency medical guide, ed. 2, New York, 1969, McGraw-Hill Book Co.
4. Lombroso, C. T.: The treatment of status epilepticus, Pediatrics 53:536-540, 1970.
5. Miller, R. H., and Cantrell, J. R., editors: Textbook of basic emergency medicine, St. Louis, 1975, The C. V. Mosby Co.
6. Solomon, G. E., and Plum, F.: Clinical management of seizures, Philadelphia, 1967, W. B. Saunders Co.
7. The wonderful human machine, Chicago, 1976, American Medical Association.

14

HEAT-RELATED ILLNESSES AND
EMERGENCIES

J. Maurice Mahan

The human body is a complex integration of systems that constantly strives to maintain a state of homeostasis. The heat regulation system of the body is sensitive and occasionally gets sufficiently out of balance to cause great discomfort and create medical emergencies.

Each year over 4000 people die from heat injuries in the United States,[7] with thousands more suffering the less serious effects of such injuries. Heat injuries can be serious, and a good knowledge of the mechanisms, signs and symptoms, and emergency care procedures is important to prevention as well as intervention.

PHYSIOLOGICAL PROCESSES

As a warm-blooded mammal, man has to adjust his heat production and loss in an effort to keep a constant body temperature of approximately 37° C (98.6° F). The body temperature, as measured rectally or orally, does not fluctuate much. The deep-body temperature remains relatively stable while skin and tissues just below the skin may vary greatly. The temperature of this outer shell is usually about 32° C (90° F). The temperatures of tissues between the internal organs and the outer shell gradually increase the further they are from the surface. The temperature of the outer shell also varies, with the head being the warmest and gradually decreasing in the trunk, hands, and feet.

Heat production

Heat is built up in the body through the internal process of oxidation of food and through external processes of absorbing heat from the environment (Fig. 14-1).

Internal production. Heat is produced within the body through the conversion of food to energy by the process of oxidation. When the food is burned, it uses oxygen and gives off carbon dioxide and heat. The heat production of most of the organs such as liver, kidney, spleen, heart, and brain is relatively constant. The heat production of the muscles can vary greatly. At rest the muscles produce little heat, but under conditions of increased exercise they produce great amounts of heat.

As an example of this, a 160-pound person working at a metabolic rate of 2 liters of oxygen a minute will produce about 7.5 kcal of excess heat a minute. (One kilocalorie [kcal] is the amount of heat required to raise the temperature of 1 kg [2.205 pounds] of water 1° C [1.8° F].) This would cause the body's temperature to rise 0.2° C (0.36° F) in 1 minute. After 10 minutes this could result in raising the body temperature from 37° to 38.9° C (98.6° to 102° F) if the body did not lose any heat.

Gaining heat from the environment. Heat can also be gained from the environment through the processes of radiation, convection, and conduction. A basic principle of physics is that heat will move from areas of high temperature to those of lower temperature. Therefore, if the temperature of the environment is higher than that of the human body, then heat will move to the body.

The body absorbs heat directly from the radiated heat of the sun or other heat source such as fire. A person exposed to bright sunlight will gain an average of 150 kcal of heat an hour. If the body did not lose any heat, this could result in raising the body temperature of a 160-pound person approximately 15.6° C (60° F) or more in an hour. The body also absorbs radiated heat from the reflection from surfaces such as water, rocks, buildings, and roofs. The ef-

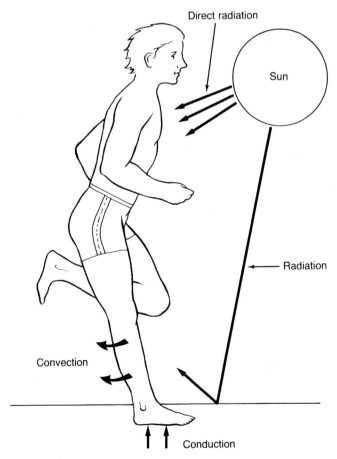

Fig. 14-1. Heat gain from environment.

fects of radiated heat are minimized by finding protection in reflective clothing or shade.

The body can absorb heat from a moving liquid or gases such as water and air through the process of convection. If the skin temperature and the air or water temperature are approximately the same, then no heat will be gained by the body. When the air temperature becomes five or six degrees warmer or the body is moving through this air, as on a motorcycle or in an open car, the effect of convection is minimized in heat gain.

Transmission of heat through solids or liquids that are not moving is produced by conduction. This is not usually a significant source of heat gain unless heavy clothing is worn close to the body.

Body heat produced internally through production of energy and/or absorbed from the external environment can significantly increase the temperature of the body. If this heat significantly raises the temperature throughout the body, it can result in serious damage to tissues and possibly death. Fortunately the body also has mechanisms that work to remove excess heat and keep the body temperature within a safe range.

Heat loss

Heat is removed from the body by the processes of radiation, convection, conduction, and evaporation (Fig. 14-2).

Radiation. The amount of heat lost by radiation depends on the amount of

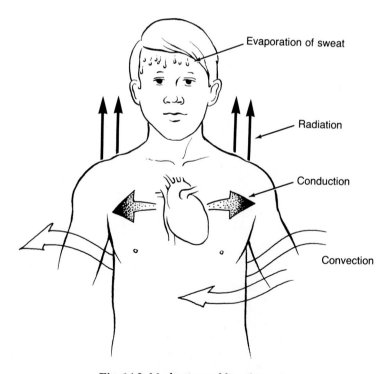

Fig. 14-2. Mechanisms of heat loss.

skin surface exposed and the differences in temperature between the skin and surrounding objects. Persons at rest in a moderate climate will lose about 60% of their body heat by radiation from the skin. As the person increases the rate of work, the amount of heat radiated will remain about the same or slightly decrease, but the total percentage lost by radiation will decrease significantly. The temperature of the air must be at least five or six degrees below the skin's temperature for loss by radiation to occur.

Convection. The blood, utilizing the process of convection, brings heat from the deep body tissues to the surface of the skin. This is similar to the process used in an automobile engine in which water is used to transfer excess heat from the engine block to the radiator, where it can be released into the atmosphere. The blood is not as efficient as the water in the automobile, since it also must transport food and waste products. In a warm environment, an increased rate of work is accompanied by a need for increased heat loss, and this is accomplished by a dilation of the blood vessels in the skin to provide more surface area for heat loss and by the increased blood flow. Unfortunately, the blood may reach its maximum capacity for transferring heat before it reaches its maximum capacity for transporting nutrients to the body tissues. Therefore the body can continue to increase its work rate and heat production with a resulting rise in body temperature. If the physical activity of the body is to continue, the work rate must be decreased to the point at which the blood can remove the heat produced through the process of conduction.

Conduction. Conduction occurs in the body when heat moves from tissues or liquids that are not moving to tissues or nonmoving liquids that are at a lower temperature. Under normal conditions conduction is a minor factor in heat loss in the body.

Under normal conditions most heat loss occurs through the processes of radiation, convection, and conduction. It is important to remember that heat passes from areas of high temperature to areas of lower temperature.

If the temperature of the surrounding environment, air and objects, is equal to or greater than that of the skin, then no heat may be lost from the body by these processes, and, in fact, the body will gain heat.

Environmental temperatures above about 32° or 33° C (90° or 92° F) cause a two-part problem for the body. The high temperatures may interfere with heat loss from the body, and, second, the high temperatures add additional heat to the body, which already is having trouble losing heat.

Evaporation of sweat. A fourth important means of heat loss is through evaporation of sweat. The amount of heat lost is directly dependent on the changing of sweat (water) to a vapor. During periods of increased work rates or high temperatures, evaporation of sweat is the most important means of heat loss, since the other three means are not able to adequately handle the removal of the necessary amounts of heat. In fact, most heat loss in these conditions is accomplished by evaporation of sweat.

The body has over 2 million sweat glands, which are distributed all over the body and are utilized in sweating as needed. By evaporation of this water (sweat) the skin is cooled and so in turn is the blood in the skin, which brings the heat from the deep body tissue. The cooling effect occurs because it takes heat to change the water to a vapor, and, as a result, heat is removed from the skin to accomplish the process. As the skin becomes cooler, the transmission of heat from the skin becomes possible, and the cooler blood when it returns from the skin to the deep body makes it possible to absorb more heat and transport it to the surface.

In understanding this mechanism it should be noted that although the temperature within the body is usually about 37° C (98.6° F) and rarely varies more than about 1° to 1.6° C (2° or 3° F), the temperature of the skin is usually about 32.2° C (90° F) and may vary as much as about 11° C (20° F). For heat loss to continue to occur, the temperature of the skin must be at least 1° C (2° F) below that of the temperature within the body. If the skin temperature rises above this point, heat exchange from the body to the environment stops, and the body temperature may rise to extremes. The skin in this case becomes a layer of insulation that works to keep the heat in.

Sweat production starts between 5 and 40 minutes after the conditions of high heat are entered, although it can begin immediately if the conditions are extreme. The rate of sweating gradually increases over a period of about ½ to 1 hour. Subsequent to this period, it maintains the same level for a time and then declines. Sweating usually starts when the skin temperature reaches about 34.4° C (94° F), but if the internal body temperature is extremely high, sweating may occur at a lower skin temperature.

Sweating is important because of its evaporation, which cools the body. Sweat that runs off the body or is wiped off is of no use in effecting heat loss. It has no cooling function unless it evaporates.

Dehydration

Even though evaporation of sweat is an important means for removing excess heat from the body, it also has some costs to the body. The sweating, which decreases the total volume of water in the body unless it is replaced, can result in dehydration. Dehydration is dangerous for two reasons. First, it makes sweating difficult or impossible because of the lack of available water for sweating, and, therefore, no evaporative cooling can occur. This results in a further increase of body heat. Dehydration also decreases the total blood volume. The decreased supply of blood has to carry the same or increased amounts of oxygen and heat, putting an extra burden on the cardiac and respiratory systems. Decrease in circulation can result in difficult breathing, nausea, muscle restriction, and increasing body temperatures.

A person walking at a rate of 3 or 4 mph in 38° C (100° F) heat can lose a liter (a quart, or about 2 pounds) of water an hour. The accumulative effects of this, without water replacement, can be serious. If a person loses as little as 5% or 6% of his total body weight by dehydration, it may become difficult to continue activities. If the dehydration increases to 10% or 12%, then the body is unable to continue to carry on many of its normal activities such as heat loss. The body temperature may increase tremendously, and severe tissue damage or death may result. Persons working and/or playing strenuously in warm temperatures must have water available to them at all times to avoid dehydration and its complications.

Salt depletion

Profuse sweating in warm environments also may, in some instances, result in a depletion of salt (sodium chloride), particularly in the individual who is not acclimatized. Decrease in salt may result in muscle cramps. Ordinarily this loss of salt by sweating may be replaced by the ordinary use of table salt with meals, and after the first day or so of acclimatization, it is not necessary to give any supplemental salt if the person is eating regular meals with salt. The percentage of loss by sweating will significantly decrease as the person becomes acclimatized.

Environmental risks

The nature of environmental risks should be especially considered with heat injuries. Environmental risks are not limited to hot tropical or desert climates. They exist in factories, shops, gymnasiums, playgrounds, cities, mines, and anyplace else where high temperature, humidity, and increased exercise rates exist.

Heat. When the environmental temperature is sufficiently high, the rate of work must be decreased to the point at which the resulting body heat can be eliminated adequately, otherwise the body will try to protect itself by forcing all activity to cease. Heat from the environment causes a dual burden because it interferes with body heat loss and may also add more heat to the body.

The movement of air around a body will work to increase the rate of heat transfer. If the air is cooler than the body, then heat loss can be facilitated by the air circulation. If the air temperature is above that of the body, then the use of fans is not advisable, since it will increase the rate of heat transfer from the environment to the person.

Humidity. Humidity also presents an increased burden because if the environment is warmer than the body, heat cannot be lost by evaporation, convection, or radiation, and therefore evaporation by sweating must occur. The rate of sweating is limited by the amount of water vapor already in the air. If the relative humidity of the air is high, the rate of evaporation of sweat is restricted, and sweating does not provide enough cooling.

TYPES OF EMERGENCIES
Heat cramps

Heat cramps will occur with sweating and low salt replacement. High environmental temperature is not a necessary precursor to this condition.

Signs and symptoms. Heat cramps are usually identified by a painful muscle spasm of the arms and legs in persons who otherwise seem to be in good physical condition. These cramps are normally the only manifestations of this condition. If any other signs and symptoms exist besides simple muscle cramps, then the problem automatically becomes classified as heat exhaustion and should be treated as such.

First aid procedures. Heat cramps are not life threatening; however, they can be painful and incapacitating. The patient should be given dilute salt and water solutions (a tablespoon of table salt to a quart of water). This is the only effective treatment for this condition. Ice may be applied to the cramped muscle to provide relief from the pain. This is often done with wrestlers. The muscles will cramp again unless water and salt are replaced.

Follow-up care. The person should continue to drink plenty of water over the next 24 hours to ensure replacement of water. Increased salt intake by tablets is not usually necessary. The person should be allowed to eat at normal meal times, and the salt used on the food should be enough to keep the salt level up. The person should continue to have cold water available during the day on demand. Water rationing should not be observed. If the person is going to continue in this strenuous activity in a hot climate, a program of physical conditioning should be instituted to prevent future occurrences.

Heat exhaustion

Heat exhaustion is the most common of the heat-related injuries and is most likely to occur during heat waves. This condition will also occur in situations of heavy muscular work in warm to hot temperatures.

Heat exhaustion may be caused by dehydration, salt depletion, or both. A normal person engaged in strenuous work or play in a warm to hot environment will sweat extensively to ensure heat loss. This sweating will often lead to water depletion equal to 1%, 2%, or even 3% of the total body weight. It is difficult to replace this much water, since the person's thirst will be quenched long before the water loss is replaced. If this condition continues over a day or more, the person will become dehydrated without knowing it.

Soldiers, athletes, and workers in hot climates, as well as infants and incapacitated adults who cannot express their need for water, may become dehydrated through this process and still be able to maintain adequate levels of salt through ingestion with regular meals. Heat loss may also occur in persons who sweat profusely but replace their water loss, but have a reduced intake of salt that does not make up for the salt lost in sweating. Occasionally persons will have both salt and water depletion because of inadequate replacement of both elements.

Even though heat exhaustion may occur from any of the causes just mentioned, its signs and symptoms will be similar, and emergency treatment should be the same for both causes, since it will be difficult for the first aider to determine the actual cause.

Signs and symptoms. Heat exhaustion is sometimes difficult to determine. The vital signs may be normal, and, in fact, the temperature is usually normal and may even be subnormal. The following should be looked for in determining if the victim is suffering from heat exhaustion:

1. The victim may experience progressive weakness, inability to work, and loss of appetite.
2. The skin is usually moist and clammy.
3. The pupils may be dilated.
4. The skin will be pale or ashen gray.
5. Temperature will usually be normal or subnormal.
6. The patient will usually be conscious; however, it is not uncommon for fainting to occur.
7. Pulse may be slightly more rapid than normal, less than 100, and weak.
8. The patient may be suffering from heat cramps.

First aid procedures. Heat exhaustion is an emergency but not usually life threatening. The correct first aid procedure is to make the patient lie in the coolest available place and to give the patient cold drinks. (The drinks should be chilled or cold to encourage the person to drink as much as possible. Warm drinks are not easily tolerated by most victims, and it is therefore difficult for them to drink enough water to be rehydrated.) Rest to decrease work rate and heat output and water replacement are the proper first aid procedures for heat exhaustion.

Follow-up procedures. The person should be taken to a hospital in case there may be other complications. Additionally, when the person returns to the same work or play conditions when the temperatures are high, adequate amounts of cool water should be available for drinking.

Heat stroke

Heat stroke is most common in tropical or semitropical climates, during heat waves almost anyplace, in hot factories, and on hot, humid athletic fields. The symptoms are caused by high body temperature, salt loss, and dehydration. The body's mechanisms for dissipating heat have *stopped working*, and a tremendous increase in body temperature will occur rapidly. *Heat stroke is a medical emergency and should be treated as a life-threatening situation!*

Heat stroke and heat exhaustion are sometimes confused, and this could result in diasastrous consequences if appropriate action is not taken. Table 2 compares the signs and symptoms of these two heat injuries.

Signs and symptoms. The signs and symptoms of heat stroke are different from those of heat exhaustion, and one should make special effort to memorize the differences. The signs and symptoms of a heat stroke are as follows:

1. Often the victim may be dizzy, weak, mentally confused, euphoric, or have a sense of impending doom before becoming unconscious.
2. The person may become unconscious, and this may occur with little warning.
3. The patient will have an exceedingly high temperature. The skin will feel hot to the touch. Rectally the temperature will be above 40.6° C (105° F) and may range as high as 42.8° C (109° F).
4. The person's skin will be extremely dry because of the stoppage of the sweating mechanisms. Even the armpits will be dry. Sweating often stops shortly before the onset of heat stroke and is usually, but not always, absent later.
5. The skin will appear flushed.
6. The pulse rate will be strong and rapid.

Table 2. Comparison of signs and symptoms for heat exhaustion and heat stroke

	Heat exhaustion	Heat stroke
Face	Pale	Red and flushed
Skin	Moist	Hot and dry
Sweating	Profuse	None
Temperature	Normal	Extremely high
Pulse	Weak and rapid	Strong and rapid
Unconscious	Not usually	Usually

First aid procedures. Since heat stroke is caused by the body's acute inability to lose heat rapidly enough, steps must be taken immediately.

1. Make immediate arrangements to have the patient transported to the nearest medical facility. The serious nature of this injury requires quick and definitive medical attention, which the first aider cannot provide. Severe neurological, circulatory, and hepatic complications may occur. Until the patient arrives at the medical facility, the first aider should do the following to preserve life.
2. All clothing should be removed and the patient placed in the coolest available place.
3. Cool the patient's body by any means possible. The most effective method for doing this is by placing the patient in an ice bath to lower the whole body temperature. Since one might not have an ice bath available, improvise anything that would help lower the body temperature: cold water, chemical cooling packs, ice from an ice chest rubbed vigorously all over the body, etc.
4. If the patient can cooperate, also give him or her *cold* drinks to aid in heat loss.

PREVENTION OF DEHYDRATION AND HEAT ILLNESS EMERGENCIES

Unlike many medical emergencies, heat-related illnesses and injuries can be avoided by relatively simple and effective means.

Reducing environmental risks. Environmental risks related to heat and humidity can be minimized by wearing appropriate clothing to allow the mechanisms of heat loss to work and to also avoid the absorption of heat by heavy, close-knit fabrics, reducing work loads (especially until the person becomes acclimatized), providing protection from the heat by shields or shade, and, when appropriate, providing circulation of air to facilitate the transfer of heat from the body to the environment.

Fluid intake. All individuals working or playing hard in high temperatures should have plenty of water, preferably cool water, to drink whenever they are thirsty. If a person is not allowed to drink whenever thirsty, then he should be replacing fluids at an adequate rate to avoid dehydration.

It is not unusual for an individual to lose 3% of the body's weight from sweating. This is about the maximum acceptable for the average adult. With weight losses above that level the individual may be on the verge of heat exhaustion or heat stroke, depending on the severity of the water depletion. It is important that persons working as well as at rest avoid dehydration and subsequent heat injuries.

Use of salt. Replacement of salt is especially important in the first few days of working in a hot environment. This can best be accomplished by the use of salt with normal meals. However, it is advisable to check to make certain the individual is eating adequate meals to replace the salt.

Acclimatization and physical conditioning. Athletes, weekend sports enthusiasts, vacationers moving from a cold climate to a warm one, industrial workers, agricultural workers, construction workers, and others who are not properly acclimated to increased temperatures and are not in appropriate physical condition are prime candidates for a heat-related injury. There should be scheduled breaks for rest and drinking of water, and, if necessary, the hours of work or hard play should be decreased for these persons. If a company moves a group of workers from a cool climate to a warm or hot one, it may be necessary to cut the work day to 4 or 6 hours for the first week or two to avoid serious problems with heat injuries.

Acclimatization is not just a psychological adjustment, it is also a physical one that results in lower skin and rectal temperatures, lower heart rate, and an increased rate of sweating with a decrease of salt intake during strenuous work or play. Acclimatization is a fairly rapid process, which usually takes from 4 to 7 days.

Physical conditioning is also important because one cannot become acclimatized to heat without working or playing strenuously in the heat. Athletes, sports enthusiasts, workers, and others should engage in moderately strenuous work at first then gradually increase this until full acclimatization is reached. It should be noted that people acclimatize to the temperature they work in and are less acclimatized to temperatures above that point. Even an athlete or worker who is in excellent physical condition at an average environmental temperature of 21° C (70° F) may suffer a heat-related emergency when exposed to playing or working at an average environmental temperature of 32° C (90° F).

SUMMARY

Heat illnesses and injuries can provide a serious threat to those who engage in strenuous physical activity in warm temperatures. For this reason it is necessary that the first aider understand the physiological processes and environmental factors associated with heat production and loss so as to be able to prevent heat illnesses and injuries. Once a person has experienced heat illness or injury, it is imperative that the first aider be able to differentiate between heat cramps, heat exhaustion, and heat stroke and take appropriate action. It is of the utmost importance to know the difference between heat exhaustion and heat stroke and to react to heat stroke as a serious medical emergency.

Through a thorough understanding of the factors relating to heat illnesses and injuries the first aider should be able to help prevent them as well as take correct and effective action when necessary.

FIRST AIDER COMPETENCIES

After studying the material presented in this chapter, the student should be able to:
- Describe how the human body gains heat from the environment.
- Describe the mechanisms of heat loss from the human body.
- Relate the effects of environmental conditions and physical activity to the production and loss of body heat.
- List the environmental conditions that will inhibit loss of body heat.
- List the signs and symptoms of heat cramps and the appropriate first aid procedures.
- List the signs and symptoms of heat exhaustion and the appropriate first aid procedures.

- List the signs and symptoms of heat stroke and the appropriate procedures for the first aider to follow.
- Differentiate between heat exhaustion and heat stroke.

REFERENCES AND RECOMMENDED READINGS

1. Clowes, G. H. A., and O'Donnel, T. F.: Current concepts—heat stroke, New England Journal of Medicine **291**:564-567, 1974.
2. Flemming, A. J., D'Alonzo, C. A., and Zapp, J. A.: Modern occupational medicine, Philadelphia, 1960, Lea & Febiger.
3. Gold, J.: Development of heat pyrexia, Journal of the American Medical Association **173**:1175-1182, 1960.
4. Knochel, J. P.: Environmental heat illness, Archives of Internal Medicine **133**:841-864, 1974.
5. Leitheard, C. S., and Lind, A. R.: Heat stress and heat disorder, Philadelphia, 1964, F. A. Davis Co.
6. Malamud, N., Haymaher, W., and Custer, R. P.: Heat stroke: a clinicopathologic study of 125 fatal cases, Military Surgery **99**:397-449, 1946.
7. Schuman, S. H.: Patterns of heat-wave deaths and implications for prevention: data from New York and St. Louis during July, 1966, Environmental Research **5**:59-75, 1972.
8. Shibolet, S.: Heat stroke: its clinical picture and mechanisms in 36 cases, Quarterly Journal of Medicine **36**:525-548, 1967.
9. Stonehill, R. B., and Keil, P. G.: Successful preventive medical measures against heat illness at Lackland Air Force Base, American Journal of Public Health **51**:586-590, 1971.

15

PSYCHOLOGICAL EMERGENCIES

Rosemary K. McKevitt

When under severe stress, people may exhibit unusual, dysfunctional, or even bizarre behavior. A first aider may intervene to lessen the severe discomfort generated by stress and help affected persons cope in more constructive ways.

Often a sudden emergency situation, such as an auto accident or fire, generates temporary psychological stress to which those involved react in various ways. On other occasions, an individual may react to prolonged psychological stress with unusual behavior that, in itself, can constitute an emergency situation. An example would be a suicide threat or grossly inappropriate or bizarre behavior that presents a danger to the patient or others. In any one of these emergency situations, an individual's actions may appear incomprehensible to those who wish to be of help to the affected person. This chapter is designed to aid readers in understanding some of the behaviors that might be problematic in a psychological emergency and to suggest ways to help.

As people develop from childhood to maturity, they require fulfillment of basic human needs related to biological sustenance and the emotional and social needs of security, love, belongingness, and the fulfillment of potential. Externally or internally generated stress may interfere with gratification of these needs and create psychological disequilibrium within the individual. People respond to stress in a variety of ways, some inborn, some learned. Throughout a lifetime, an individual develops a repertoire of coping mechanisms and strategies to help maintain and reestablish psychological equilibrium. In emergency situations, anxiety increases markedly. Coping mechanisms that usually work for the individual are temporarily ineffective in decreasing anxiety.

Psychological emergencies result from either acute or chronic psychological disequilibrium in a patient. Four varieties of psychological emergency situations will be considered:

1. Emergency situations in which the patient perceives a threat of bodily injury
2. Emergency situations in which the patient sustains a loss of a significant person
3. Suicide threats or attempts
4. Emergency situations in which the patient is demonstrating psychotic behavior

197

Generally, the nature of the psychological emergency is evident on the basis of what first aiders observe or what others tell them has happened. Knowledge of the precipitating event is particularly helpful in psychological emergencies, since patients' behaviors in different emergency situations may appear somewhat similar. It is also important to keep in mind other reasons for unusual or confused behavior in an individual, such as drug reactions, head injuries, stroke, diabetes, epilepsy, and many other medical conditions.

THE PATIENT PERCEIVING THREAT OF BODILY INJURY

In time of an emergency, human coping mechanisms are often taxed to the limit. Major stress occurs suddenly, and individuals perceive themselves to be in acute physical danger. Severe psychological disequilibrium results from this threat to body integrity and basic security. Those involved may see physical evidence of the threat around them, the flames of a fire, for example, or the high winds and rain of a hurricane. Even after the actual threat has passed, the psychological disequilibrium may persist as they view the aftermath: a wrecked automobile, debris from an explosion, or injured people around them. All of these serve to emphasize the severity of the threat and to evoke fear and anxiety. On some occasions, those individuals experiencing acute psychological disequilibrium may also have sustained major or minor physical trauma, which further emphasizes their own vulnerability.

It is important for the person administering first aid to understand that the psychological disequilibrium accompanying an emergency situation may make a patient less aware of physical injuries. Sometimes patients' acute anxiety and fear of death cause them to deny the seriousness of their conditions. For this reason, direct efforts must be made to identify and care for the patient with previously undetected trauma. The confidence of the helping person and the initiation of competent first aid measures generally decrease patients' anxiety and foster their acceptance of the need for care.

What patients do and say generally indicates the degree of their psychological disequilibrium. Requesting the name of the individual and asking for a brief description of what has happened will elicit sufficient information to allow an immediate assessment of functioning. The observation of the patient's nonverbal as well as verbal behavior will generally indicate the severity of psychological disequilibrium.

Signs and symptoms

Mild disequilibrium. Mild disequilibrium is generally characterized by the increased alertness and attentiveness of the individual. The person is able to focus on the emergency situation and generally talks freely and extensively about it. Restlessness, talkativeness, repetitive questioning, eagerness to help, and, on occasion, joking are signs of mild psychological disequilibrium. One may frequently observe this minor disequilibrium among bystanders viewing an auto accident. They are generally eager to describe the accident from their perspectives and question each other about details of the event. Intervention to help people experiencing mild disequilibrium is usually unnecessary. Unless the incident is personally traumatic in some way, the sharing of experience among those involved is generally sufficient for the expression of feelings and the mobilization of usual coping strategies. If the questions or talkativeness of someone experiencing mild psychological disequilibrium interferes with ongoing emergency care, redirection of these individuals into other activities is usually effective.

Moderate psychological disequilibrium. Patients experiencing moderate psychological disequilibrium tend to manifest fight or flight behaviors. One individual may act inappropriately aggressive, arguing loudly and threatening to strike someone; another may run from one activity to another, giving orders and directions but not staying to see if anyone is carrying them out; a third may withdraw, sit passively, and become less responsive. Moderate psychological disequilibrium is often accompanied by physiological reactions. Patients generally have increased pulse and respiration rates and may experience increased perspiration, trembling, crying, nausea, vomiting, and possibly fainting. They usually have a short attention span and find it difficult to concentrate. Perception is narrowed, and the patient tends to focus on only selected aspects of what has occurred or what is currently taking place in the immediate environment. This selective inattention may also cause the person to misperceive and fail to comprehend what others are saying. This is of particular significance if the person is attempting to follow directions, aid others, or perform unfamiliar tasks.

Severe psychological disequilibrium. A person experiencing severe psychological disequilibrium may manifest some of these same behaviors. Generally, however, behavior appears even more extreme. The individual may exhibit severe agitation, pacing constantly, unable to remain in one place. Conversely, the withdrawn patient may appear almost unreachable, sitting silent and seemingly apathetic or huddled in fear. Verbally and nonverbally, the patient's behavior indicates confusion and disorganization. Communication may be disjointed and difficult to understand, or the person may repeat phrases or sentences over and over again. Perception is even more restricted, and little of what others say to the affected person may be understood.

Panic. At its most severe, temporary psychological disequilibrium becomes panic in which the affected individual is overwhelmed by the fear and anxiety generated by the threatening situation. The individual in panic has lost the ability to control behavior. He or she may remain motionless as though frozen, cry uncontrollably, or flee irrationally from the perceived danger.

First aid

It is of prime importance that those rendering emergency care understand that the unusual behaviors evidenced in an emergency situation are the result of psychological disequilibrium rather than overdramatization or intentional uncooperativeness on the part of the patient. Reactions in a crisis are determined by past experience and a lifetime of coping successfully and unsuccessfully with stress. They cannot be wholly predicted for any one individual in a given emergency situation. A nonjudgmental attitude is essential in establishing a helping relationship with a patient who is experiencing the discomfort and pain of a psychological emergency.

A calm, confident approach is most helpful to patients experiencing moderate or severe psychological disequilibrium. Encouraging patients to describe stressful events in their own words and to express the related feelings will generally help them to come to terms with what has happened. Talking and crying are two of the most effective ways of alleviating the discomfort that patients experience. Overactive patients may be given a simple task to perform to help direct their activity into more useful channels and enhance their feelings of control and usefulness. Aggressive patients may sometimes be diverted into useful activity after they have had the opportunity to be heard by a nonjudgmental listener who refrains from arguing yet avoids insincere placating.

More active intervention is often necessary to help withdrawn patients. Talking quietly to them, describing what you think they might be feeling, and giving them the opportunity to agree or disagree can be successful in encouraging them to emerge from their withdrawn state. Nonverbal modes of communication are often more effective than verbal in reaching these patients. An arm around the shoulders may convey concern and a willingness to help. Holding the patient's hand as you talk may help the individual to focus on what is being said. A familiar person such as a close friend or member of the family is usually more successful in communicating with a withdrawn patient than a stranger. If such a person is available and able to help, he or she should be involved. In providing help for withdrawn patients, first aiders must attempt to *explicitly* convey the message that they sincerely want to understand and help. The message should be repeated as often as possible by a variety of verbal and nonverbal means.

Supportive measures are necessary if the patient experiences physiological reactions. The prime purpose is to make the patient more comfortable and to avoid further complications or injury. Specific first aid measures for reactions such as vomiting or fainting are described elsewhere in this book. Other symptoms are uncomfortable for the patient but can be alleviated only by reducing the psychological disequilibrium. One additional reaction that is not uncommon in individuals experiencing psychological stress is hyperventilation or overbreathing. Hyperventilation can be identified by the patient's rapid respirations and such subjective sensations as shortness of breath, weakness, dizziness, numbness of extremities, and feeling faint. It can eventually lead to loss of consciousness or convulsions. Through rapid breathing, the individual has decreased the level of carbon dioxide in the body, thus precipitating the other symptoms, which tend to reinforce the rapid breathing pattern. First aid is aimed at intervening in this cycle by increasing the patient's respiratory intake of carbon dioxide. This is most easily accomplished by encouraging the patient to breathe into a paper bag. As the carbon dioxide increases in the bag from exhalation, the patient receives proportionately more carbon dioxide on inhalation, thus increasing the carbon dioxide in the body and breaking the hyperventilation cycle.

Some of the first aid measures described above are helpful in aiding a person experiencing panic. In addition, the first aider must actively intervene to provide the controls the patient has lost. A person in panic is virtually helpless, unable to perceive and evaluate the surrounding reality. Someone in a panic flight needs to be protected from inadvertently fleeing into more danger. More than one person may be needed to provide the controls, but it is important to avoid threatening the patient further. Striking or dousing a panic-stricken person with water are likely to increase the threat and aggravate the situation. If possible, the individual should be removed to a less stimulating environment where one or two people can provide care. A confident, matter-of-fact approach is most effective. A person in panic is seldom able to comprehend the words that a helping person is saying, but the rate of speech, tone of voice, and nonverbal messages may be understood. As the person becomes more receptive, the interventions previously described can be helpful. It is important to recognize that panic is an extremely overpowering reaction to stress. If unchecked, it can be communicated to others as well as lead to injury or exhaustion for the involved individual.

Follow-up care

As patients begin to respond to psychological first aid, their usual coping mechanisms come into play. At this point they may be able to indicate what will be most helpful to them. Perhaps a particular family member or other individual may be contacted to further aid each patient. Some people may feel somewhat embarrassed about their behavior during an emergency and need to be reassured that most people have strong emotional reactions to emergencies and that their actions were understandable. Such individuals may wish to help in some way and can be assigned tasks within their ability at this time.

Delayed reactions are not uncommon in psychological emergencies. Individuals may appear to cope well with the immediate emergency and experience the symptoms of psychological disequilibrium at a later time. Generally, such delayed reactions are more common among people who are actually involved in an emergency and narrowly escape injury rather than those who happen on the scene after the crisis has occurred. For this reason it is wise to keep uninjured accident patients under observation for several hours after the accident or ensure that someone remains with them during this time. If other people or a medical team assume responsibility for care, the patient's status and need for specific first aid measures should be communicated to them.

In considering the degrees of psychological disequilibrium that patients might experience, recognize that first aiders are not immune to these same reactions. The surprise element of many emergencies and the feeling that one "should be doing something" add to the stress. The inexperienced first aider, in particular, is likely to experience psychological disequilibrium. It can be helpful for individuals to recall emergency situations in the past and attempt to remember their specific reactions and the particular coping mechanisms they utilized in regaining emotional equilibrium. Most people have several conscious techniques for reducing anxiety in the course of daily living, talking the situation over briefly with someone else or perhaps sitting quietly for a moment and consciously relaxing tense muscles. Some of these may be appropriate for emergency situations as well. In addition, practicing first aid skills in a variety of realistically simulated situations can help individuals gain confidence in their ability to handle emergencies and can aid them in anticipating their own reactions. First aid rules and routines are designed to help people establish priorities of care in stressful situations.

THE PATIENT SUSTAINING THE LOSS OR THREATENED LOSS OF A SIGNIFICANT PERSON

Many emergencies result in serious injury, illness, or death. Relatives or close associates of patients have understandably strong emotional reactions to these events. Many of their reactions may be similar to those previously described. However, other reactions may occur that are specifically related to the loss or threatened loss of a significant person. The grieving process has been identified through observation of many people experiencing loss. Some of the first studies by Erich Lindemann[8] included survivors of those killed in the Cocoanut Grove nightclub fire in Boston some years ago.

Through observations and interviews with relatives of those who died in the fire as well as other people who had experienced recent bereavement, Lindemann identified both common and unusual grief reactions. Subsequent interviews enabled him to describe "grief work," the process through which individuals resolved the loss. Others have extended Lindemann's work and defined stages in the grieving process. It is significant also that although grief is most often associated with death, similar reactions are common with other kinds of loss such as the end of a close relationship or sudden and severe loss of self-esteem.

Signs and symptoms

The grieving process, as described by Engel,[3] progresses through several stages over a period of several months or a year. People administering emergency care are likely to observe relatives and close friends of victims experiencing reactions related to the first two stages.

First-stage reactions. The initial reactions of survivors center around shock and disbelief. There may be desperate attempts to revive or aid the victim, to deny the seriousness of the situation, or to discount reports of the tragedy. A period of dazed numbness may follow as the person attempts to cope with the loss. Occasionally, intellectual acceptance is evident while the emotional reaction is delayed. During the first stage, denial is the dominant coping mechanism as the individual attempts to reject or delay full awareness of the loss.

Second-stage reactions. The first stage of grieving is followed by sudden awareness of loss. Overt emotional reactions dominate this stage. Crying is the most common expression of emotion, communicating feelings of profound grief, anger, and helplessness.

Somatic symptoms, such as a physical sensation of emptiness, are common in acute grief. Individuals interviewed by Lindemann sometimes described somatic sensations occurring in waves, lasting from 20 minutes to an hour, which were characterized by a feeling of tightness in the throat, choking and shortness of breath, an empty feeling in the stomach, exhaustion, and weakness. Sighing respirations were an overt sign of these subjective sensations.[8]

Survivors may express anger toward those viewed at fault in causing the severe injury or death or sometimes even toward those who have attempted to help. The anger may be turned inward by the individual experiencing the loss and become mixed with strong feelings of guilt. The individual may think he could have prevented the accident or that he has failed the patient in some way. Often individuals experiencing the loss of a person close to them feel abandoned, and sometimes they feel angry toward the person who has died for having left them. These feelings are often confusing and worrisome to the survivors who do not realize that such feelings are a normal part of the grieving process.

First aid

The grieving person is in need of immediate psychological support. Family members or close friends are often best able to provide support if they are available. During the denial stage of grieving, the individual should not be forcefully confronted with the reality of the loss nor should the helping person make statements that would reinforce the rejection of reality. Answering questions honestly but empathically is most helpful, as the individual gradually becomes able to accept what has occurred. If the patient is seriously ill or injured, cautious hope can be conveyed without misleading friends and relatives about the patient's condition. Do not attempt to make a prognosis or promises of recovery. Transportation should be arranged for family and friends who wish to accompany the ill or injured person to medical care.

Ventilation of feelings during the second stage should be supported. Expressions of anger as well as those of sadness and grief need to be accepted. Although anger may seem irrational and unjustified in the situation, attempts to argue or defend an opposing position should be avoided. Encouraging and supporting the grieving individuals to talk about what has happened and express their feelings promotes progress through the normal grieving process.

Follow-up care

Efforts should be made to enlist the aid of friends or family of the grieving person, since grieving is a social as well as an individual phenomenon. The relationship of the person to the patient must be made clear to those assuming responsibility for care of the patient. Provision for waiting in privacy should be obtained if the person cannot remain with the patient, and a certain staff member should be designated to be responsible for keeping the family informed. The aid of clergy or professional staff should be enlisted as available for the family, particularly if reactions seem unusually severe. If the patient dies, the grieving person will generally proceed through subsequent stages of the grieving process during the next several months or a year. Continued support during this period is important in helping the person accept the loss and reorganize interpersonal relationships.

THE PATIENT THREATENING OR ATTEMPTING SUICIDE

Many factors contribute to self-destructive behavior in an individual. Most potentially suicidal patients are suffering from depression that may be related to recent bereavement, loss of self-esteem, or prolonged physical illness. A disrupted family life, economic distress, or social isolation are often a part of the patient's problem. Some have a history of alcoholism or other drug dependence. Less than a fourth of all suicidal patients are actively psychotic and unable to evaluate reality. In general, women are more likely than men to threaten or attempt suicide; however, more men than women are victims in completed suicides. For both men and women, the greatest number of suicides occur when the patients are in their forties, although the rate for men continues high for older age groups. Suicide is also a leading cause of death in the adolescent and young adult population. Suicide ranks third among leading causes of death from ages 14 to 24 years[10] and second among causes of death among college students.[4] Suicide attempts are more common among younger age groups with the greatest number occurring when patients are in their twenties or thirties.

Signs and symptoms

There is a prevalent myth that those who threaten suicide do not commit suicide. Actually, a large percentage of those who attempt or commit suicide have spoken overtly or covertly of their intentions. Some have given nonverbal cues such as giving away prized possessions. Four out of five people who commit suicide have previously attempted suicide.

Many people contemplating suicide manifest signs of depression. Subjectively, they feel sad, helpless, and hopeless. Ordinary tasks become increasingly difficult as their attention span decreases, and a pervading sense of fatigue predominates. There are generally changes in social functioning as the depressed person withdraws from activities and relationships. Decreased sexual activity is common, as well as decreased appetite and weight loss. Depressed individuals may complain of various physical ailments. One of the most frequent problems is insomnia, especially early morning awakening.

First aid

Direct, immediate response to an overt or covert suicide threat must be made. If a person clearly states, "I am going to kill myself," it can be fatal to assume he or she is not serious. An appropriate direct response might be, "Do you mean you have been thinking of suicide?" followed by "What has been upsetting you that's led you to thoughts of harming yourself?" If the hint is more subtle, such as "I won't be around after next week," it is imperative to establish exactly what the individual means by the comment. If, in either case, the individual has been considering suicide, follow-up questions should be directed toward the patient's elaboration of the suicidal plans. If the person has a carefully considered plan, has chosen a mode by which to commit suicide, and has immediate access to that means, there is generally a high suicide potential. A fourth factor is the lethality of the chosen method of committing suicide. Suicide by shooting oneself with a gun is a more immediate and certain lethal mode than ingesting drugs. Other factors being equal, there is a higher suicide risk if the person has chosen a highly lethal mode of suicide.

A high-suicide-risk patient *should not be left alone.* Since active and direct intervention is the most appropriate response to suicide threats, first aid is directed toward preventing the patient from harming himself. Means of self-injury must be removed and the patient's physical safety ensured. Direct action not only circumvents the patient's immediate plan, but it also communicates the fact that someone cares.

Verbal interchange with a suicidal person should be built on the understanding that ambivalence is nearly always present. The helping person has a powerful ally in the patient's own will to live. Communication with the patient should explicitly convey the message of caring and hope that solutions to the patient's problems can be found. The helping person needs to convey a willingness to listen and understand. The establishment of even a beginning relationship with the patient can be helpful to one who feels alone and has chosen death as a way of coping with his or her situation.

Finally, the attitude of the helper is important. Suicide is an anxiety-provoking thought for many people. Some react with anger, believing that the person threatening or attempting suicide merely seeks attention. Some feel uncomfortable discussing suicide with one who has indicated his or her intent, particularly if they are relatives or friends of the person. Others have strong moral or religious views related to suicide. It is essential that the helping person remain accepting and nonjudgmental in aiding the suicidal person. The individual may be able to explore the suicidal intent and find alternative solutions to current problems in counseling with mental health personnel. In the emergency situation, the aim is to establish rapport and intervene to preserve the life of the patient.

Follow-up care

Referral to mental health personnel is essential for any person threatening or attempting suicide. Some cities have suicide prevention centers with personnel experienced in dealing with suicide crisis. Community mental health centers, psychiatrists, college mental health and counseling services, and crisis centers are resources in this type of emergency. General hospital emergency room personnel can provide both physical and psychological care in the case of attempted suicide.

If there is high risk of immediate suicidal action or if there has been an attempt, the patient should be immediately accompanied to professional care. All pertinent information about the patient's suicidal behavior must be conveyed to those assuming responsibility for care. Close friends or family can often be involved to reaffirm to the patient that he or she is a valued person. These individuals as well as the patient may need support in coping with their own anxiety and guilt related to the patient.

In the event the patient completes the suicidal act, the family and close friends need special help in proceeding through the grieving process. Suicide still carries a social stigma in many communities, and shame may be combined with the family's grief. In many instances, the survivors become preoccupied with thoughts of what they might have done to prevent the patient's death. As in the normal grieving process, recognition, expression, and ventilation of these feelings are preliminary steps in resolving the loss.

THE PATIENT WHO DEMONSTRATES PSYCHOTIC BEHAVIOR

Markedly unusual or inappropriate behavior can have its roots in a variety of medical conditions or can be induced by various drugs. Prolonged psychological stress can precipitate a psychotic state in which patients misperceive or misinterpret the reality around them. When their behavior becomes disruptive and disturbing to others or when it is evident that they cannot meet their basic safety needs, a psychiatric emergency ensues. Immediate first aid is necessary to protect the patient and to ensure psychiatric care.

Signs and symptoms

Often a family member or friend of the patient can provide information useful in evaluating an emergency. They may describe the patient's recent behavior, provide information about past and current psychiatric treatment, and perhaps identify an event that precipitated the patient's current episode of psychotic behavior.

This history is often significant in differentiating patients who need immediate medical first aid from those for whom psychological first aid is more appropriate.

Initial observation of the patient yields behavioral cues to the dominant mood of the patient, which may be fear, rage, excitement, or apathy. Psychotic patients may manifest many of the symptoms of acute anxiety and psychological disequilibrium described previously. Some patients suffer from delusions, convinced that others wish to harm them or that peculiar things are happening to their bodies. A few hallucinate, hearing voices no one else can hear. Confusion, disorganization, vagueness, and memory gaps are most characteristic of the patient who has some organic condition involving the brain such as arteriosclerosis. Complete withdrawal and mutism may be evident in patients' behavior or aggressive hostility and destructiveness. A few may seem to be on a high, talking incessantly, laughing, and constantly moving. Although the behaviors vary widely, the meaning is generally that the patient is severely threatened by external or, more often, internal stresses. Psychotic behavior is the patient's way of coping with overwhelming stress.

First aid

The basic approach in providing first aid to psychotic patients is calm, reassuring firmness. Renshaw[12] suggests several initial steps: first, introduce yourself and define your role. One might say simply, "My name is _____. You seem to need some help." Second, personalize the contact by asking the patient's name and subsequently using it. Third, define the problem in a simple statement. For example, in the case of a confused, wandering patient in a potentially dangerous environment one might say, "It isn't safe for you to stay here."

After initial contact, the first aider should try to elicit the patient's view of the situation. A comment such as, "You seem upset. What has happened?" may let the patient know the helper wants to understand. Generally there is time even in an emergency situation to talk with the patient to allay fear and begin to establish a basis for trust.

Delusional patients may try to convince the helping person that their delusions are real. First aiders should neither agree or disagree with patients' delusions. Agreeing or playing along with patients' delusions often only reinforces the threat; disagreeing may evoke anger or aggression. If pressed for a response, the helping person may simply state that he understands that the patient truly believes what he is describing. The first aider should try to respond to the *feeling* that the patient is conveying. The feeling associated with many delusions is fear.

The overactive patient presents a different kind of problem. Incessant talking and activity provide a cyclic stimulating effect. Such patients should not be encouraged to talk but should be removed to an environment less stimulating. A calm, matter-of-fact, firm approach is most successful with overactive patients.

In talking with patients, the helping person must give a simple explanation of the plan of action. Patients need to be told where they are being taken, without deception. Sometimes it is helpful to reassure patients that they will be safe and that a member of the family or a friend may accompany them.

As a last resort, physical restraint of the individual may be necessary to protect the patient or others. If physical restraint is used, it must be unequivocal to avoid harm to the patient or to those attempting to help. Patients react in diverse ways to physical restraint. For some, it has a calming effect as they recognize that someone else is able to provide the control they lack at the moment; for many it is an additional threat that must be resisted. For this reason, physical restraint should not be attempted unless there is a sufficient number of well-trained people to effectively restrain the patient, who may react in self-defense as though literally fighting for life. Legal authorities should be involved if there is risk of harm to the patient, bystanders, or the first aider.

Follow-up care

There are legal implications in taking patients to emergency care when they either do not comprehend the action or do not want to go. For this reason, it is important to involve legal authorities or a relative of the patient who can assume at least temporary responsibility for treatment of the patient until the individual can make decisions.

First aiders should describe as accurately as possible what they observed the patient doing and saying in the emergency situation. Such information is helpful to the mental health or medical care team providing immediate treatment for the patient.

SUMMARY

Providing first aid in psychological emergencies requires more than specific communication skills on the part of the helping person. It requires warmth and genuine concern for patients who are emotionally unable to cope with their current situational stress. It also requires a nonjudgmental attitude on the part of the first aider and the ability to quickly establish some sort of helping relationship. It entails the risk of involvement on the part of the helping person who, in a sense, shares his own strength with a patient who temporarily feels weak and helpless.

As an overall guide in dealing with psychological emergencies, five general rules may be followed:

1. Use simple, direct communication.
2. Explicitly convey the wish to help and the desire to understand.
3. Encourage the patient to talk about what has occurred.
4. Support the patient's existent coping skills.
5. Involve family or friends to support the patient.

An exception to the third rule should be made for overactive patients, for whom talking would perpetuate the stimulation and compound the problem. An exception to the fifth rule would be necessary when the patient's friends or family are emotionally unable or unwilling to be supportive. Finally, first aiders must remember that no one is immune to the stress of an emergency situation. By anticipating the effects and by developing appropriate understanding and skill, individuals can confidently provide effective psychological first aid.

FIRST AIDER COMPETENCIES

After studying the material and practicing the techniques presented in this chapter, the student should be able to:

- Describe the behaviors that may be demonstrated by patients during specific psychological emergencies.

- Describe and demonstrate, in a simulated situation, appropriate intervention in the psychological emergencies included in this chapter.
- Give a simple explanation of possible reasons for patients' behaviors in psychological emergencies.
- Review psychological emergency situations that they have experienced or that others describe to identify the type of psychological disequilibrium in each case and to describe the appropriate intervention.
- Discuss how they have reacted when under sudden, temporary stress, and anticipate the effect of various psychological emergencies on their ability to provide first aid.

REFERENCES AND RECOMMENDED READINGS

1. Aguilera, D. C., and Messick, J. M.: Crisis intervention—theory and methodology, St. Louis, 1974, The C. V. Mosby Co.
2. Aldrich, C. K.: Some dynamics of anticipatory grief. In Schoenberg, B., et al., editors: Anticipatory grief, New York, 1974, Columbia University Press.
3. Engel, G. L.: Grief and grieving. In Folta, J. R., and Deck, E. S., editors: A sociological framework for patient care, New York, 1966, John Wiley & Sons, Inc.
4. Farberow, N. L., and Shneidman, E. S., editors: The cry for help, New York, 1965, McGraw-Hill Book Co.
5. Francis, G. M., and Munjas, B.: Promoting psychological comfort, Dubuque, Iowa, 1968, William C. Brown Co., Publishers.
6. Grollman, E. A.: Suicide: prevention, intervention, postvention, Boston, 1971, Beacon Press.
7. Knight, J. A.: Suicide among students. In Resnick, H. L. P., editor: Suicidal behaviors: diagnosis and management, Boston, 1968, Little, Brown & Co.
8. Lindemann, E.: Symptomatology and management of acute grief. In Parad, H. J., editor: Crisis intervention: selected readings, New York, 1965, Family Service Association of America.
9. Mahoney, S. G.: The art of helping people effectively, New York, 1967, Association Press.
10. Monthly vital statistics report: summary report, final mortality statistics, 1973, 23:11, suppl. 2, Public Health Service, Health Resources Administration, Washington, D.C., 1975, U.S. Department of Health, Education, and Welfare.
11. Murphy, G. E., and Robins, E.: The communication of suicidal ideas. In Resnick, H. L. P., editor: Suicidal behaviors: diagnosis and management, Boston, 1968, Little, Brown & Co.
12. Renshaw, D.: Psychiatric first aid in an emergency, American Journal of Nursing 72:497, 1972.
13. Rusk, T. N., and Edwards, B. J.: Psychiatric emergencies. In Sproul, C. W., and Mullanney, P. J., editors: Emergency care: assessment and intervention, St. Louis, 1974, The C. V. Mosby Co.
14. Stengel, E.: Suicide and attempted suicide, New York, 1974, Jason Aronson, Inc.

16

▼▼

OBSTETRICAL AND GYNECOLOGICAL EMERGENCIES

Alexander Franco and J. Robert Wirag

There is a group of emergency situations involving problems that are unique to women. Problems related to pregnancy are regarded as obstetrical emergencies, and problems related to the genital tract of females are regarded as gynecological emergencies.

OBSTETRICAL EMERGENCIES

The average length of pregnancy is about 266 days. Within this span of time there may be a wide range of signs and symptoms that make it difficult to differentiate between what is normal or expected and what is abnormal. The signs and symptoms may range from nausea, vomiting, and mood changes in the early stages of pregnancy to the more serious complications involving severe hemorrhage and shock secondary to abortion (spontaneous, criminal, or therapeutic) or impending childbirth (premature or full-term).

Abortion

Abortion involves the expulsion of the products of conception from the uterus. Sometimes this occurs naturally and is called a *spontaneous abortion.* At other times the pregnant woman may intentionally attempt to end her pregnancy by herself by using mechanical devices or chemical douches (induced abortions), or illegal attempts may be made to produce an abortion by unqualified, unlicensed, incompetent persons (criminal abortion).

Other descriptions of abortion include "threatened," "incomplete," and "therapeutic" (induced to save the life of the mother or in cases in which congenital malformations are suspected).

Signs and symptoms. In cases of spontaneous abortion the woman may describe the passage of "tissue" or an actual embryo or fetus. Occasionally this may occur during a bowel movement and be precipitated by straining. In cases involving the possibility of an induced abortion, it is not unusual to find the woman with a temperature elevated above 38° C (100.4° F) caused by infection introduced by chemicals or mechanical devices used in a prior attempt to cause abortion. In addition to cramping pain expressed by the woman, one can expect to find hemorrhage from the vaginal tract ranging from slight to severe. If the hemorrhage is severe, it could lead to hemorrhagic shock because of fluid loss. Other visible signs may include vomiting, abdominal distension, dehydration, rapid heartbeat, and labored breathing. Most cases of abortion, regardless of the cause, will occur at less than 20 weeks of gestation.

First aid procedures. The following procedures are primarily aimed at maintaining vital functions while arranging for transportation to medical care.

1. Use a sanitary napkin or absorbent cloth to cover the vaginal opening to collect any blood that may be present.
2. Care for shock. Maintain an open airway.
3. Keep the woman quiet but permit her to assume a position of comfort. Physical activity may increase the bleeding.
4. Collect any tissue that may have been discharged from the uterus through the vaginal opening. It will be helpful for the medical diagnosis.
5. Transport without delay to medical facility.

Ectopic (tubal) pregnancy

An ectopic pregnancy (Fig. 16-1) means that the fertilized ovum is developing away from its usual location. Fertilization of the ovum occurs in the fallopian tube, and, after a period of a couple of days, the fertilized egg reaches the endometrial cavity, where implantation occurs. Sometimes the fertilized ovum is implanted in the fallopian tube. Survival of the developing embryo in the tube is limited because of a lack of nutrients essential to maintenance of the placenta and fetus. Usually by the second or third month of pregnancy, spontaneous abortion (tubal abortion) through one end of the fallopian tube will occur, or the tubal wall will rupture (rupture tubal pregnancy), resulting in intraabdominal hemorrhage.

Signs and symptoms. In most cases involving an ectopic pregnancy, the woman will have experienced the usual symptoms of pregnancy, including a history of missed period, nausea, faintness or dizziness, breast swelling and tenderness, and intermittent vaginal spotting. If tubal rupture has not yet occurred, the patient will usually have experienced intermittent pain in the lower part of the abdomen,

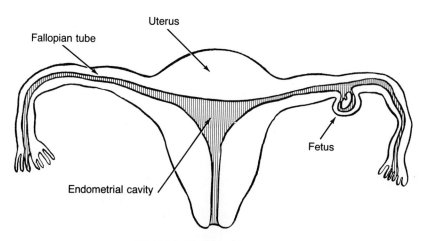

Fig. 16-1. Ectopic pregnancy.

sometimes localized to one side. Although heavy bleeding is rare, there is usually mild, intermittent bleeding.

If tubal rupture has occurred, abdominal pain is usually sudden and may radiate to the shoulder on the affected side. Internal bleeding could be severe, with a large amount of blood being accumulated within the abdominal cavity. If this is the case, the woman may appear in shock with low blood pressure, weak and rapid pulse, and pale and clammy skin.

First aid procedures. When a woman complains of pain in the lower abdomen with bleeding from the vaginal opening, a tubal pregnancy or a ruptured tubal pregnancy must be suspected. Since the treatment for an ectopic pregnancy is surgical, arrangements must be made to transport the woman to a medical facility without delay.

1. Use a sanitary napkin or suitable cloth to cover the vaginal opening to collect any blood that may be present. Try to keep the woman calm by providing reassurance that, to the extent possible, everything is being done to get her to qualified medical personnel.
2. Prepare to transport the woman in a reclining comfortable position (usually more comfortable with the head elevated). However, if the patient is in shock, the head should be kept level with the rest of the body to avoid loss of consciousness by improving circulation to the brain.
3. Care for shock.
4. Continually check vital life signs for changes in respiration and circulation. In cases involving respiratory and circulatory collapse, cardiopulmonary resuscitation must be started immediately.

Placenta previa

The usual site of implantation of the fertilized ovum and subsequent development of the placenta and fetus is in the upper portion of the uterus. On occasion the placenta may be attached in the lower part of the uterus and cover all or part of the opening between the uterus and the vagina (Fig. 16-2). Implantation of the placenta in this region is referred to as *placenta previa*. In the early stages of pregnancy, placenta previa usually does not present any problems. However, in the later stages of pregnancy, physical changes are taking place in preparation for delivery. At this time, at or about the thirty-seventh week of pregnancy, the placental attachments may be torn, and hemorrhage may begin.

Signs and symptoms. The amount of bleeding from the vaginal opening may vary. Usually the woman will note that the onset of bleeding was sudden and without pain. Depending on the amount of blood lost, shock may or may not be present. Also, labor may or may not be present.

First aid procedures. Assess the patient's general condition. A sanitary napkin can be used to cover the vaginal opening to collect the discharge. Psychological first aid is important at this time. Care for shock and prepare to transport the woman in the supine position to a medical facility without delay. Medical attention is essential to control hemorrhage and prevent fetal death. Signs of labor plus bleeding from the vaginal opening increase the urgency to obtain medical attention.

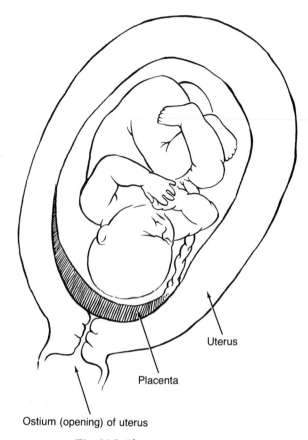

Uterus

Placenta

Ostium (opening) of uterus

Fig. 16-2. Placenta previa.

Abruptio placentae

Premature separation of the normally implanted placenta is referred to as *abruptio placentae*. Although the cause is unknown, the extent of the separation may be slight to complete detachment and may occur anytime from the twentieth week of pregnancy to the expected time of birth.

Signs and symptoms. The principal symptoms include bleeding in varying amounts from the vaginal opening and pain. In placenta previa there is usually bleeding without pain, but in abruptio placentae there is bleeding with pain of varying degrees. If medical attention is not obtained immediately, maternal hemorrhage may result in shock and death to the fetus because of lack of oxygen. Follow the same first aid procedure described for suspected placenta previa.

Vaginal hemorrhage

Bleeding of unknown origin is certainly a cause for concern and warrants medical investigation to render a diagnosis and begin treatment. In the nonpregnant female only severe hemorrhage demands immediate, emergency medical attention. However, if the woman is known to be or suspected to be pregnant, any

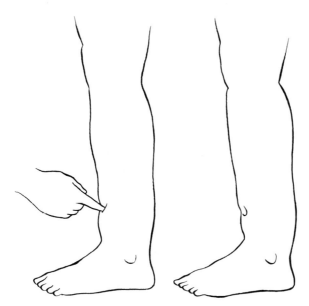

Fig. 16-3. Pitting edema: when pressure is applied with finger, it makes depression that tends to remain after finger is removed.

amount of bleeding from the vaginal area should be regarded as an emergency, and arrangements should be made to have the condition evaluated by medical personnel without delay. In general, bleeding after the twenty-fourth week of pregnancy may be caused by anomalies and/or injury of the placenta and uterus, diseases and/or injury to the cervix and vagina, or benign or malignant tumors of the cervix or body of the uterus.

Preeclampsia and eclampsia

Eclampsia is an extremely dangerous complication of pregnancy, appearing after 24 weeks of gestation, which is characterized by convulsions, loss of consciousness, and coma. The cause of eclampsia is unknown; it is always preceded by preeclampsia, which is characterized primarily by an elevated blood pressure and by the accumulation of fluid in the body. Patients with preeclampsia usually have certain warning signals indicating that convulsions may be imminent. These signs and symptoms may include the presence of a severe headache, blurring of vision, epigastric (upper middle area of abdomen) pain or discomfort, and further elevation of blood pressure, which usually is above 160/110 mm Hg.

Signs and symptoms. Hopefully the pregnant woman is under obstetrical care and has been taught to recognize certain physical changes warranting medical attention. One might expect to find evidence of edema (fluid retention), especially puffiness of the face and eyelids and, perhaps, swollen legs characterized by pitting edema. *Pitting edema* refers to the depression that remains after finger pressure has been applied to the swollen area (Fig. 16-3). However, most pregnant women have some degree of leg edema, and it is not necessarily an abnormal finding.

If preeclampsia has gone unrecognized and an eclamptic seizure begins, one can expect to note that the convulsion usually begins with twitching of the corners of the mouth followed by a generalized total body muscular contraction lasting about 20 or 30 seconds. The episode may resemble that of grand-mal epilepsy, and the patient may progress from a semicomatose state to profound coma. After the initial convulsion, the body muscles may alternately relax and contract for a few seconds with the mouth opening and closing rapidly. Breathing may be arrested during the convulsion. There is always the risk of successive convulsions, which present a grave danger to the woman because of increased stress, resulting in cardiac failure and death. Also, successive convulsions can present a serious danger to the fetus.

First aid procedures. If one is fortunate in recognizing the signs and symptoms of preeclampsia, the woman should be referred at once to a medical facility for attention by an obstetrician. These patients usually have an acute startle reflex, and loud noises may precipitate convulsions.

If an eclamptic seizure is expected or underway, the same general care should be provided as if attending to an epileptic seizure. These procedures include:
1. Protect the woman from additional injury. If possible have her lie on a padded surface.
2. Maintain an open airway.
3. If available, suction should be used to prevent the aspiration of vomitus, saliva, and nasopharyngeal secretions.
4. If necessary, perform mouth-to-mouth ventilation or cardiopulmonary resuscitation.
5. Transport the woman to a hospital at once.

Impending childbirth

In most cases, women experience an uneventful pregnancy, and childbirth occurs as a normal physiological process in the presence of medical and nursing personnel. On occasion, however, there may be circumstances that lead to complications and thus interrupt the expected normal process. Some of these unexpected emergencies have already been discussed. Perhaps there was an error in estimating the expected time of delivery, or the onset of labor may occur more rapidly than anticipated without a medical facility readily accessible, or the expecting mother may be involved in an accident that stimulates the premature onset of labor. Regardless of the cause, it is important to recognize an impending childbirth and prepare oneself to assist in the delivery process. The procedures that follow are emergency procedures only and are not intended to substitute for medical care after the delivery.

Labor. Labor is a series of contractions of the uterus so that the contents of the uterus (developed fetus and supporting tissue) can be discharged through the vagina to the outside world. When the contractions are approximately 2 minutes apart and the woman is in pain and pushing down with each contraction, birth of the child will occur at any time.

Delivery procedures
1. Preparation
   a. Every attempt should be made to protect the woman from embarrassment, especially if the delivery will occur in a public place.

    b. Newspapers or other absorbent materials should be placed beneath the woman's buttocks and close by.

    c. Remove any underclothing that may interfere with the delivery.

    d. Position the woman on her back, knees bent, and legs spread wide apart (Fig. 16-4). This should add to the woman's comfort and permit the attendant access to the vaginal opening.

    e. If water is available, thoroughly wash hands.

    f. Do not administer medication or stimulants.

    g. Provide reassurance.

2. Supplies: Ambulances or rescue vehicles should have a childbirth kit on board. If one is not available, every attempt should be made to obtain the following:

    a. Towel

    b. Scissors

    c. String

    d. Bulb syringe

3. Delivery (Fig. 16-5)

    a. Examine the vaginal opening. The baby's head will usually be visible with each contraction and recede when the contraction stops.

    b. If the exposed area of the baby's head is less than the size of a 50-cent piece, there may be sufficient time to reach a hospital, if it can be reached in less than about 20 minutes. If the exposed area of the baby's head is larger than a 50-cent piece, delivery may occur any minute.

    c. Encourage the woman to breathe with panting breaths and to relax as much as possible between contractions.

    d. The contractions will increase in frequency and intensity. There will also be increased pain, and the woman may feel she has to move her bowels. This is normal because of the pressure of the baby's head on the rectum. If a bowel movement does occur, cover it to prevent contamination of the baby and the attendant's hands.

    e. Prepare to receive the baby in a suitable container lined with towels. *Do not* reach into the birth canal and *do not* pull on the baby; simply guide the baby out.

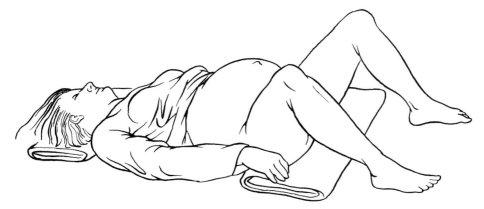

Fig. 16-4. Position for delivery.

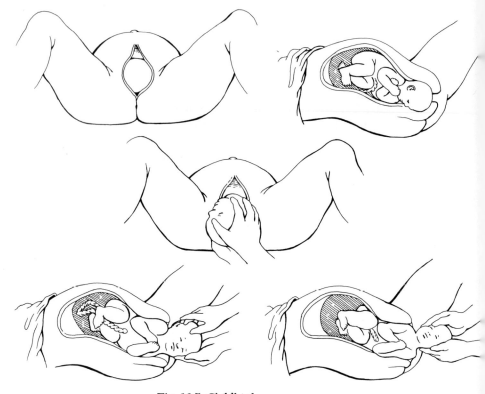

Fig. 16-5. Childbirth sequence.

f. At this point the bag of waters may or may not have been broken. If the bag has broken, the child will emerge quickly. If the bag of waters has not broken and the baby's head is exposed outside the birth canal, tear the bag with your fingers. This will prevent the baby from aspirating any of the contents as it takes its first breaths.

g. You may expect tissue to be torn in the vaginal area as the baby's head begins to emerge. You may prevent extensive tissue tear by applying gentle pressure on the baby's head to prevent it from exploding from the vaginal opening.

h. Usually the baby's head will be face down. Gently support the head to keep the face away from the blood and other fluid from the bag of waters. Check to see if the umbilical cord is wrapped around the baby's neck. If it is around the neck, gently remove it to prevent strangulation.

i. At this point the shoulders should appear either spontaneously or with the next contraction, followed by the birth of the rest of the body.

4. Resuscitation

a. As soon as possible, help the infant to breathe. If a bulb syringe is available, use it to remove mucus from the baby's mouth and nose. If a syringe is not available, elevate the baby's feet and lower the head to help drain the mucus. Use a cloth or your finger to remove mucus. Be careful. The baby will be slippery.

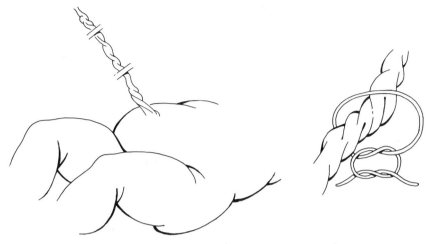

Fig. 16-6. Procedure for tying off umbilical cord.

    b. If crying does not occur spontaneously, rub its back, spank the buttocks, or tap the bottom of its feet. If breathing does not begin, administer mouth-to-mouth resuscitation (covering baby's mouth and nose) at the rate of a breath (in puffs) every 3 seconds. If available, use a piece of gauze over the baby's mouth to minimize possible respiratory infection.

    c. When breathing begins, wrap the baby in cloth to keep it warm.

5. Umbilical cord

    a. If the mother and infant are to be transported without delay to the hospital, there is no need to cut the cord. The baby should be placed in a position assuring that an open airway will be maintained in transit and that any traction on the cord is avoided.

    b. If the mother and child cannot be transported immediately to the hospital, the baby should be separated from the mother by tying and cutting the cord. The umbilical cord is a ropelike structure, about 20 inches long, that provides the lifeline that circulates blood between the developing baby and the placenta. After birth occurs and breathing begins, the umbilical cord is useless.

    c. Since there is usually no urgency to cut the cord, the materials that will be used should be sterilized by boiling or soaking in alcohol for at least 20 minutes.

    d. The first tie should should be made 4 to 6 inches from the baby's navel and the second tie about 8 to 10 inches from the baby (Fig. 16-6). Make the cut between the ties. It is best to leave the first tie far enough away from the baby (4 to 6 inches) so that if necessary the baby can receive transfusion. The cord can be cut shorter later by the doctor.

6. Afterbirth

    a. Usually within 5 minutes or so after the baby is born, blood will flow from the vagina, and the cord will advance. This signals the separation

of the placenta from its attachment in the uterus and, when discharged, is called the afterbirth.
  b. *Do not* pull on the cord to hasten delivery of the afterbirth.
  c. Save the cord and placenta for examination by hospital personnel.
  d. After the placenta has been expelled, gently massage the uterus by placing your hand or the mother's hand over the lower part of her abdomen. Massaging will stimulate the uterus to contract and help control bleeding.
  7. After delivery
  a. Remove all soiled materials.
  b. Cleanse the vaginal area.
  c. Place a sanitary napkin or folded towel over the vaginal opening and ask the mother to close her legs.
  d. Keep both mother and child warm.
  e. The baby will be covered with a white, slippery, protective coating. Do not attempt to wash off.
  f. Comfort mother and child and transport them to a hospital for follow-up care.

Please note that this discussion focused on the uncomplicated delivery. If complications should occur at any time in the delivery process, transport the mother at once to the nearest hospital or doctor's office.

GYNECOLOGICAL EMERGENCIES

The female genital area is subject to a broad spectrum of conditions involving pain and discomfort resulting from trauma, infection, and/or endocrine disturbance. In this section attention will be directed to pelvic pain, genital injuries, and the most common lower genital tract infections. In most cases gynecological emergencies are not life-and-death situations. However, all cases should receive medical consultation and, if necessary, treatment.

Pelvic inflammatory disease

Pelvic inflammatory disease is usually the result of an acute infection of the pelvic organs. The causative organism is usually bacteria from a gonorrheal infection or from infection after delivery or abortion. Usually the only complaint is pain and tenderness in the lower abdominal area. However, the woman may complain of discharge from the vaginal opening. There may be fever, nausea, and vomiting. Typically, the woman will be bent at the waist with both hands pressing against the lower abdomen.

Minimize physical activity, and transport the woman in a semireclining position to a hospital or doctor's office for medical evaluation and treatment.

Genital trauma

A wound or injury to tissue in the genital area, internal or external, may have occurred by accident or by sexual assault, or it may have been self-induced. The extent of the injury and the circumstances surrounding the accident will determine the urgency with which medical attention is necessary. Tissue damage may be the result of direct trauma from a kick, a piece of machinery, a blow from a sharp instrument, or from a straddle injury such as may occur in climbing a fence.

Injuries due to blows received from blunt objects may result in severe pain and marked swelling of tissues in the external genitalia. The application of cold packs may help reduce the swelling. Although bleeding after an injury to genital tissue is usually self-limiting, it can be controlled by direct pressure. Sometimes tissue damage has been self-induced. Young children may accidentally cut themselves with a sharp toy or introduce an object into the vaginal opening. Also, violent or unusual techniques of masturbation may result in swelling or bleeding of vaginal, clitoral, or urinary tissue.

Trauma from sexual assault may cause damage ranging from slight to severe, depending on the age of the female assaulted and the violence with which the assault took place. Seldom is sexual trauma sufficient to cause tissue lacerations. Bleeding, therefore, is seldom evident, but when present it may be severe enough to require sutures.

In the presence of pain and/or bleeding, arrangements should be made to obtain medical attention. The entire vaginal area should be examined by medical personnel so that an associated separate vaginal injury is not overlooked.

Lower genital tract infections

Lower genital tract infections involve the vulvar and vaginal tissues. Although they are seldom severe enough to require urgent treatment, they can be exceptionally distressing to the woman because of severe itching and burning of inflamed tissue and perhaps a discharge from the vaginal opening. *Vaginitis* is the general term used to refer to an inflammation of the vaginal tissue, which may be caused by a number of different infectious organisms, friction irritation, or allergies of one sort or another.

Until the services of a physician can be obtained, temporary relief from the burning and itching may be provided by following these procedures:
1. Sit in a tub of cool water or apply cool wet compresses over the vulva.
2. Use mild soap when washing the vaginal area.
3. Avoid tight-fitting panty hose and any other tight clothing.
4. Wear cotton panties, rather than those manufactured from a synthetic fabric.
5. Douche with solution of a quart water with 2 tablespoons of white distilled vinegar.

SUMMARY

There is a wide range of problems or concerns unique to girls and women that deserve special attention. The foregoing discussion focused on the more important emergencies encountered by both pregnant and nonpregnant females.

The first aider must recognize the girl's or woman's anxiety and embarrassment often associated with gynecological and obstetrical problems. Special precautions must be made, therefore, to protect her privacy and to provide assurance that measures are being taken in her behalf. Attention must also be paid to the psychological aspects of the emergency involving the anxiety associated with the expectant mother's thought of losing her child.

Some of the situations discussed, such as vaginal discharge and sudden pain, occur without provocation and are bewildering to both the patient and to the first aider. In other cases involving trauma caused by an external blow resulting in bruising and/or tearing to genital tissue, the first aider must take steps to control hemorrhage as well as attend to the psychological needs of the person.

In all cases the first aider with some knowledge of common obstetrical and gynecological emergencies must attend to both the physical and psychological needs of the person. Vital signs must be continuously monitored, and respiration and circulation must be adequate. Hemorrhage must be controlled, and shock must be cared for. Spotting or bleeding without pain must not be regarded lightly and passed off as insignificant. Anything unusual demands further attention and medical evaluation. The principal role of the first aider in the overall management involves attention to the immediate physical and psychological needs of the person and the expeditious transfer to qualified medical personnel.

FIRST AIDER COMPETENCIES

After studying the material and practicing the techniques presented in this chapter, the student should be able to:
- Describe the following obstetrical emergencies and outline the appropriate first aid for each type of emergency: spontaneous abortion, ectopic pregnancy, preeclampsia and eclampsia, vaginal hemorrhage, and placenta previa.
- Describe under what conditions it would be necessary for the first aider to attend an impending delivery.
- Describe the characteristics of labor that would indicate that childbirth is imminent.
- Outline, in order, the impending delivery procedures.
- Demonstrate the correct position to place the mother in for an impending delivery.
- Outline the procedures for attending an impending delivery.
- Describe the major symptoms for the following gynecological problems, and outline the appropriate first aid procedures: pelvic inflammatory disease, genital trauma, and lower genital tract infections.

REFERENCES AND RECOMMENDED READINGS

1. Barber, H. R. K., and Graber, E. A.: Quick reference to OB-GYN procedures, Philadelphia, 1969, J. B. Lippincott Co.
2. Fitzpatrick, E., and Reeder, S. R.: Maternity nursing, ed. 12, Philadelphia, 1971, J. B. Lippincott Co.
3. Haynes, D. M.: Medical complications during pregnancy, New York, 1969, McGraw-Hill Book Co.
4. Iorio, J.: Childbirth: family centered nursing, ed. 3, St. Louis, 1975, The C. V. Mosby Co.
5. Oxorn, H., and Foote, W. R.: Human labor and birth, ed. 3, New York, 1975, Appleton-Century-Crofts.
6. Sproul, C. W., and Mullanney, P. J., editors: Emergency care: assessment and intervention, St. Louis, 1974, The C. V. Mosby Co.
7. Stephenson, H. E.: Immediate care of the acutely ill and injured, St. Louis, 1974, The C. V. Mosby Co.

Application of emergency care skills and principles

17

PREVENTION AND CARE OF
ATHLETIC INJURIES

Guy S. Parcel

Athletic activities (including varsity sports, intramural athletics, physical education classes, and unorganized sporting activities) constitute a major source of injuries among school-age children and young adults. Because athletic activities present a high-risk factor for injuries, individuals responsible for the conduct and supervision of these activities should be prepared to provide emergency care for the injured.

The American Medical Association's Committee on Medical Aspects of Sports has cited five areas that warrant attention: (1) conditioning, (2) coaching, (3) medical supervision, (4) equipment, and (5) officiating. Within these considerations lie the peculiarities of sport.

- The athlete is highly motivated and may mask an injury or attempt to return to the game prematurely.
- The pressure to win tempts the parent and/or coach to take chances with the safety of the motivated athlete.
- The performance requirements of sport can convert a minor injury into a disability (for example, a sprained thumb on a quarterback).
- The setting produces unusual circumstances that tax the judgment of the first aider (for example, what do you do with the face mask of a helmeted football player who needs an airway but who could become a quadriplegic if the helmet were removed?).

Consequently, the principles of prevention and care in this chapter must be visualized in a variety of contexts to do justice to the profound complexity of sport.

In addition to the basic fundamentals, the first aider should know what types of injuries are most likely to occur in specific activities, anticipate measures required for the management of these injuries, and have an awareness of the consequences of continued participation by an injured player. Coaches, athletic trainers, teachers, and others responsible for the supervision of athletic activities must also provide a safe environment for the participants and take the necessary steps to prevent injuries whenever possible.

In this chapter the role of the first aider is extended beyond providing immediate and temporary care to include methods of injury prevention and injury management. The material is organized so that general principles of injury prevention and management are presented first, and then attention is focused on specific problems involved in athletic injuries. The purpose is to provide the first aider with additional information and skills so that he or she is better able to prevent and care for injuries in the high-risk area of athletic activities.

PREVENTION OF ATHLETIC INJURIES

Athletic injuries do occur, but it would be a grave mistake to accept all injuries as an inevitable part of athletic activities. Properly conducted injury prevention programs can reduce the number and severity of injuries. The effectiveness of an injury prevention program was demonstrated in intramural lacrosse at the United States Military Academy as indicated in the data shown in Table 3. On analyzing the injury statistics in intramural lacrosse in 1968, those involved thought that the injury rate was much too high and that the injuries sustained were too severe for the activity. Before the 1969 season, the injury prevention program was intensified and strictly applied. The resulting injury statistics in 1969 showed a dramatic 67% reduction in the incidence of injuries and a decrease in the severity of injuries. This reduction reflects a concentrated effort to correct those factors suspected of causing the injuries the previous year.

Prevention procedures

The success of an injury prevention program depends on planning, coordination, and careful supervision. Regardless of who has responsibility for the overall program, everyone concerned, including the participants, can make a contribution to prevent injuries. General principles and methods of athletic injury prevention are presented within the following areas of concern.

Supervision. Competent supervision is of prime importance in the conduct of any athletic activity at all levels. Individuals supervising athletic activities should have a knowledge of the sport, the rules and regulations, and the inherent dangers involved in the sport. Supervisors should have foremost in their minds the welfare and safety of the participants. Coaches and officials should be carefully trained to try to prevent accident situations from arising. All competitive situations must be kept under control, and the supervisors must be constantly on the alert to take proper measures to prevent injuries.

Facilities. Playing areas should be free of all hazards that might lead to or contribute to the cause of injuries. In addition, playing areas should be continuously surveyed to prevent any new hazards from developing. Playing surfaces should be smooth, clean, and cleared of foreign objects. Whenever regula-

Table 3. Injuries sustained in intramural lacrosse at the United States Military Academy in 1968 and 1969

	1968	1969
Number of injuries	67	22
Percentage of participants injured	13.6	04.1
Percentage of participants hospitalized	2.6	00.4
Number of knee surgery cases	8	0

tion standards cannot be met, the desirability of allowing participation should be seriously questioned.

Equipment. An activity should not be conducted unless adequate, proper, and safe equipment can be provided for all participants. Discard and replace any broken or worn-out equipment. Protective equipment worn by the participant should be individually fitted, and personal equipment should not be exchanged or swapped among participants. Instruct participants on the proper care and use of equipment. For example, throwing a helmet to the ground runs the risk of weakening or damaging its protective ability.

Cost is often a major factor to consider when purchasing equipment. As with other commodities, you get what you pay for. Cheap products are usually inferior in quality. When buying equipment, quality should never be sacrificed to save money. The money saved may be lost to medical expenses at a later date. It is a common practice to hand down equipment to beginners or young players. This often leads to improper fits and inadequate protection and may contribute to injury. Avoid this practice, and provide the proper equipment at all levels of competition.

Health examination and fitness screening. The value and desirability of preseason health examinations have been well and widely accepted by physicians, athletic directors, and coaches. The examination may be conducted by a team physician or a school physician, or each participant may be examined by his or her own family physician. The exact format or procedure will differ from one situation to another, but the following points should be kept in mind:

1. The initial examination should be conducted well in advance of any participation.
2. A complete history including previous injuries and illnesses should be obtained.
3. The examination should determine fitness for specific activities. For example, an individual unfit for contact sports may be able to participate in activities such as track or swimming.
4. Dental, visual, auditory, medical, neurological, orthopedic, and emotional and psychiatric surveys are all an integral part of the examination.
5. Special attention should be focused on previous injuries or surgery to determine the status of recovery.
6. Individuals found to have defects, weaknesses, or health problems should be restricted, assigned to an activity that would not aggravate the condition, or they should have the problem corrected before participation.
7. All injuries occurring during the season must be reevaluated before returning to participation.

In addition to the health examination conducted by the physician, coaches, athletic trainers, and physical education teachers can establish a mechanism for determining an individual's physical fitness for specific activities. This can be accomplished by surveying the participants with a simple questionnaire to obtain information that would indicate the need for additional evaluation. Individuals with suspicious histories should be called in and evaluated for joint stability, flexibility, and muscle strength. Individuals having a weakness or problem that might contribute to injuries should be restricted or assigned to safer activities. A file can be maintained and updated as an individual's fitness status changes. Through this mechanism, conditions that are missed by the physician or conditions developing after the health examination can be picked up and evaluated.

Conditioning. Poor physical condition has been frequently identified as a contributing factor to the cause of athletic injuries. Each sport requires a different level and type of physical conditioning. Any conditioning program must be specifically designed to meet the needs and demands of the particular sport. The major components of conditioning are endurance, strength, flexibility, coordination, and reaction. The amount of emphasis placed on each component depends on the specific sport activity.

Cardiovascular conditioning stresses the respiratory and circulatory systems to increase the individual's endurance and delay the onset of fatigue. When a player is tired, he or she takes short cuts, makes mistakes, and increases the chances of getting injured. Endurance conditioning is important early in the season and can be accomplished through distance running or interval training

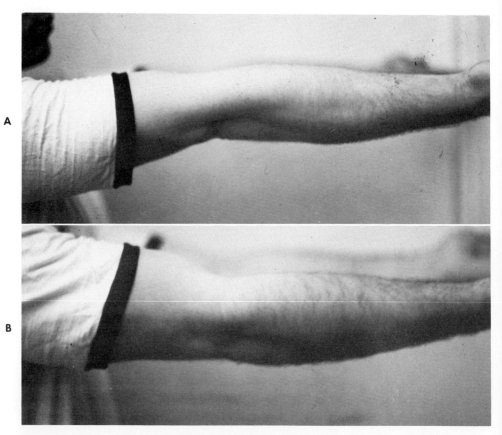

A

B

Fig. 17-1. Degrees of joint flexibility. **A,** Hyperflexibility of elbow joint. **B,** Restricted flexibility of elbow joint.

such as wind sprints. Muscular endurance is increased by stressing the muscles with high repetitions and low resistance and can be accomplished through calisthenics and weight training.

Muscular conditioning is important to prevent joint and muscle injuries. Strength may be increased by exercising particular groups of muscles with a high resistance. Muscular conditioning should be specific for the body part and specific for the body type. Some individuals are flexible, whereas others have tight muscular development with some limited flexibility (Fig. 17-1). Loose-jointed individuals may be more susceptible to joint injuries, and they should concentrate on strengthening exercises. Individuals with tight muscular development may be more susceptible to muscle and tendon injuries and should concentrate more on stretching and flexibility exercises.

Training is used to improve an individual's ability to perform. Stress is placed on certain body parts or functions to stimulate adaptation. Methods used to produce stress must be carefully planned and executed to stay within the limits of safety. Improper or excessive stress may damage parts of the body or contribute to causing an injury.

Reporting of injuries. The cause of injuries must be identified if future injuries are to be prevented. Any injury prevention program must include on-the-spot reporting of all injuries with special attention given to cause. Fig. 17-2 shows an example of a simple injury report form that can be filled out at the time of the injury. By collecting, summarizing, and analyzing injury data, factors responsible for causing athletic injuries can be identified. Then steps can be taken to eliminate or modify these factors to prevent injuries.

ATHLETIC INJURY REPORT

DATE OF INJURY | HOUR

NAME OF INJURED CADET *(last, first, MI)* | COMPANY | CLASS | NAME OF SPORT INVOLVED

TYPE OF ACTIVITY *(Check one)*
☐ INTRAMURAL
☐ PHYS ED CLASS ☐ FREE TIME ACTIVITY
☐ CLUBS ☐ CORPS SQUAD

POSITION PLAYED

CONDITION OF FIELD
☐ DRY ☐ WET ☐ HARD

WEATHER
☐ RAIN
☐ COLD ☐ HOT

BODY PART AFFECTED
☐ HEAD ☐ CHEST ☐ HAND ☐ HIP
☐ NECK ☐ ARM ☐ FINGER ☐ ANKLE
☐ SHOULDER ☐ ELBOW ☐ THIGH ☐ FOOT
☐ BACK ☐ WRIST ☐ KNEE
☐ *(Other)* ....

NATURE OF INJURY
☐ LACERATION ☐ DISLOCATION
☐ BRUISE ☐ FRACTURE
☐ STRAINED MUSCLE ☐ RE-INJURY
☐ SPRAIN
☐ *(Other)* ....

HOW INJURY OCCURRED - DESCRIBE

....
Signature of Reporting Official or Cadet in Charge

SECTION BELOW TO BE COMPLETED FOR REFERRALS TO U. S. ARMY HOSPITAL ONLY

TO BE COMPLETED BY TRAINER - SUSPECTED INJURY

....
Signature

TO BE COMPLETED BY PHYSICIAN - DIAGNOSIS

....
Signature

After completion, forward to Director of Physical Education.

USMA FORM 2–178 *(Edition of 3 Nov 65 is obsolete)*
13 MAR 68

ARMY-WP-2500-5256-68

Fig. 17-2. Sample of athletic injury report.

Policies for prevention program

Any athletic activity should include plans for an injury prevention program. In summary, the following policies are suggested for a good athletic injury prevention program:

1. A program of medical examination and screening to determine physical capabilities of participants
2. Individuals who demonstrate physical weakness reconditioned before participating in vigorous sports
3. Sports programs well organized and properly supervised by a responsible and well trained staff
4. A well-planned program of preseason physical conditioning
5. An adequate level of knowledge and skill of the sport acquired by the participants
6. A well-designed warm-up program carried out before each practice and contest
7. Protective equipment provided with proper fitting for all participants
8. Good playing conditions present for practices and contests
9. Care provided for injuries when they do occur
10. An accurate injury reporting system
11. A good reconditioning program to bring the injured participant back to normal strength before being permitted to return to participation
12. A rescreening process to evaluate an injured participant before being permitted to return to participation

MANAGEMENT OF ATHLETIC INJURIES

Because of the nature of athletic activities, injuries will occur even though preventive steps have been taken. Attention then must be focused on proper injury management. A basic principle of first aid to keep in mind when caring for an injured athlete is *do not cause further harm.* Improper handling, getting the player up too soon, or telling the injured player to run it off will often cause further injury. When a player is injured, go to his or her assistance and calmly determine the extent and nature of the injury. If the injury is not serious, allow the player to get up or refer to further medical care before allowing return to competition. If the injury is serious or is questionable, the player should not get up until it is determined what procedures are necessary to safely transport the injured player.

The first stage of the examination of an injured player should include a history of how the injury occurred. If the player is conscious, let the player tell you about the history, how it happened, where it hurts, and how he or she feels. If the player is unconscious, you may obtain a history concerning the injury from other players or from observers at the time of the injury. This brief history can give you clues as to exactly what the injury is and will save time in eliminating or ruling out certain conditions.

The next step is to physically examine the individual to determine the extent and nature of the injury. Because some injuries are more serious or more life threatening or may provide more complications, it is recommended that a certain order be given to the inspection for the various types of injuries. Check first to be sure that the injured individual is breathing. Sometimes this can be done quickly because it is obvious that the individual is breathing. Then check quickly for serious bleeding. Again, this possibility can be quickly eliminated by observation. Examine next for head and spinal injuries. Observe carefully for the possibility of heat stroke or heat exhaustion.

The foregoing conditions can be life threatening and require immediate attention, therefore they rank high in priority in your inspection. Many of these conditions can be determined quickly, and then you can continue your inspection for the types of injuries that are more common in athletics. These are, in the recommended order, fractures, dislocations, sprains, strains, contusions, and wounds. In any injury situation, a condition may exist that may greatly complicate the seriousness of even a minor injury.

Once you have determined the nature and severity of the injuries, the next step is to carry out the appropriate first aid. The specific first aid procedures are outlined in other chapters. Most of these procedures will apply to the care of athletic injuries. Any special consideration will be included in the discussion of specific athletic injury problems in this chapter.

Fig. 17-3 is a conceptualization of what happens to the body when an athletic injury occurs. Not all injuries will fit this model, but most musculoskeletal injuries, which account for the majority of athletic injuries, will follow a pattern similar to the vicious cycle of injury. Trauma sets off a chain reaction of events and changes in the body to produce a cycle of degeneration and impairment of the injured part. When an athletic injury takes place, there is usually a rupturing of blood vessels, which results in hemorrhaging into the tissue or joints. This results in effusion (swelling) and leads to inflammation. The inflammatory action causes pain, which, in turn, causes muscle spasm in an attempt to protect the injured area from further pain. If the injured part were used or moved, it would

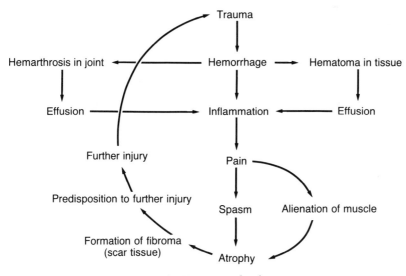

Fig. 17-3. Vicious cycle of injury.

cause increased pain; therefore the body alienates the muscles involved. As a result of this alienation, the muscles are not used, and atrophy (degeneration of tissue) begins to develop. Atrophy results in decreased strength and efficiency, therefore predisposing the injured part to further injury, causing increased pain or starting the whole cycle over again.

If athletic injury management is to be successful, the vicious cycle of injury must be broken and controlled. Although treatment and therapy beyond the scope of first aid will be necessary, first aid care plays an important and essential role. Proper first aid care immediately applied at the time the injury occurs will contribute greatly to controlling hemorrhaging and reducing pain.

An additional role of the first aider is to provide follow-up care for all athletic injuries by referring the injured player to a physician or appropriate medical personnel. Also, those having positions such as coach or athletic trainer should be sure that an injured player is physically fit before returning to an athletic activity. Experience and data have indicated that many athletic injuries are re-injuries of previous injuries. It is of extreme importance to stop this cycle of injury-reinjury whenever possible.

SPECIFIC PROBLEMS

The preceding section of this chapter presented general guidelines to be applied for the prevention and care of athletic injuries. In this section, attention is focused on specific methods of injury prevention and care for problems most likely to occur in athletic activities.

Knee injuries

In many athletic activities, the knee joint is one of the parts of the body most vulnerable to serious injury. Preventive programs can be effective in reducing the frequency and severity of knee injuries. The responsibility for an effective prevention program must be accepted at all levels. The director, physician, athletic trainer, coach, and athlete all play a role in the prevention of injuries.

The usual knee injury occurs when the player is caught off guard, his foot is fixed to the ground, and a twisting or shearing force is imposed through the momentum of another player. When the player is off guard and his foot is fixed, the knee is unprotected by the muscles, and the entire strain must be accepted by the ligaments. The number of knee scars evident in any group of young men is mute testimony to the frailty of these ligaments.

Prevention. In addition to the actual mechanics of forces that damage structure of the knee joint, certain physiological factors may be predisposing to knee injuries. In some activities flexibility is considered desirable, but in contact sports, too much flexibility, as evidenced in hyperextensibility of the knee joint (Fig. 17-4), is considered a possible predisposing cause of knee injury. An individual with excessive laxity in the knee joint should be encouraged not to play contact sports or to attempt to compensate by strengthening supporting musculature.

The muscles that support the lower extremities provide the first line of defense against forces that might damage structures of the knee joint. Important supportive muscles include the hip abductors, which run from the pelvis to the femur and lift the leg to the side; the hip flexors, which run from the crest of the

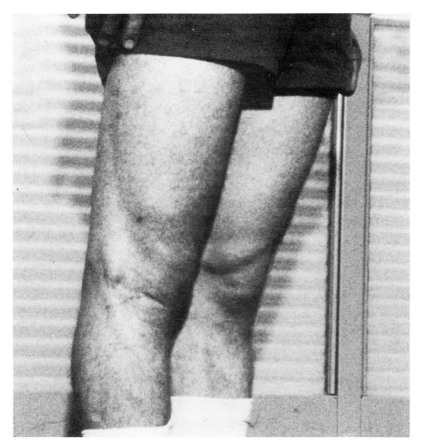

Fig. 17-4. Hyperextensibility of knee joint.

pelvis to the femur and lift the leg upward; the quadriceps, which run from the pelvis and the upper femur to the knee cap, where it forms into a tendon and inserts on the tibia, and functions to extend the lower leg; the hamstrings, which run from the pelvis and the upper femur to the tibia and flex the lower leg; and the calf muscles, which run from the lower end of the femur to the heel bone and aid in flexion of the lower leg. To provide maximum protection and support to the knee joint, all of the muscle groups must have a high level of strength and endurance. Weakness in any of these groups may be a contributing factor to injury when the knee is in a stress situation. Muscle weakness may result from faulty posture habits, injury, or inactivity.

Poor posture, such as abnormal curvatures of the spine and pelvis tilts (Fig. 17-5), should be detected and corrected before participating in athletic activities. Muscular imbalance resulting from poor posture places stress and strain on the knee joint, causing instability of the pelvic girdle and contributing to increase the chances of injury.

Exercise program. Injury to the lower extremity that causes limited use for even a short period of time results in atrophy of the affected muscles. Unless this

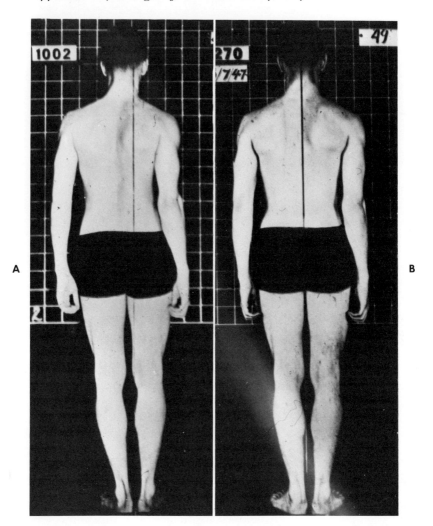

Fig. 17-5. Spinal lateral curvature **A**, before, and **B**, after, corrective exercise program.

residual muscle weakness is corrected, the individual is highly susceptible to re-injury. To break this cycle of injury-reinjury, it is necessary to engage in specific conditioning exercises to increase the strength and endurance of the muscles that support the knee joint.

Three years of continuous research at the United States Military Academy produced a program of exercises to recondition muscles that support the knee. This program is used each summer by the Knee Strength Development Squad, which is made up of new cadets with a history of knee injuries and muscle weak-nesses. This program has demonstrated that it is effective in increasing strength and endurance and has contributed to preventing reinjury.

The first exercise in the series is stool stepping. Individuals step up and down, fully extending the leg. Time should slowly be increased to a maximum of 5 minutes of stepping with each leg.

The quadriceps can be strengthened by extending the lower leg with an iron boot and weight on the foot. The suggested progression is:

1. Five repetitions of ⅓ maximum weight
2. Five repetitions of ⅔ maximum weight
3. Five repetitions near maximum weight
4. Ten repetitions ⅔ maximum weight
5. Twenty repetitions ⅓ maximum weight

This progression enables the individual to get complete extension with the lighter weight, provides a heavy resistance to increase strength, and provides many repetitions to increase endurance. Another exercise for the quadriceps is the leg press on the universal gym. Follow the same progression as with the iron boot. A third exercise for the quadriceps is the knee bend with weights across the shoulders. To protect the knee from hyperflexion, a bench is used to stop the buttocks as the upper legs become parallel to the floor. The same progression as the iron boot can be utilized by changing the amount of weight held across the shoulders. A fourth exercise for the quadriceps can be accomplished by fixing the feet at one end and coming to an erect position by contracting the quadriceps. Start with ten repetitions and increase each workout. Another exercise for the quadriceps can be done without any equipment. Stand against the wall in a squatting position and slowly push up and back, taking about 8 seconds to complete a repetition. Start with ten repetitions and increase to three sets of ten repetitions.

To exercise the hamstrings, pulley weights can be used in a prone position, flexing the lower leg. Use the same progression as with the iron boot. To exercise the calf muscles, place the front part of the foot on a board 2 inches thick, holding a weight across the shoulders, and extend upward. To exercise the hip flexors, use an iron boot with weight and bring the knee up, flexing at the hip. The hip abductors can be exercised by lying on the side, stabilizing the pelvic girdle, pointing the toe, and lifting up. Resistance can be increased by wearing a heavier shoe. This may also be accomplished by using the pulley weights and lifting the leg sideward.

Isometrics are used to supplement the isotonic exercises. For the quadriceps, the individual attempts to extend his leg against a fixed object for 6 seconds. This can be repeated at different angles. For the hamstrings, the individual flexes the lower leg against a fixed object. Do these repetitions, 6 seconds each, at each angle.

This exercise program for the muscles that support the knee joint can be used for reconditioning after an injury has occurred and as a prophylactic means of preventing new knee injuries. By keeping the musculature strong, it is hoped that the knee will be better protected and able to sustain force without damage. Any conditioninng program should be conducted well in advance of the season. Once the season begins, the prevention of knee injuries depends on sound training and coaching methods, good equipment, game control, proper injury management, and good judgment.

Training. Sound training means that methods used to assist the players to improve ability to perform do not subject them to undue danger or harm. Proper warm-up before every game, practice, or workout is important to injury prevention. Warm-up should include stretching exercises to prevent muscle strains, agility drills to stimulate alertness and coordination, and interval training to maintain endurance. It is important to avoid practices that contribute to knee injuries, such as the duckwalk, which can actually damage structures of the knee joint; avoid contact too early in the season before players become conditioned; avoid contact after fatigue; and avoid unequal competition.

Taping. To this date there has been no brace, pad, or other mechanical gimmick designed that can prevent injuries to the knee. Taping the knee may be effective in preventing reinjury to the knee, provided the musculature is strong and the original injury is minor. Taping a knee to allow a recently injured player to continue playing with muscle atrophy or joint instability is strongly discouraged. If knee ligaments or cartilages have been torn, the knee should not be taped, and the athlete should not continue playing. An athlete who attempts to continue playing with a torn ligament or cartilage runs the risk of further damage to the knee or may decrease the chances for a good surgical repair.

Management. Proper injury management is often the key to a speedy and successful recovery from trauma. The original injury to a knee must be kept from becoming more serious. To be effective, injury management should include immediate care on the field, follow up care in the training room, medical examination, reconditioning, and evaluation before returning to activity. When a player receives a knee injury, it should be evaluated on the spot to determine the severity of the injury. If the injury is suspected to be serious, apply ice or cold packs and an elastic bandage for compression, and assist the player from the field. Remove the injured player from the field to the training room, physician's office, or hospital for more specific evaluation. After referral to the physician and medical care, be sure that the athlete is ready before he or she returns to active participation. Keep in mind that inactivity of the injured part results in atrophy and muscle weakness. This can be measured and evaluated. If there is muscle weakness, do not allow the athlete to return until strength is brought back to normal by reconditioning exercises.

It is difficult to foresee all the factors that cause or influence an injury to the knee. It may be true that knee injuries will always be a part of athletic activities, but the number and severity of knee injuries can be reduced through a comprehensive injury prevention program, including:
1. The elimination of individuals unfit for contact sports
2. Development of strength and endurance in the muscles that support the knee joint
3. Reconditioning of the musculature after injury or to correct poor posture
4. Sound training methods
5. Good control and good officiating
6. Modification of field and equipment
7. Proper injury management

Head injuries

Injuries to the head in athletic activities may range from minor contusions to severe cerebral concussions. The specific nature of these injuries and the appropriate first aid care is presented in Chapter 12. Since head injuries may result in permanent neurological impairment and even death, it is essential that preventive steps be taken by those supervising the activities as well as the participants. The procedures listed here should be followed to prevent head injuries:

1. If protective head gear is required in a sport, obtain the best equipment available on the market. Quality should not be sacrificed to save money.
2. Fit each player individually, and inspect equipment frequently to ensure a proper fit. For example, the suspension of a football helmet will sometimes loosen up so that the player's head comes in contact with the hard shell, eliminating the protection of the helmet.
3. Replace all worn-out or damaged head gear.
4. If a player comes out of a game or practice with a head injury, do not allow the player to return until he or she has been examined and cleared by a physician.
5. Screen participants for any history of head injuries, and eliminate those with questionable histories from contact sports. In a study conducted by Dickinson, the following statement indicates the importance of previous head injury history: "A significantly greater percentage (40%) of athletes injured during the 1966 football season had a history of previous concussive episodes than the expected frequency (10% to 20%) of athletes with prior histories that comprise an intact football squad. It would certainly appear that the young man who has sustained one cerebral concussion is more likely to sustain more. . . ."[4]

Neck injuries

Not all neck injuries are serious, but the potential for serious complications and even death resulting from an injury to the neck requires careful attention to this type of injury. The complex structures of the neck, including the spinal cord and spinal nerves, make it especially vulnerable to serious injury. The most common types of injuries to the neck include strains, sprains, and fractures. When examining an injured player for a neck injury, first check for the possibility of a fractured vertebra. Follow the first aid procedures presented in Chapter 12 for musculoskeletal injuries.

Before participation in contact sports such as football, wrestling, and soccer, participants should engage in exercises for the neck muscles to provide protection from injury. Coaches and physical education teachers should carefully examine sport skills and techniques for possible risk of neck injuries. For example, in football, spear tackling and blocking techniques using the head as a battering ram are dangerous practices and may lead to serious neck injuries. When such dangers are identified, they should be eliminated or altered to reduce the risk of injury. Establish ahead of time procedures to be followed if a serious neck injury does occur in a sport activity.

Heat injuries

A more detailed discussion of heat emergencies is presented in Chapter 14, but special reference is made in this chapter as to the importance of preventing heat injuries in sport activities.

Heat is a by-product of producing energy during physical activity. As the body temperature rises, the excess heat must be dispersed into the environment to regulate body temperature. The primary mode of temperature regulation during physical activity is usually by means of the sweating mechanism. The participant in sports activities may get into trouble with heat problems if the sweating is too excessive or if the body is unable to cope with high environmental temperatures. The three major types of heat injuries include heat cramps, heat exhaustion, and heat stroke. Specific signs, symptoms, and first aid procedures for each type are presented in Chapter 14.

Sports activity can be identified as a high-risk area for heat injuries because physical activity is often strenuous, and activities frequently take place in a hot or humid environment. On the other hand, since most sports activities are planned activities, it is possible to greatly reduce the risk of serious problems by applying proper precautions to prevent heat injuries.

Athletes should go through a conditioning program before the season and actual competition. The well-conditioned athlete is better able to cope with thermal stress. Practice should take place under conditions similar to actual conditions of competition. For example, if the first few football games of a season are to be played on hot September days, players should be exposed to working in a hot environment so that the body has an opportunity to become naturally adapted to heat. It is therefore essential to provide for gradual acclimation to hot-weather activity.

Restricted water intake during workouts may deplete sufficient water in the body. Water lost by perspiration should be replaced during exercise in the heat. It is dangerous to withhold water from athletes during physical activity, and there is no good reason to conduct such a practice. It is also hazardous and useless for players to use rubberized sweat suits or other clothing that prevents normal temperature regulation. The use of such devices should not be permitted in warm-environment sport activities.

The following suggestions are offered to help coaches prevent heat exhaustion and heat stroke during hot weather athletic activity:

- Require a careful medical history and checkup before the beginning of practice.
- Schedule workouts during cooler morning and early evening hours in hot weather.
- Acclimate athletes to hot-weather activity by carefully graduated practice schedules.
- Provide rest periods of 15 to 30 minutes during workouts of an hour or more in hot weather.
- Supply clothing that is white to reflect heat, comfortable to permit heat escape, and permeable to moisture to allow heat loss by sweat evaporation.
- Furnish extra salt and water in recommended amounts during hot weather.
- Watch athletes carefully for signs of trouble, particularly athletes who may not report discomfort.
- Remember that temperature and humidity are the crucial factors. Measuring the relative humidity by use of a sling psychrometer on the field is advantageous in this regard. Heat exhaustion and heat stroke can occur in the shade.
- Alert the hospital emergency room medical and nursing staff of the pos-

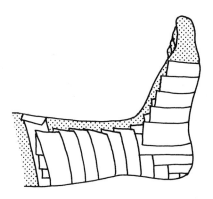

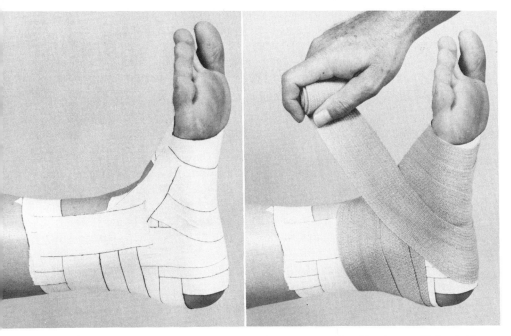

Fig. 17-6. Open basket weave tape procedure applied to sprained ankle. (From Klafs, C. E., and Arnheim, D. D.: Modern principles of athletic training—the science of injury prevention and care, ed. 4, St. Louis, 1977, The C. V. Mosby Co.)

sibility of heat illness among athletes before an emergency occurs so that they are prepared to care for a stricken athlete.

- Know what to do in case of such an emergency. Be familiar with immediate first aid practices and prearranged procedures for obtaining immediate medical care, including ambulance service.
- Outlaw the hazardous warm-weather use of rubberized apparel or other dehydration devices by players.[2]

Ankle injuries

One of the most common injuries in sport activities is a sprain to the ankle joint. The ankle joint, formed by the articulation of the tibia and fibula with the talus, is supported by the ligament structures. Ankle sprains result from a stretching and/or tearing of these ligaments, which is usually caused by forcing the joint beyond its normal range of motion. Most sprains will occur to the lateral side of the ankle as a result of the foot being forcefully turned inward.

Injury management for ankle sprains includes the first aid procedures outlined for sprains in Chapter 11. This includes application of ice, a pressure bandage, and elevation of the ankle. For ankle sprains, a special type of pressure bandage can be applied to give some support to the joint. The open basket weave (Fig. 17-6) is applied with strips of adhesive tape, leaving a gap in the front of the leg and foot to allow for swelling. An elastic bandage is applied over the open basket weave to help control swelling. The elastic bandage should not be kept on overnight. All ankle sprains should be referred to medical care to determine necessary treatment and to evaluate for possible fracture.

Dental injuries

Any injury to the teeth or supportive tissue should be referred to dental medical care. If a tooth is fractured or displaced, the tooth or fragment should be taken to the dentist along with the injured person. Mouth protectors have proved to be effective in preventing dental injuries and should be used in all contact sports or activities in which impact is possible. There are different types of mouth protectors; however, the custom-made and mouth-formed types are considered to provide better protection than the stock variety (not fitted to the individual mouth). Proper fit is important; therefore mouth protectors should be fitted under the supervision of a dentist.

ATHLETIC EMERGENCY PROCEDURE

For a number of years, the National Federation of State High School Associations and the AMA Committee on the Medical Aspects of Sports have recommended that a physician be present at all athletic games and readily available during practice sessions. However, with the many sports events at all levels, it is not always possible for a physician to be present. This necessitates clear-cut arrangements to reach immediately a designated physician or medical facility in case of emergency.

The five cardinal points to be stressed in successful emergency care, particularly when a physician cannot be present, are:

- *First aid* should be available at the scene with well-trained personnel to administer it.
- *A communication system.* A nonpay telephone with a direct outside line should be available at all times at the field or field facility so that a physician or ambulance may be called if necessary.
- *Quality emergency care facilities.* They should be available at the hospital level, including excellent staff and equipment.
- *Notification.* The facility to which the injured player is being transported should be informed of the player's condition as part of the emergency care so that necessary personnel and equipment will be available when the player arrives.
- *Transportation.* Well-equipped emergency vehicles should be available, staffed by emergency medical technicians equipped to provide all necessary life support at the scene and during transportation.

The plan of action just specified should be carefully worked out in advance with the responsibilities of all concerned—athletic trainer, coach, and others—precisely defined. When an emergency occurs, those involved can function as an informed and efficient team.

When there is a school physician or the community health department provides school health services, the medical people involved should share in the planning. Where no such arrangements exist, the school administration may approach the local medical profession through the county medical society or hospital staff.

The important thing is to have a clear understanding on the part of everyone—schools, allied medical personnel, and physicians—of exactly what will be done in emergencies and who is to be responsible for carrying out the various tasks involved. When this is the case, athletes and their parents will have assurance that everything will be done to protect the health and welfare of a player who may be injured.[2]

FIRST AIDER COMPETENCIES

After studying the material presented in this chapter, the student should be able to:
- Outline and explain procedures for the prevention of athletic injuries.
- Describe the examination procedures for an injured player and indicate what types of condition should be given highest priority.
- Outline the vicious cycle of injury, indicating the sequence of events, and explain the role of the first aider in regard to athletic injury management.
- List and explain steps that can be taken to attempt to prevent knee injuries in sports activities.
- Describe the emergency management procedures for knee injuries.
- List recommended procedures for preventing head injuries, neck injuries, heat injuries, and dental injuries in sports activities.
- Outline and explain the emergency management procedures for ankle injuries and dental injuries in sports activities.
- Develop a plan of action to establish responsibility and determine athletic emergency procedures for sports activities.

REFERENCES AND
RECOMMENDED READINGS

1. Abbott, H. G., et al.: Preconditioning in the prevention of knee injuries, Archives of Physical Medicine 50:326-333, 1969.
2. Craig, T. T., editor: Comments in sports medicine, Chicago, 1973, American Medical Association.
3. Craig, T. T., editor: Current sports medicine issues, Washington, D.C., 1974, American Association for Health, Physical Education, and Recreation.
4. Dickinson, A. L., and Schramel, J. E.: The incidence of graded cerebral concussions in intercollegiate football. In Proceedings of the Eighth National Conference on the Medical Aspects of Sports, Chicago, 1967, American Medical Association.
5. Earle, A. S.: Inflatable splint for ski injuries, Journal of the American Medical Association 192:1094-1096, 1965.
6. Evaluation of mouth protectors used by high school football players, Bureau of Dental Health Education and Bureau of Economic Research and Statistics, Journal of the American Dental Association 68:117-128, 1964.
7. Fundamentals of athletic training, Chicago, 1971, American Medical Association.
8. Klafs, C. E., and Arnheim, D. D.: Modern principles of athletic training, St. Louis, 1973, The C. V. Mosby Co.
9. Man, sweat and performance, Ruther, N.J., 1969, Becton Dickinson & Co.
10. Novich, M. M., and Taylor, B.: Training and conditioning of athletes, Philadelphia, 1970, Lea & Febiger.
11. Olson, O. C.: Prevention of football injuries, Philadelphia, 1971, Lea & Febiger.
12. Rawlinson, K. B.: General treatment rules: contusions, strains, sprains, Scholastic Coach, Sept., 1968.
13. Schneider, R. C., and Kriss, F. C.: Decisions concerning cerebral concussions in football players, Medicine and Science in Sports 1:112-115, June, 1969.
14. Snook, G. A.: Head and neck injuries in contact sports, Medicine and Science in Sports 1:117-123, Sept., 1969.
15. Sports safety, Washington, D.C., 1971, American Association of Health, Physical Education, and Recreation.

18

‸‸‸

BANDAGING TECHNIQUES

Guy S. Parcel

Bandaging is a basic first aid skill used in emergencies involving trauma. Wounds, burns, and musculoskeletal injuries usually require bandaging as one of the first aid procedures.

Bandages have two basic functions: (1) to hold a dressing in place or (2) to immobilize or support a body part. Material that is soft and pliable can be used as a bandage. Almost any technique for application is satisfactory provided the bandage performs its intended function and does not cause any additional harm. Every bandage must be checked to be sure that it is not cutting off the normal circulation of blood, does not interfere with breathing, and does not cause pain or excessive pressure. Especially with injuries or burns involving swelling, it is important to continuously check bandages to make sure that they are not becoming too tight.

DRESSINGS

A bandage should never come in direct contact with a wound or burn. Dressings are used to perform the functions of controlling hemorrhaging and protecting wounds and burns. Because of the possibility of infection, a dressing should be sterile (free from germs). Some methods for improvising a sterile dressing are discussed in Chapter 7. However, in most cases it is better to leave the wound or burn open until a commercially prepared sterile dressing can be obtained. The exception, of course, is in the case of serious bleeding when the stoppage of hemorrhaging has priority over preventing contamination.

There are several different types and sizes of commercial sterile dressings. Most are made of gauze and are wrapped in sealed paper to maintain sterility. Some have a special coating to keep them from sticking. These are especially helpful for burns or wounds secreting fluids. A special type of dressing is kept moist in its package. This type is good to place on abdominal wounds with exposed intestines. The dressing should be large enough to extend an inch or more beyond the edges of the wound. When removing the dressing from its package, be careful not to contaminate it before applying it to the wound. Grasp it by a corner and carefully place it over the wound, keeping it from touching anything else. If it slips or falls, throw it away and use another dressing.

A compress is a special dressing that is attached to a bandage. A Band-Aid is an example of a compress. The gauze pad serves as a dressing and the adhesive tape as a bandage. Larger compresses are available that use gauze or cloth for bandages. Never use fluff cotton or cotton balls as a dressing because the fibers can get embedded in the wound and can be difficult to remove.

TYPES OF BANDAGES

Several different types of bandages are prepared commercially. Adhesive tape usually comes in rolls and in a variety of widths. It can be cut to almost any size to meet particular needs. It is best applied directly to the skin because it sometimes slips when applied over clothing or other material. Special caution must be taken when wrapping tape completely around a body part because it is easy to get it too tight and cut off circulation. Roller bandages are made of gauze or other cloth material and come in a roll in a variety of widths. Some roller bandages are elastic and can be used as compression bandages for sprains, strains, and contusions. Because of the elasticity, it is extremely important to make sure that the elastic bandage is not cutting off circulation. A triangular bandage is made of cloth (usually cotton) and is usually large enough to be adapted for use on almost any part of the body.

APPLICATION OF BANDAGES

If commercial bandages are available, they can facilitate the application of bandages. However, the improvisation of bandages is usually easy, and almost any cloth material can function just as well as commercial bandages. Shirts, handkerchiefs, slips, towels, sheets, pillowcases, napkins, ties, and scarves are but a few examples of readily available material that can be used for a bandage.

Performing the intended function (holding a dressing or supporting a body part) and not causing additional harm are the most important considerations. The type of knot tied and the neatness and attractiveness of the bandage are less important. Most texts suggest a square knot be tied to secure a bandage, but unless time is not a factor, the type of knot is not really important. Be careful of where a knot is tied. Avoid tying a knot directly over an area that would cause pain or pressure on a nerve, compress a blood vessel, or rub against bare skin. When applying a bandage to the extremities, leave the fingers or toes exposed. Watch for swelling, change in color, coldness or loss of feeling, or tingling in the toes or fingers. Loosen any bandage that appears to be too tight.

Roller bandages

When using a roller bandage, first select the appropriate size. Fig. 18-1 shows the correct way to hold the roller bandage for application. This position allows the first aider to let the bandage roll off the roll while maintaining a secure grip. Fig. 18-2 shows the technique for securing the first loop of a roller bandage. Make a loop leaving a corner exposed, and fold the corner over, covering it with the second loop. Circular loops can be made with the roller bandage on body parts that are even in size, as shown on the bandage applied to the hand in Fig. 18-2.

On joint areas a figure-eight pattern can be used to apply a roller bandage. As shown in Fig. 18-3, the roller bandage is looped around the foot and passed across the instep and around the back of the ankle. The bandage is moved for-

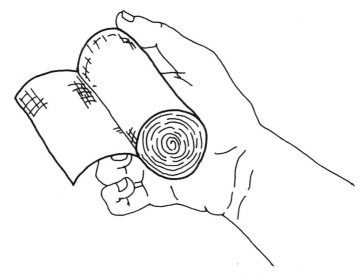

Fig. 18-1. Position for applying roller bandage.

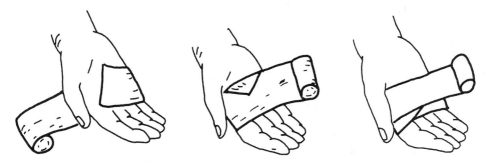

Fig. 18-2. Roller bandage applied to hand.

ward across the instep and then under the foot, forming a figure-eight pattern. By repeating the figure-eight pattern the foot and ankle can be covered to support a dressing, support the joint, or to apply a compression bandage.

Body surfaces that increase in size make it difficult to use circular loops. Spiral loops make it easier to apply the roller bandage and keep it from slipping. As shown in Fig. 18-4, the roller bandage is applied by angling the loops in a spiral fashion, overlapping about a third of the width of the bandage.

With a little ingenuity, roller bandages can be applied to almost any body area. In Fig. 18-5, a roller bandage is applied to cover the entire top of the head. Several loops are made around the head, and then the bandage is folded at a right angle and passed across the center of the head. Each subsequent fold is lightly angled and overlaps the previous fold. Finally, the bandage is passed around the head and tied to hold the folds in place.

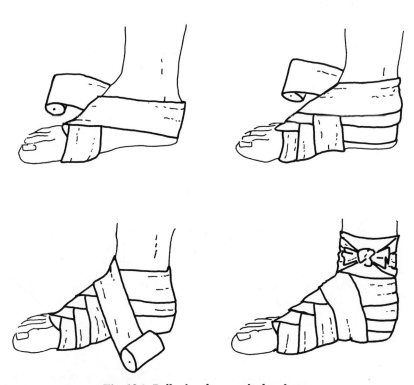

Fig. 18-3. Roller bandage applied to foot.

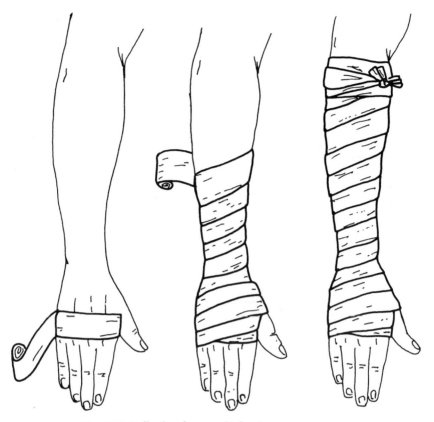

Fig. 18-4. Roller bandage applied to lower arm.

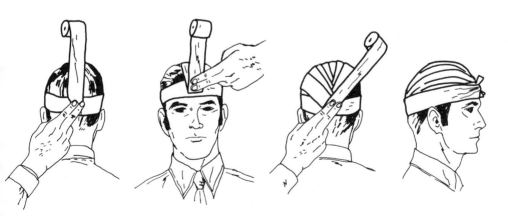

Fig. 18-5. Roller bandage applied to head.

Triangular bandages

One of the most useful bandages used in first aid is the triangular bandage. It is especially helpful for covering entire body parts and larger surfaces. Fig. 18-6 shows a triangular bandage applied to a hand. The hand is placed in the lower third of the bandage with the fingers pointing toward the point and the wrist located toward the base. The point is folded over the top of the hand, and the two tails are looped in opposite directions and tied around the wrist. A triangular bandage can be applied in a similar manner to a foot.

To apply a triangular bandage to the head (Fig. 18-7), make one fold of approximately 2 inches at the base and place the bandage over the head with the point resting in back. The two tails are passed around the head, crossed in back by the neck, brought forward, and tied at the forehead. The point hanging down in the back can be pulled up and tucked under the two tails. This type of bandage can be used to hold a large dressing in place, but it may not be possible to get the top area firm enough to secure a small dressing.

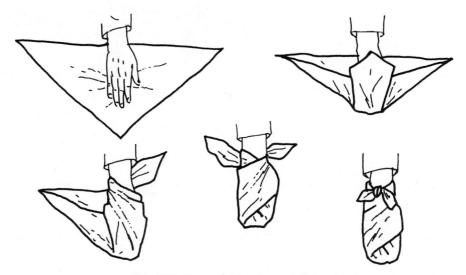

Fig. 18-6. Triangular bandage applied to hand.

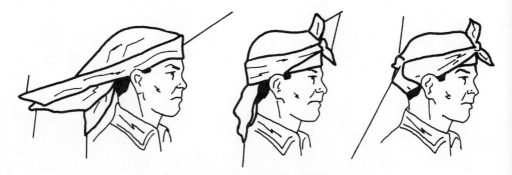

Fig. 18-7. Triangular bandage applied to head.

An arm sling is used for a variety of injuries: immobilization for fractures, strains, sprains, or subluxations, or elevation for a wound in the hand or lower arm. A triangular bandage provides an effective means of applying an arm sling. Placement of the bandage is shown in Fig. 18-8. The point is extended beyond the elbow and one tail placed over the opposite shoulder. The tail extended below the arm is lifted up over the arm, behind the neck, and tied to the other tail. The knot should be tied to the side of the neck so that it does not put any pressure on nerves or blood vessels. The tail of the bandage can be folded over and pinned or tied in a knot to prevent the elbow from slipping out of the sling.

The fingers should be exposed beyond the edge of the sling so that circulation can be monitored. The arm should be kept in a horizontal position unless it is painful in that position or the arm needs to be elevated to assist with the control of bleeding. If the arm is allowed to hang down for long periods of time, it may become uncomfortable because of increased blood pressure. There usually is no need to rush when applying a sling. Be careful to limit the movement of the injured part and protect it from any additional harm or pain.

Cravat bandages

The many possible uses for a triangular bandage can be extended by folding it into a cravat bandage. This is accomplished by folding the point to the mid-

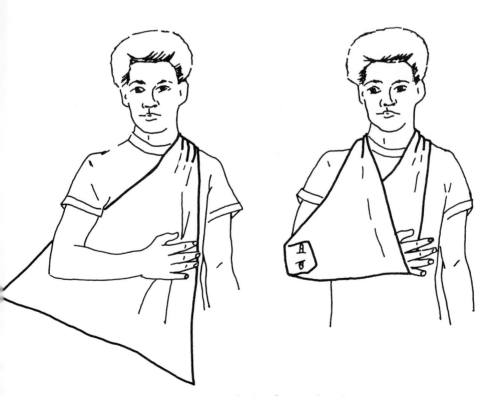

Fig. 18-8. Triangular bandage used as sling.

point of the base as shown in Fig. 18-9, *A*. Continue to fold (Fig. 18-9, *B*) until the desired width is obtained.

Fig. 18-10 illustrates the application of a cravat bandage to the lower leg. The area is uneven; therefore the first loop of the bandage is applied at an angle. One end of the bandage is wrapped upward and the other down the leg. After the desired area is covered, the ends are wrapped forward across the bandage and tied together over the central part of the bandage. A similar procedure can be used to apply a cravat to an elbow (Fig. 18-11). This type of bandage can be used to hold a dressing in place as well as to help support the joint.

Application of a cravat to the hand to hold a dressing or support the wrist requires a figure-eight wrap (Fig. 18-12). The bandage is first placed across the palm of the hand. One end is wrapped under the hand angled toward the wrist, wrapped over the wrist on the little finger side, and across to the other side of the hand. The other end is wrapped in a similar manner going across the wrist on the thumb side. This procedure is repeated a second time, making a figure-eight pattern. The final step is to tie the two ends together around the wrist.

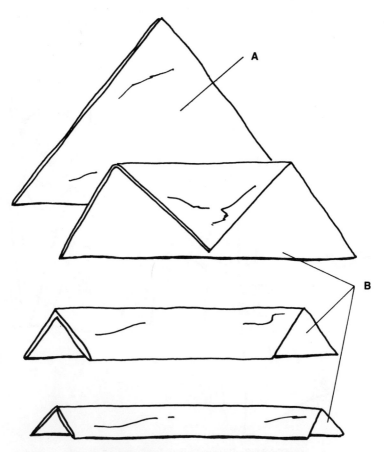

Fig. 18-9. Procedures for making cravat bandage.

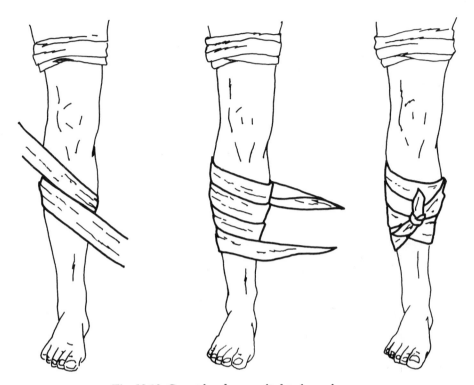

Fig. 18-10. Cravat bandage applied to lower leg.

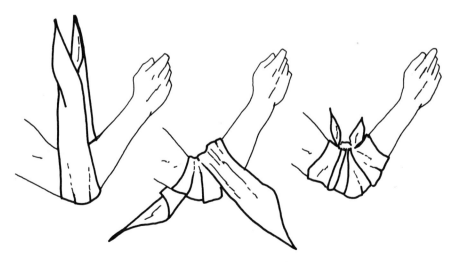

Fig. 18-11. Cravat bandage applied to elbow.

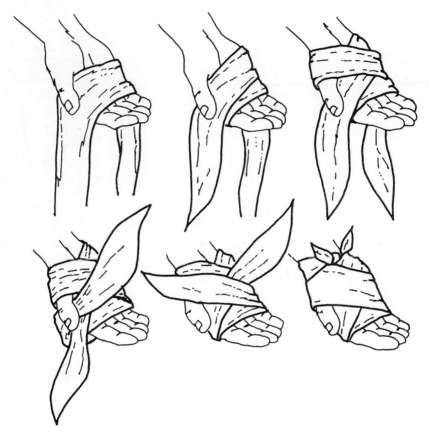

Fig. 18-12. Cravat bandage applied to hand.

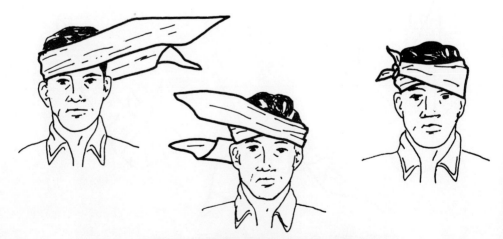

Fig. 18-13. Cravat bandage applied to head.

Except for the top part of the scalp, a cravat bandage is easily applied to hold a dressing on the head (Fig. 18-13). Fold the cravat to the desired width, wrap around twice, and tie in place. A long cravat can be adapted to support the lower jaw or to hold a dressing in place on the side of the head or lower jaw area (Fig. 18-14). Place the cravat under the jaw with one end longer than the other. Wrap over the top front of the head and across the two ends at about the position of the temple area. Wrap the ends in opposite directions around the head and tie on the opposite side. The knot should be a bow or slip knot so that the patient can quickly untie the bandage in case of vomiting or coughing up material. The patient should be shown where the knot is and how to release it.

Cravats can also be applied to large body parts as shown in Fig. 18-15. A large cravat is applied to the shoulder by making a loop under the armpit, crossing the two ends over the shoulder, wrapping one end under the opposite armpit, and tying across the chest. A similar procedure can be used to apply a cravat to a hip area. Wide cravats can be used for chest and rib injuries. When applying a cravat around the chest, tie the bandage at the end of an exhalation. If tied when the chest is expanded, it may slip loose when the patient exhales.

Dressings covering the eyes can be effectively held in place with a cravat bandage (Fig. 18-16). To protect the injured eye, it is a good procedure to also cover the other eye. This will help to restrict eye movement and possible further damage. The bandage should be tied loosely to prevent any pressure on the eyes. Tie to the side of the head and never directly over the eye.

Combinations of cravat and triangular bandages can be utilized to cover more difficult areas. Fig. 18-17 illustrates a triangular bandage tied to a cravat to cover a shoulder area. The cravat is tied around the neck and armpit on the opposite side. The point of the triangular bandage is wrapped around the cravat.

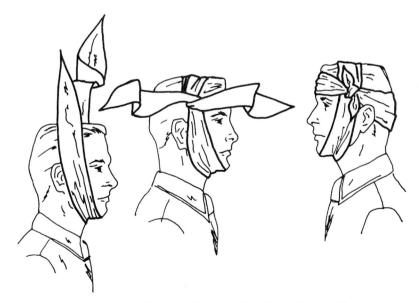

Fig. 18-14. Cravat bandage used for facial injuries or fractured lower jaw.

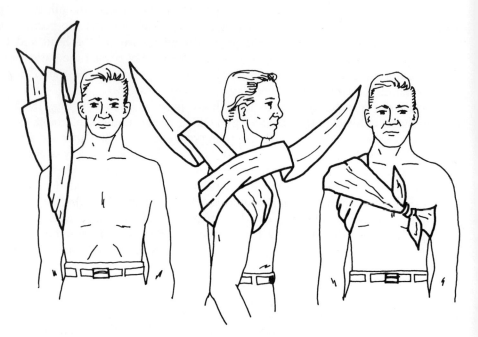

Fig. 18-15. Cravat bandage applied to shoulder.

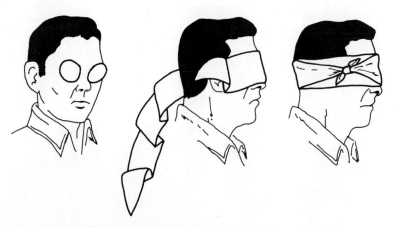

Fig. 18-16. Cravat bandage used to hold dressings over eyes.

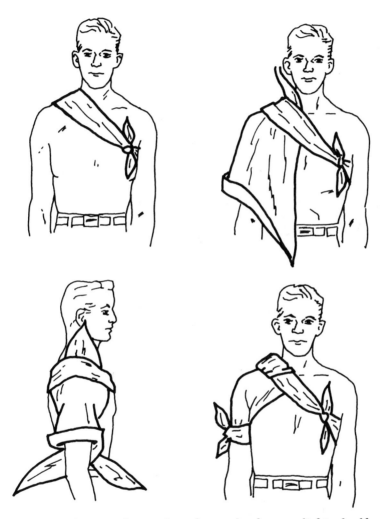

Fig. 18-17. Combination of triangular and cravat bandages applied to shoulder.

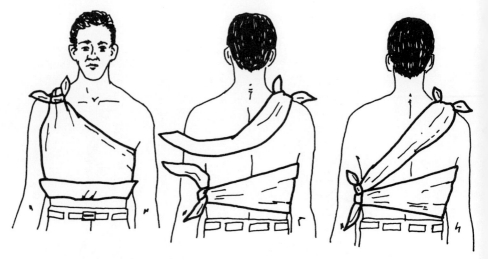

Fig. 18-18. Combination of triangular and cravat bandages applied to chest.

The ends are wrapped around the arm and tied in place. In Fig. 18-18, a triangular bandage to cover the chest is held in place by tying a cravat to the point, with the two ends tied together around the trunk.

SUMMARY

The bandaging procedures for specific body parts were selected to illustrate the application of bandaging techniques. Numerous additional types of procedures can be devised to meet specific injury problems. The three types of bandages are roller, triangular, and cravat. The basic wrapping techniques are circular, spiral, and figure-eight. An almost endless number of bandages can be applied using various combinations of types of bandages and wrapping techniques. The important criteria are that the bandage performs its functions and does not cause any additional harm or discomfort. Practicing bandaging techniques will develop the skills and confidence that will make things go smoothly in an actual emergency.

FIRST AIDER COMPETENCIES

After studying the material and practicing the techniques presented in this chapter, the student should be able to:
- Differentiate between the functions of bandages and dressings.
- Explain the criteria for acceptable bandaging techniques.
- Demonstrate the application of roller, triangular, and cravat bandages to hold dressings in place and to immobilize or support body parts.

19

▼▲▼

TRANSPORTATION AND EXTRICATION TECHNIQUES

Guy S. Parcel

Emergency care efforts to move the injured or ill should be carefully planned and executed so that transportation and extrication techniques will contribute to their well-being and not cause additional or unnecessary harm.

One of the most common errors made during an emergency situation is the unnecessary or dangerous movement of an injured or ill patient. During an emergency there is often an almost overwhelming drive to move people as soon as possible without thinking and taking time to survey the situation. Unfortunately, the result is often additional pain and harm to the patient and sometimes even death. The purpose of this chapter is to prepare the first aider to plan and carry out effective emergency care procedures involving the movement of individuals experiencing sudden illness or injury.

TRANSPORTATION

Transportation, in the broadest terms, involves all action taken to move individuals from the present location of an accident or illness to appropriate medical facilities to obtain treatment and follow-up care. The involvement of the first aider in this process is limited to three general activities: (1) making arrangements for professional ambulance or rescue personnel to transport patients, (2) assisting professional personnel with transportation procedures, and (3) carrying out transportation procedures when professional services cannot be obtained and it is necessary to move patients to protect them from immediate danger to their lives. The following general procedures should be applied when transportation becomes a necessary part of emergency care:

1. Plan exactly what has to be done before any action is taken. Call for a professional ambulance or rescue personnel. Obtain any special equipment needed to carry out the transportation procedures.
2. Administer all necessary first aid needed to stabilize the patient's condition.
3. Carry out the transportation procedures in an orderly and unhurried manner so as not to cause further harm or aggravation of the patient's condition.

Unassisted transportation techniques

The first set of transport problems to be discussed will deal with those patients who are not seriously injured. Examples of such injuries are moderate sprains, wounds in which the bleeding has been brought under control, moderate burns that present no immediate life hazard, fainting, heat exhaustion, and similar cases.

Walking assist. The most elementary form of transport is the walking assist (Fig. 19-1). In this procedure, part of the patient's weight burden is assumed by the first aider. The patient's arm is placed across the back or waist, depending on what is most advantageous at the time. The key to the effectiveness of this procedure is not to impose any added forces or strains on the injured part but rather to give the injured person a sort of walking crutch. Do not pull or tug at the patient's arm across your shoulders, since this may be a source of discomfort to the patient.

Fireman's carry. This carry is useful for moving a person rapidly from a hazardous environment, such as fire. An advantage of this carry is that it leaves

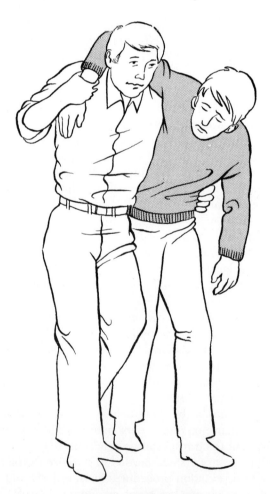

Fig. 19-1. Walking assist.

one arm free while you are in the process of moving with the patient (Fig. 19-2).

1. Kneeling at the head of the patient, place your hands under the arms and on the sides of the patient.
2. Raise the patient to an upright position.
3. Bend at the waist and hoist the patient across your back and shoulders.
4. Center the patient.
5. Bring one arm around the legs of the patient.
6. Secure the arm of the patient by grasping it with the arm that you brought around the legs.

This carry was developed for rapid transport of the injured from hazardous situations. It should not be used on patients who have serious injuries, particularly those of an abdominal nature, unless it is absolutely necessary.

Packstrap carry. Possibly the most useful all-around carry is the packstrap

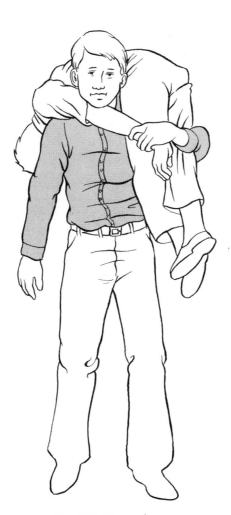

Fig. 19-2. Fireman's carry.

carry (Fig. 19-3), which is especially effective because tension is maintained along the vertical axis of the body. This cannot be done with the fireman's carry or the walking assist. The steps for the packstrap carry are as follows:

1. Place your body parallel to that of the patient.
2. Pull the patient's arms across your body so that they cross. The forearms are parallel as they lie across your chest.
3. Pull the patient up off the ground and on your shoulders, and then inward close to you.
4. If the patient is on the ground, come to your knees and balance the patient, then rise to your feet and walk.
5. If the patient is already standing up, then simply raise the body high enough so that the patient's feet clear the ground and then proceed toward your destination.

Saddleback carry. An alternative to the fireman's carry that is especially useful when involving removal from bodies of water such as pools or at the beach is the saddleback carry (Fig. 19-4). This carry is strongly advised when a large differential exists between the strength of the transporter and the weight of the patient. The carry works because the center of gravity of the patient lies in the

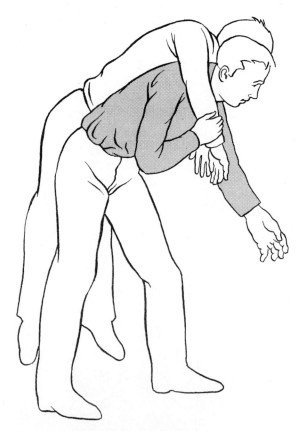

Fig. 19-3. Packstrap carry.

low of the back, resting on the buttocks. This removes most of the strain of carry from the muscles, letting the patient rest passively. It is performed as follows:

1. Stand perpendicular to the patient.
2. Bring the patient to the level of your hips.
3. Slip your arm under one shoulder of the patient as you bring one of the patient's arms across your neck.
4. With your other hand, grasp the bottom thigh near the knee.
5. Ease the patient onto your lower back and pull toward you. The body may be balanced to provide the most comfort for both of you.

Blanket drag. The last of the unassisted carries is the blanket drag (Fig. 19-5), which is valuable because it maintains a constant pull along the long axis of the body and helps prevent the movement of possibly fractured bones. In addition to blankets, small rugs, sheets, bedspreads, coats, or other apparel may be used to move the patient. The drag is a simple and easily applied technique. A firm grasp of the material being used is made at the head end of the patient, and a slow tension is exerted on the material to prevent jerking the patient in any way. Then simply drag the patient to a safe place.

All of these techniques can be performed by one person to move a patient.

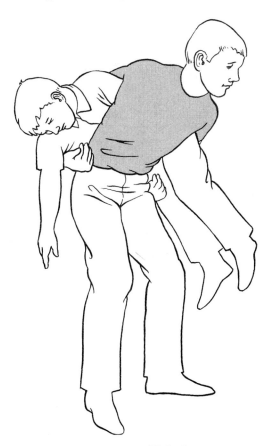

Fig. 19-4. Saddleback carry.

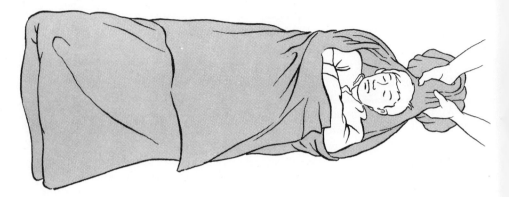

Fig. 19-5. Blanket drag.

However, none of these carries are intended to be used for severely injured individuals.

Assisted transportation techniques

Any type of transport of patients involving more than one person must first begin with a variety of lift. The lift is used to position the patient in such a way that a litter of some sort may be used, or so that the patient may be repositioned so that one of the nonlitter multiperson carries may be used. The key problems of lift are coordination and teamwork. An improper lift can do severe damage to a patient, particularly when spinal injuries involve serious fractures. Improper lifting may also cause low-back injury and muscle strain to the individual doing the lifting.

The best way to avoid undesirable occurrences is to remember the following three steps: preparation, position, and smooth execution.

1. *Preparation.* Analyze exactly what must be accomplished and what is the best way to do it. Are there sufficient personnel to move the patient based on his or her height and weight? Are the injuries incurred properly cared for? Is the area that you are working in cleared of any obstacles and extraneous observers that could interfere with your movement once you have begun? Is the litter properly prepared for the patient, and is it secure in its present position? If a positive answer is obtained for all of these questions, then proceed to step 2.

2. *Position.* After everyone involved with the lift has been instructed in what to do, they should take their respective places in relation to their functions. Special care must be taken to ensure that all injured parts are given proper support when moved. The litter should be placed as close to the patient as possible to minimize the distance of the move.

3. *Smooth execution.* All movements should be smooth and fluid. Jerky and unsure motions can only add to a patient's anxiety and may increase the danger of traumatic shock. Damage to surrounding tissue from musculoskeletal injuries may be increased if the handling is rough. The best way to achieve the capability of smooth execution is through constant practice as a team with one person

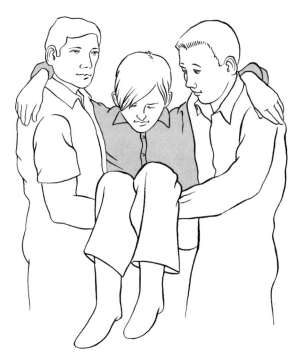

Fig. 19-6. Two-man carry.

designated as the squad leader. This individual assumes the responsibility for cueing all the other members of the team in their movements.

A standard practice is to count a cadence to initiate the lift or movement. A simple and effective cadence would be, *"Ready, one, two, three, lift."* An alternative and shorter cadence might be, *"Prepare to lift, lift."* In either case it is important to remember that all those who are involved in the operation must know fully what is expected of them and when to perform their stated tasks. The number of people involved with a lift may vary from two to five. The optimal number is four. This permits one person to be responsible for a major quadrant of the body, that is, the legs, hips, chest, and the head. Most of the lifting force should be applied at the region bordered by the hips and torso, since this is where most of the patient's weight is likely to be found.

The *safe* way to lift an object is with the lifter's back straight and the main lifting thrust emanating from the strong muscles of the upper leg. This is true regardless of how you are lifting a patient—singly, in a group, or using an appliance such as a stretcher. There usually is no need for a first aider to ever have back strain from lifting a patient. If the patient cannot be lifted properly with the personnel available, then additional help is indicated.

Two-man carry. The two-man carry (Fig. 19-6) is used with a patient who is conscious and is able to cooperate in some way with the rescuers. The key to the carry lies with the formation of a seat by the carriers. It is formed by crossing hands and using an interlocking grip about the wrists. The patient sits in the seat that is formed and places his arms around the necks of the carriers. It is not designed to be used with anyone displaying signs of serious injuries.

Four-man lift and carry. The four-man lift and carry is designed for short-distance transport when there are injuries that require constant support and extremely gentle care.

1. All those participating form a line on the same side of the patient. This facilitates forward motion and makes turns relatively simple to execute.
2. The rescuers come down to their knees.
3. Hands are slid under the patient. Each team member takes a major portion of the body, giving special consideration to the injuries in question.
4. At the command of the person previously designated as the leader of the team, the patient is brought to the level of the waist of the team members.
5. A check is made to be sure that the support is proper and uniform over the patient's body.
6. After the command is given, the team will stand up completely.
7. All movements should be smooth and coordinated. The decisions to stop, turn, or change speed should be given only by the group leader. If the patient is to be carried any distance or if travel is over rugged terrain, then a stretcher or stretcher substitute should be prepared.

Litters

The safest way to transport a patient with an injury is on some variety of litter. Litters are designed with specific uses in mind. For spinal injuries the use of either a backboard or orthopedic stretcher is recommended. For narrow, confined spaces such as an elevator or a tight, winding staircase, a chair or Washington (chairlike) stretcher is indicated. When patients must be moved from hard-to-reach places such as mountainsides, caves, pits, or from the tops of multistory buildings, then a Stokes or navy basket litter is required. The cot-style ambulance litter is a common type due to its versatility and the comfort it affords the patient in most cases. It may be raised or lowered vertically to the level of the patient, making transfer of the patient easy. Both ends of the litter may be raised; the upper (head) end is raised to help relieve some of the stress of heart conditions and gives comfort for certain head and chest injuries.

Possibly the litter most commonly found on the scene of most emergencies is the army litter. It consists of two poles with a pliable material, such as canvas, attached. It is easily stored in either a folded or rolled position, depending on the style. The folded model has the added feature of two collapsible bars at the foot and head ends of the litter, which give increased rigidity to the litter and allow for less patient movement. Because of its compactness and durability, it is commonly found at the scene of large-scale disasters, since quantities are stored in emergency supply facilities.

The army litter is one of the easiest types to improvise; two stout poles, of sufficient length in relation to the patient, and a blanket may be handily folded into a litter (Fig. 19-7). This may be done in two ways. One method is to place each pole at the edge of the blanket and to roll the blanket around the pole several times. The weight of the patient against the poles will tighten the grip of the

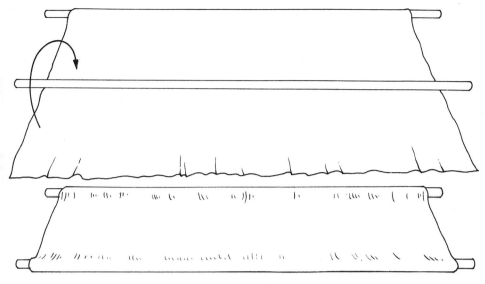

Fig. 19-7. Pole-and-blanket stretcher.

cloth around the surface of the pole and secure it. An alternative to the rolling method is to fold the blanket over the poles so that the patient will lie on the overlapping folds and make it snug. Each method is equally effective, the choice being governed by the situation presented at the time.

If there is no quantity of fabric available, shirts or jackets may be substituted. Usually two or three will be required along with the poles. Fasteners, such as buttons and zippers, should be secured so that the poles are held together. This form of improvised litter is possibly the one kind that can be made under the most primitive of conditions.

If a situation should arise in which two poles or similar substitutes should not be present, just a blanket or suitable material may be placed under the patient and used to transport him. It will, however, require a minimum of four individuals to perform the task. After a blanket has been placed under the patient, the persons performing the transport roll the edge of the blanket toward the patient. After it is rolled about 2 inches from the body of the patient, it is slowly pulled outward to remove any slack that could jar the patient on lifting. After the slack has been removed, then the lifting procedures may be carried out.

The problem of orthopedic injuries, particularly those of the vertebral column, deserves special discussion, since their handling is of critical importance to the future health and recovery of the patient. The traditional appliance for transport has always been a fracture or back board (Fig. 19-8). It is a rigid wood surface that is reinforced to prevent any bending or twisting of the patient. Along the edges of the board are handholds and fittings for straps to secure the injured to the board. The unfortunate aspects of the fracture board are twofold: first, the patient must be raised off the ground so the board may be placed underneath. As a result, a minimum of six people are required to perform the task. The need for so many personnel may yield the device ineffective under many circumstances. Even if the

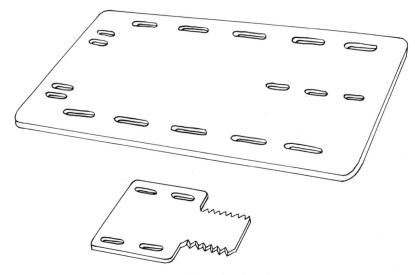

Fig. 19-8. Backboard and neckboard.

number of personnel is satisfactory, the act of lifting may cause the very injury that you are trying to prevent.

To eliminate the need for the movement of the patient and also reduce the manpower requirements, it is preferable to use an orthopedic stretcher. It functions by splitting in half longitudinally. Each half may be adjusted for the height of the patient. They are then placed under the injured patient on each side of the body and connected by means of two threaded knobs at the head and foot of the patient. The effect is similar to that of a clamshell scoop. The head is supported by means of a pliable material that is connected to one of the halves of the unit and may be adjusted to fit the desired width. It is usually secured by Velcro closures. The straps for holding the patient onto the litter are also found in a pouch contained within the head support. Only two people are required for the placing, lifting, and carrying of a patient on this type of stretcher.

In areas where the terrain is rough or where a patient must be first extricated from a height or depth at which there are no convenient ways of removal, a Stokes basket (Fig. 19-9) is almost always necessary. This unit consists of a metal frame over which a wire mesh, like chicken wire, is fitted. The advantage of the Stokes over other litters under the described conditions is that due to its strength, it may be raised or lowered by rope or cable without any other support equipment if necessary. Once the patient is properly strapped in, the stretcher and the patient become one unit. Even if the unit should twist or be upended, the patient is secure. This property makes it useful for both cave and mountain rescues. Recent developments in the manufacturing process have resulted in a new type of Stokes that is constructed of fiberglass or plastic. An advantage to this is the elimination of any corrosion problem and the elimination of any danger from charged electrical apparatus. In most instances, the use of a Stokes will be accompanied by the need for some type of rescue operations. As a result, the Stokes is not usually found

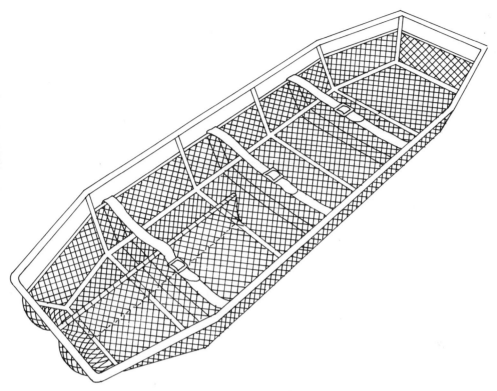

Fig. 19-9. Stokes basket.

in many locations; it is frequently brought by fire companies, ambulances, or rescue squads when they respond to a call.

Another type of litter that is not usually readily available under most conditions, but is very useful, is the chair or stair litter. The chair litter consists of a foldable rigid frame. Frequently, it will have wheels on it so that it may double as a wheelchair. On narrow or exceptionally angled staircases, an ordinary straight litter cannot be used. Under these circumstances the patient is seated in the chair and securely strapped. He may then be rolled or carried down the stairway with the greatest degree of comfort for him and ease for the people doing the transporting. If conditions warrant, a half back board may be used in conjunction with the chair litter.

It is possible to improvise substitutes for the orthopedic and chair stretchers. The main requirements for the orthopedic stretcher are flatness and rigidity. Some possibilities include doors, surfboards, benches, ladders, boards, and window shutters. In some cases padding and straps will be needed to secure the patient. For a chair litter, a rigid straight-backed chair is the logical substitute. Do not use a plush or soft chair, since they afford little or poor support and are usually bulky and hard to manage. Do not let the arms of the transportee dangle. Arms should be secured at the waist with the aid of available materials.

As a rule, the transportation of a patient by one of the devices previously discussed will require more than one person. This means that certain problems result when a carrying team is faced by obstacles, doorways, or staircases. There are a few general guidelines that may be of some help. First, make a survey of the ground that has to be covered and familiarize yourself with it. Where are there depressions that may cause tripping or injury to you? After this has been done, remove any of the obstacles that you are able to move. These would be items such as furniture, rugs, or tools or implements that may be scattered about outside. Plan ahead for impediments that cannot be moved. If the route to be traveled is a long or tedious one, or if the patient is extremely heavy, then plan where you will want to rest and/or change carrying positions.

EXTRICATION

The removal of an injured person from a confined environment often requires specialized equipment and training. The first aider should make all possible efforts to obtain the services of professional rescue personnel.

A knowledge of extrication procedures has become essential so that lifesaving aid may be given to victims of accidents that involve entrapment in automobile wreckage or other structures. Often the delay in waiting for trained rescue crews would be more than the injured person or persons could tolerate. Many lives can be saved, injuries reduced, and fears and anxieties relieved by all concerned if the first aider can gain safe access to the victims of accidents and provide needed care while awaiting the arrival of fire department, police, and rescue squad personnel. Extrication involves:

1. Gaining safe entry to the person(s)
2. Giving lifesaving emergency care
3. Disentanglement
4. Preparation for removal
5. Actual removal

Objectives of rescue

The first objective of the first aider in a situation involving rescue and extrication must be to *gain access* to the patient in a manner not only safe to the injured persons but safe to the first aider as well. Gaining such access may involve the removal of windows with a knife, in which the rubber molding is cut and the window removed; smashing of glass, using caution not to cut those inside or outside the car by covering the patients with a blanket beforehand; or removal of a door. In each instance, it is important that the first aider keep a calm and clear head and critically analyze the situation quickly but effectively to determine the quickest, safest, and most effective way to reach the injured, given existing equipment, experience, and circumstances.

Once access has been gained, the next objective of rescue is to give whatever *emergency care* is needed and can be given under existing circumstances. External bleeding must be stopped quickly or internal bleeding recognized by shocklike and other symptoms, with effective care given immediately. An open airway must be obtained and resuscitation provided for injured patients who are not breathing or are breathing inadequately. Unfortunately, cardiopulmonary resuscitation is not effectively performed in an automobile. After emergency care has been given, more general care can be given after a careful examination. This would include the splinting of fractures, not to mention other procedures such as emotional care which will be vital in almost every situation, and should always be provided to the best of the first aider's abilities.

The third step in effective rescue and extrication is the *disentanglement* of individuals from any material that is restraining them. This may involve the cutting of metal impaled within the patient's body or cutting a seat belt that has become defective in the accident and is restraining the patient. In more involved situations it may be necessary or advisable for the first aider to wait for the arrival of more trained personnel for this step. For example, sometimes only a rescue squad will have the equipment for this procedure, or a surgeon may have to be summoned to the scene in rare instances for emergency surgical amputation to free the victim from entanglement. Again, common sense and logical thinking as well as wise use of available knowledge and tools on the first aider's part will go a long way in helping such individuals.

Once disentanglement has been accomplished, the fourth step of rescue, *preparation for safe removal,* becomes of primary concern. This involves making sure the patients are properly packaged—bandaged, splinted, and all necessary care given so that movement will not endanger their life or cause additional harm. The most appropriate means for removal must be investigated. This may involve an exit different from the entrance that the first aider used in gaining access to the injured. This step may involve the removal of windows, doors, or seats, or waiting for the arrival of a rescue squad to remove the automobile's roof or other structures in automobile accidents. In a swimming pool, this step implies that before removal, a spine board, surfboard, or other such object has been obtained and placed under the patient with a possible spinal cord injury.

The fifth and last step in emergency rescue and extrication is to *remove the injured in a safe and deliberate manner.* This step does not represent a race unless serious injuries or complications threaten life, and thus it must be done quickly but as carefully and safely as possible. Once again, common tools that a first aider may have in an automobile tool kit or in a car, such as a hacksaw, screwdriver, or crowbar, can be used effectively in providing a safe and efficient exit for the patient's removal. The importance of a good pair of scissors cannot be overemphasized. An object such as an ordinary wrench or crowbar can be effectively used to smash glass, using caution not to cut those inside the car or oneself. Unfortunately, a crowbar is rarely effective in prying open a smashed-in door. When many people are available, rescue should represent a team effort, using each one's best talents and knowing what each is doing to provide an effective coordinated effort and avoid injuries and wasted efforts.

Additional suggestions

On arrival at an automobile accident, flares should be placed immediately to prevent additional accidents. Caution must be used by the first aider, who may become a victim by being struck by cars when attempting to cross a highway or give other aid. Extreme care must be used to ensure that you are not injured by broken glass, metal fragments, or other sharp objects, which, if you are excited, you may easily overlook. Care must be taken when electrical wires or broken street lights are involved, which may fall on those below. Water rescues must never be attempted by entering the water unless you are sure that you will not also become a victim. The old adage of *"reach, throw, row, and go"* is appropriate here. Care must be taken to control traffic and crowds, which may cause harm through well-meant but misguided efforts.

When arriving at an accident, any and all necessary equipment should be summoned *at once* and not called only after less extensive rescue equipment has proved to be ineffective in getting the injured extricated or rescued. Again, time delays must be avoided as much as possible, particularly in those cases such as surgical emergencies for which even with effective care given, time will determine the outcome and thus becomes of vital importance.

Several flashlights should be carried along with flares. Flashlights can be used to examine the injured or the wreckage in a dark situation. They can be used to warn and direct traffic before the arrival of the police. As part of a complete first aid kit, it is also useful to carry change, to call for help, and blankets, which can be used for those who are in shock, with low body temperatures, or to cover the injured while glass is being broken to protect them from additional injury.

FIRST AIDER COMPETENCIES

After studying the material and practicing the techniques presented in this chapter, the student should be able to:

- Explain the role of the first aider in planning and carrying out transportation and extrication procedures.
- Outline the general procedures for transportation of the injured or ill.
- Demonstrate unassisted transportation techniques.
- Explain under what conditions the following techniques can be used: walking assist, fireman's carry, packstrap carry, and saddleback carry.
- Demonstrate assisted transportation techniques, including lifts and carriers, as a team member and as a team leader.
- Explain the specific uses and limitations of the various types of litters.
- Describe under what circumstances a first aider should get involved in extrication procedures.
- Identify specific sources and groups in the community that provide specialized services and equipment for rescue and extrication.

REFERENCES AND
RECOMMENDED READINGS

1. Curry, G. J., editor: Immediate care and transport of the injured, Springfield, Ill., 1965, Charles C Thomas, Publisher.
2. deGravelles, W. D., Jr., and Kelley, J. H.: Injuries following rear-end automobile collisions, Springfield, Ill., 1969, Charles C Thomas, Publisher.
3. Emergency care and transportation of the sick and injured, Committee on Injuries, Chicago, 1971, American Academy of Orthopaedic Surgeons.
4. First aid for soldiers, Washington, D.C., 1970, Department of the Army.
5. Grant, H., and Murry, R.: Emergency care, Washington, D.C., 1971, Robert J. Brady Co.
6. Gurdjian, E. S., et al.: Impact injury and crash protection, Springfield, Ill., 1970, Charles C Thomas, Publisher.
7. Shires, G. T., editor: Care of the trauma patient, New York, 1966, McGraw-Hill Book Co.

20

COMMUNITY PLANNING
FOR EMERGENCY MEDICAL SERVICES

John G. Bruhn and James A. Williams

EMERGENCY MEDICAL SERVICES: A NATIONAL CONCERN

Disability and the loss of life from sudden catastrophic illness and accidents is one of the most visible and critical areas in health care in the United States. Each year there are about 55,000 traffic deaths and 2 million highway injuries, 200,000 of which result in permanent disability. In addition, each year there are more than 64,000 deaths and 9.3 million nonfatal injuries from nonhighway accidents, 250,000 of which are permanently disabling.[1,2]

Currently accidents kill more people in the productive age groups up to 39 years than any disease and are the fourth largest cause of death after that age. The costs of accidental death, disability, and property damage are estimated at about $29.5 billion a year.[1] Some studies have demonstrated that 15% to 20% of accidental highway deaths could be avoided if prompt, effective medical care were available at the scene of the emergency, on the way to the hospital, and in the hospital.[15,32]

A sudden medical emergency is another category of unforeseen events that benefit from prompt effective medical care. These include, for example, coronary occlusions, cerebrovascular strokes, diabetic crises, precipitous miscarriages or deliveries, suicidal and homicidal attempts, drug and alcohol crises, and battered children and spouses. The American Heart Association estimates that approximately 10% to 20% of prehospital coronary deaths could be prevented if proper care were administered at the scene and en route to a medical facility.[11]

The approach to emergency medical services in many communities in the United States is to provide rapid ambulance service from the scene of an emergency to a hospital. Often the personnel operating the ambulance are not trained to give on-the-scene emergency care or to assist in stabilizing the patient while en route to a hospital. Ambulances, in addition, are often not equipped to provide on-the-scene or in-transit emergency assistance and may lack communications equipment to inform the receiving hospital that a patient is on the way. This approach to emergency medical services is referred to as "load and go," and it is practiced at considerable risk to the patient. There is increasing concern among laymen and health professionals that more efficient and economical ways of providing emergency medical services must be planned and developed.

The purpose of this chapter is (1) to describe the process whereby communities may plan and develop more efficient and economical ways of providing emergency medical services; (2) to discuss the issues that facilitate and impede the planning, development, and implementation phases of an emergency medical services system; (3) to present an overview of the components of a functioning emergency medical service system and their interrelationships; and (4) to present an example of a county and a regional emergency medical services system.

EMERGENCY MEDICAL SERVICES AS A SYSTEM

A medical emergency is an unforeseen event affecting a person in such a manner that a need for immediate medical care (physiological or psychological) is created. The term *emergency medical services* (EMS) refers to all of the services used in responding to the perceived individual need for immediate medical care. Many human and physical resources are employed in a predetermined sequence over the entire time period encompassing the medical emergency. These resources and their joint or individual responses to medical emergencies in a defined geographic area make up a community EMS system.[16] There are no firm rules for establishing the geographic boundaries of an EMS system. A system may encompass a neighborhood, a metropolitan area, a county, or a region, depending on population density, trade and hospitalization patterns, and political or natural boundaries. A functional community, for the purposes of the emergency medical services system, can be defined only at the local level. Geographic boundaries of the system will need to be specified in the planning process.

An emergency medical services system should include the following components irrespective of its geographic boundaries: (1) accessible transportation; (2) trained personnel; (3) continuous communication; (4) hospital readiness; (5) an organization or agency that will be responsible for operating or coordinating the system; and (6) an emergency medical services council, which will serve as an advisory group to the organization operating the system. Ambulances should be located geographically for maximum utilization and should be accessible to citizens in need through a 911 telephone number, 24 hours a day, and dispatched by a trained emergency communications dispatcher. A maximally equipped ambulance should arrive on the scene of the emergency within 5 minutes. Trained, full-time emergency medical technicians (EMTs) must be transported to the scene of an emergency, and, to administer care effectively on the scene and en route to the hospital, they must have the necessary radio and telemetry equipment to communicate with physicians. A communication network must be established between emergency vehicles and medical facilities in different cities. Such a communication network is essential for individual emergencies as well as community disasters. The ambulance should proceed safely to the nearest hospital, which has been prepared to receive the patient. The hospital should be alerted as to the nature of the incoming emergency to adjust workload and minimize the disruption of ongoing activities. These components need to be coordinated by an emergency medical services council, which would help secure the cooperation and involvement of community agencies and health facilities in planning, providing care, education, training, and funding (Fig. 20-1).

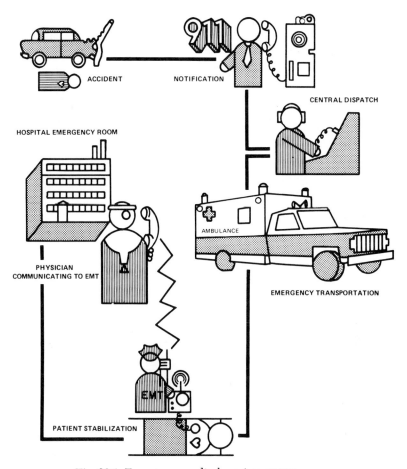

Fig. 20-1. Emergency medical services system.

COMMUNITY RESPONSIBILITY FOR EMERGENCY MEDICAL SERVICES

Many communities lack one or more of these components and therefore do not have a coordinated system for providing emergency medical services. One of the reasons underlying the failure of many communities to develop a coordinated system for providing emergency medical services is the unanswered question, "Whose responsibility is it?" In communities where changing the status quo is required, one individual or group must see the program as a personal responsibility and devote energy to seeing it implemented. However, an emergency medical services system cannot work unless the organizations, agencies, and facilities that contribute to the system recognize the need to improve emergency services and actively participate in the planning process. Indeed, there must be broad citizen support for developing the best available type of emergency services for a community. The citizenry must acknowledge that emergency services, like fire and police protection, are a public responsibility and that the improvement of all of these services requires citizen financial support. Every community has unique needs, and therefore all communities do not need the same type of emergency medical service systems. The quality, effectiveness, and efficiency of emergency medical services in a community, however, reflect the degree of interest and support of citizens in emergency medical services.

PLANNING FOR COMMUNITY EMERGENCY MEDICAL SERVICES
The setting for community EMS planning

Several assumptions underlie this discussion on community planning for emergency medical services. The first is that the geographic community most viable as a unit for EMS planning is a city or county. In areas where individual local governments have insufficient medical or financial resources to develop an EMS system, it is reasonable that a group of contiguous local governmental units can enter into a mutual agreement to plan and operate a multicounty or regional EMS system.

A second assumption underlying this discussion is that a major change in the community is necessary.[30] This means that the prehospital phase of emergency care is clearly inadequate and that ambulances are insufficiently equipped and staffed to initiate treatment at the scene. Other components of an EMS system, such as communication, may be missing, or linkage between the various institutions attempting to deliver emergency medical services may be inadequate. It is assumed that the changes needed to establish a flexible and coordinated EMS system will require (1) the reallocation of resources and personnel and (2) a rethinking of the responsibilities and participation of the public in this aspect of health care. This will involve the providers of health services as well as the political and economic leaders of the community. Therefore a broad-based community planning organization is necessary to design an appropriate EMS plan for the community and to develop the necessary community support for the adoption of the EMS plan by the unit of local government to operate the system.[19]

A final assumption is that the optimal size and type of city or local government unit to plan and operate an EMS system ranges from several thousand to several hundred thousand in population. It is in communities of this size range, either the free-standing cities or the mosaic patchwork of independent suburbs around larger urban complexes, that vast numbers of people now live without adequate emergency medical services. Larger cities will find the community planning process useful if there are still avenues, even though seldom used, whereby citizens can participate in the planning and decision making processes.

Larger urban complexes are often committed to professional planning departments within large administrative bureaucracies for the design of any community change. The strategies for developing a community planning process in such areas are complex and will not be dealt with in this discussion. Most of these cities have already made commitments to operating EMS systems because of the sheer magnitude of providing emergency care to the massive population.

Small communities or rural areas, on the other hand, have entirely different problems. Because of sparse population and limited economic resources, these communities are frequently in a crisis over health care in general. Inadequate hospitals and a shortage of physicians and other health manpower make it difficult to focus on only the one issue of emergency medical services. Yet studies[1] show that rural areas have up to 400% greater fatalities from survivable medical emergencies because of these inadequacies. The community planning approach to the health care issue in general would be a more fruitful method of dealing with these problems in rural areas. In this way, the EMS system would be a part of the larger issue of health care for all the citizens in the affected areas. Many of the comments on planning and organizing EMS systems in this section will also be relevant to the issues of planning for the total health care system in rural communities.

The community planning process

The selection of an approach to planning and community change is critical in planning for an EMS system. The tone and style of the whole effort, the avenues for community participation, and the specific strategies available to be used in implementation are determined by that choice. The choice should be based on the type of change necessary in the community and on the characteristics of the community under consideration.[7]

There are numerous planning models available, each implying a basic theoretical approach as to what a community is and how change can be brought about.[19] Most of these models can be categorized either as (1) the community planning (or participatory) approach, or (2) the professional planning (or expert) approach. There are circumstances in planning for community change in which the expert approach to planning may be the most effective.[22,31] Experience has shown, however, that in most communities, planning for emergency medical services should be *community* planning. Since the delivery of excellent emergency medical services requires a flexible and coordinated system, the planning process should involve key persons from every component or institution in the community that will become a part of the EMS system.[16] This approach necessitates the creation of a broad-based community planning organization that will take responsibility for designing the plan and guiding its implementation.[9,19]

The community planning approach views the community as a social system, in which many processes are already in existence that can bring about change.[5,17] Too frequently, planning for emergency medical services has been isolated from the community as a whole. Intelligent and expert planning efforts have produced plans that were out of step with the various institutions and components necessary for an EMS system to function. By beginning with the *people*, instead of with the *problem*, this mistake can be avoided. Using this approach, the community, through its people, has the opportunity to participate in creating a plan that reflects the unique characteristics of that community in its very fabric.

Another important characteristic of the community planning approach is that it helps avoid the error of viewing the plan (or the planners) as *initiating* a change process.[17] This point is particularly critical in planning for emergency medical services, in that the institutions and persons currently providing health services in a community are already involved in trying to deliver emergency care, no matter how inadequate. They will be the first to resist efforts to change that do not involve them and that are not at least understanding of their efforts in the past. What must be considered is the climate of the community—that difficult-to-measure blend of geography, history, personalities, institutions, organizations, behaviors, and priorities that make up any community.[8,10]

It is difficult not to overemphasize that the EMS plan be the *product* of processes that are moving toward change and not the initial step in a change process. The people affected by the proposed change must participate *from the first* in the planning and continue throughout the implementation of the plan.[19] Viewing the whole community as a social system in which change processes are going on all the time keeps the context of the community uppermost for those doing the planning and ensures that the elements of the EMS plan reflect the community's understanding of itself and represent what is reasonable, appropriate, and possible.[25]

It is axiomatic that the longer the delay in involving the community in the planning process, the more difficult will be the eventual decision to implement the plan. This has been proved true in planning for emergency medical services.

The basic resource for any change in a community is the people who make up the community.[18,23] People grow and develop through participation in the processes that bring about change. They are enabled to develop an image of themselves as capable and competent and able to make a difference in the future of the community. The key is the development in the minds of a significant number of people of "we" instead of "they" when viewing the community and its needs. "We are responsible for the future of our community." This is the participatory process that must be constantly and systematically renewed in every community.[29] No better opportunity is available than to participate in the community planning process for creating an EMS system.

Steps in community planning for EMS

Preplanning phase. The planning for EMS becomes a part of the change processes in a community when a person or a group decides that they will initiate or accept responsibility to move forward on the problem. They may have voluntarily identified emergency services as a problem warranting their personal involvement, or they may have been designated formally by some sponsoring body as a task group to study and report. Frequently, the formal appointment by a city council, a community council, medical society, or civic organization is the result of considerable preliminary investigation by persons who are concerned about the levels of services. The management of this preplanning phase greatly influences the success of the subsequent planning effort.[8,10,19]

The first activities at this informal and exploratory stage are (1) to increase the possibility of sustained interaction by increasing the communication linkages between people in the community who will become vital to the planning process and (2) to increase levels of information on the problem.

The small, informal core group that is frequently found in this early stage can best begin its work by tapping into the stored experiences in the community on the problem around EMS. This means a survey, but one not aimed at the facts and figures. Stored in the memory of the institutions, services, and organizations of a community, and particularly in some persons who have been involved in EMS, are collected memory fragments of problems, concerns, efforts, feelings, disappointments, and frustrations. Sampling this storage is important because no single person or organization will be in possession of the total picture.

This first survey is really a people survey or *people* identification. Who has the problem, who says it is a problem, what do they feel is the magnitude of the problem? What have been the past attempts to work on it, if any? Has anyone in a position of authority listened in the past? Why is the problem surfacing now? Who are the key people who must be involved if this problem is to be solved? Who should contact the key people? These and other similar questions will help penetrate the levels of concern in the community and begin linking people together.

People tend to talk to people like themselves and therefore selectively limit their knowledge of a community. Any one person's total knowledge of the history of his community will have many gaps, even though he may have held positions of responsibility. For this reason, the deliberate effort to move through the community and take a survey of the stored experiences and feelings built up around EMS over the years is a vital step to be taken before beginning the formal planning process. Some of the initial contacts should include:

1. Those currently attempting to provide ambulance services
2. Health professionals who work in hospitals, such as registered nurses, laboratory technicians, licensed vocational nurses, and physical therapists
3. Physicians who most frequently respond to emergency situations and have been identified as interested in emergency medical care
4. Law enforcement, fire, and public safety personnel who routinely see extreme emergency situations and may be acutely aware of the magnitude of need
5. Citizens who are aware of the larger scene in the state, who have occasion to travel outside the community, or who may have come from other cities where EMS systems are operating
6. Patients and their families who may have experienced the inadequacy of current emergency services firsthand
7. Key persons in education, human services, communications, or business who have shared the concern in the past
8. Members of high-risk populations who have a high percentage of emergencies, such as youth, the elderly, people in industry, or the poor

During the preplanning phase some members of the core group should begin the task of becoming lay experts in EMS. They should read the basic works, study successful EMS systems, review the legislation, and, if at all possible, visit a successful working EMS system in a community of comparable size.

As a part of the stored experience of the community there also is a need for the objective data that are in health department and hospital records, for example, morbidity and mortality rates and the numbers, types, and locations of medical emergencies. These data would be used to support the developing picture in the community and as background information. The more detailed survey and analysis of health data will come later when the formal planning organization is functioning.

The preplanning and exploratory phase ends with the formation of a formal community EMS planning organization that can carry forward the participation planning process.

Developing the community EMS planning organization. Constituting the EMS planning organization from the informal groupings identified in the preplanning phase is a critical step in sustaining the community EMS planning process.[19] Determining auspices or sponsorship for any planning body is important. The simplest approach is to realize that there are two useful avenues open to those wishing to establish a community EMS planning organization: the mandated and the ad hoc.

The mandated planning organization is a committee or council appointed by a unit of local government with a specific mandate to study and plan the EMS system and make recommendations for action. Most frequently it will represent the interests in the community that are currently in power, and the motives for the formation of the committee may be complex. The key to its effectiveness is whether it also represents the health and human service interests and is composed of people who are willing seriously to examine the problems of emergency medical services in the community. The mandated committee can develop a subcommittee or a task force structure and initiate the community planning process by broadening its membership. Once it has established its ability to do this, then the techniques described below are possible.

All other ways of setting up a group to study and plan for EMS, from the more formal community council or medical society committee to the most informal grouping of concerned citizens, would be ad hoc planning organizations. These organizations initially have no formal link with the unit of local government, which must eventually make the decision to adopt the EMS plan and commit funds for implementation.

The ad hoc community EMS planning organization will be described here. The purpose of the ad hoc community planning organization is to develop a workable EMS plan for the community that will be implemented. This requires mobilizing the support of the preplanning phase into a series of task forces to work on the details of the EMS plan and continuing the process by identifying other persons who have knowledge in EMS or other skills and involving them on the various task forces.

The ad hoc organization has the advantage of great flexibility, but flexibility can become a liability unless adequate structure is developed immediately.[24] Very early, the ad hoc community planning organization needs to develop an identity with a name, a working structure of task forces, a statement of purposes and procedures, and a list of people to work on various aspects of the problem. If the ad hoc planning organization can be adopted by a strong agency or organization in the community, such as the medical society or the board of health, its task of becoming legitimate will be easier.

A community EMS planning organization works well with a steering committee of twelve to fifteen people highly committed to the development of an EMS system. These individuals become the chairpersons and cochairpersons of six planning task forces—communication, personnel and training, transportation, hospitals and medical care, organization and financing, and community education—one for each major component of a functioning EMS system. Each task force, in turn, recruits interested and concerned persons to do its planning task. These are persons who are competent in the area of the task and who have access to persons professionally active in that component of the proposed EMS system.

The steering committee, composed of the chairperson and one or two members of each task force, monitors the planning process and keeps a focus on the goals. The steering committee's task is to coordinate the various task forces and keep them working simultaneously and to see that no vital area is missed or that no task force falls seriously behind the pace of the planning process. The steering committee has the task of taking the final reports of each task force and weaving them into a coherent EMS planning document.

The first task of the steering committee, after setting up its membership, purposes, and the task force framework, may be to plan an area-wide EMS conference or workshop as a means of establishing the community planning process. An essential strategy is to gain sufficient public exposure to give the EMS planning organization higher visibility in the community. An EMS planning conference or workshop is an excellent way of consolidating the early gains, getting sufficient exposure, uncovering additional support, and initiating public education. If the conference is planned on a participatory model with small groups working on specific tasks, it can become the means of organizing the needed EMS planning task forces.[25]

Once the task force structure has been set up, simultaneous planning activity can begin. The task forces should arrange to meet regularly with specific target dates set for reporting on progress. The chairpersons of the task forces should meet as the steering committee at regular intervals to monitor progress and to allow each chairperson to keep abreast of the work of other task forces. All task forces should begin by doing the following:

1. *Study.* Send for and review materials on EMS system, standards and specifications, and funding requirements. Review EMS operations elsewhere, particularly those in cities of similar size and resources.
2. *Survey.* Examine the emergency facilities in hospitals and ambulance services and analyze health data relative to EMS. Develop detailed reports on the capabilities and limitations of existing facilities, communications, and personnel resources.
3. *Visit.* Make an on-site study of a functioning EMS system in a city of comparable size.
4. *Involvement.* Each task force should expand its membership to include as many people in its area of concern as are willing to participate.

This initial phase of task force activity is aimed toward the first major decisions: the minimum needs and standards for the EMS system in the community. Once these decisions have been made, it is possible to begin work on the planning document, outlining the eventual EMS system and including the number of personnel and vehicles, the levels of training, the communications equipment and dispatching required, the demands to be made on the treatment facilities, and the proposed organizational structure within the unit of local government. If these decisions have been made as the result of task force activity that has included persons from every sector of the community, the likelihood is great that the plan will be adequate as well as realistic.[18]

Those responsible for the planning process should avoid the error of planning too small. This has caused some communities to settle for a system less adequate than necessary or even to give up trying to solve the problem. The EMS plan should first detail the kind of system necessary to provide excellent emergency medical services for the community, then look at the costs and resources. Then it can become a matter of phasing the new service into existence, rather than settling for an inadequate service or giving up entirely if the cost seems to exceed the available funds. Determination to see the full EMS plan in operation provides the motivation to explore many sources of funding.

Production of the EMS planning document. The production of a planning document is the turning point in the community planning process. The document should demonstrate the results of the study of the community's needs, provide a detailed description of a workable EMS system, and identify the major tasks necessary for implementation.[26]

Specific attention in the EMS plan should be given to the recommended minimum standards of service and how these were determined. This should include the minimum number of personnel required and their training, vehicles and equipment specifications, communication system needs, and provisions for adequate emergency treatment at local hospitals. The plan should make a specific recommendation for setting up an organizational structure within the unit of local government to operate the EMS system and show that alternatives were examined.

Assessment of existing financial resources compared to the requirements of the proposed EMS system will usually be discouraging. In the planning document, strategies for funding should be explored, including grants from federal or private sources, local tax revenues, revenue-sharing funds, fund raising in the local community through public and business-industrial sources, assessments of surcharges on public utilities, and others. Expertise on funding schemes and options open to local governments should be sought. A detailed budget of start-up and annual costs should be included. Finally, a proposed implementation schedule with a timetable should complete the plan.

The document should be written by the steering committee of the community EMS planning organization. The contribution of each task force will be a detailed report, which provides the following information for the steering committee:

1. *Communication task force:* a survey of the existing communications capability and equipment; an outline of the requirements in design, manpower, and equipment to create the necessary links to support a fully operational EMS system; a determination of the costs

2. *Personnel and training task force:* an assessment of manpower resources and needs; establishment of the procedures for selection of personnel; design of the training program and plan to oversee the selection and training of ambulance and dispatching personnel

3. *Transportation task force:* an inventory of available equipment and a determination of the geographic area and desired response times to determine the number and location of vehicles; specification of the types of vehicles to be used; costs of vehicles and equipment; determination of utility of other forms of emergency transport, including air and water; assessment of nonemergency patient transportation needs

4. *Hospital and emergency health care task force:* a survey of the extent of need and current demand for emergency medical services; an estimate of the demand to be created by EMS, and a determination of the capability and limitation of local hospitals to meet the estimated demands of an EMS system; involvement of health care professionals, physicians, and others in planning and in training of EMS personnel

5. *Organization and finance task force:* a determination of the cost of provid-

ing the planned EMS services, identifying the appropriate organizational structure in the community's local government to operate the EMS system, and organization of a coordinating and planning body (EMS Council) to perform the diverse functions necessary to maintain the EMS system; recommendations of means of financing the costs of the EMS system

6. *Community education task force:* development of a campaign to inform the public about EMS: the needs, the problems, and the solutions; when the EMS plan has been adopted and implemented, information for the public about the functions of EMS in their community, how to use it, what to expect, what it can and cannot do; when the EMS system is operational, initiation of activities toward increasing the number of emergency-trained citizens in the community and reducing the incidence of medical emergencies in high-risk groups

The planning document should also include guidelines for the implementation of the EMS plan. There are numerous tasks and activities, such as hiring and training EMS personnel, that must be planned and completed before the first vehicle can run. These activities are the responsibility of the organization that will operate the EMS system and can be begun only after the decision has been made by the unit of local government to adopt and implement the plan. However, the planning document should list these activities, indicate how they may be completed satisfactorily, and who might be designated as responsible for each task.

In moving toward implementation, a schedule should be established with individuals or departments designated as responsible for each of the following items:

1. Plan the training program for ambulance and dispatch personnel.
2. Outline day-to-day operational procedures, including response to complaints.
3. Establish personnel selection procedures and criteria.
4. Write a personnel manual with standards, pay scales, job descriptions, rights, and expectations.
5. Arrange for medical review of the performance of personnel.
6. Detail a public information program to carry forward the work begun by the task forces.
7. Negotiate agreements with agencies who will cooperate to make the system possible, including hospitals and public safety and social service agencies.
8. Arrange for maintenance contracts on equipment and locate sources for expendable supplies.
9. Work out a continuous and standardized record-keeping system that will ensure availability of accurate patient records, maintained from entry to discharge.
10. Set up billing and collection procedures and methods of financial control.
11. Arrange for receiving, installation, and testing of all equipment. The unit of local government will routinely use its own bid procedures to purchase vehicles and medical and communication equipment.
12. Develop disaster plans in cooperation with the other public safety agencies, enabling the EMS system to function satisfactorily in the event of mass casualties, natural disaster, or national emergency.

13. Provide agreements for mutual assistance with neighboring EMS systems.
14. Set up an independent evaluation and reporting procedure to use in up-grading the service and planning for expansion as needed.

Finally, a key recommendation of the planning document should be for the organization of a permanent coordinating and advisory body, an EMS Council. Ideally, the unit of local government to implement the EMS plan will appoint many members of the community planning organization to form the EMS Council. The work of the task forces can be handed over to the EMS Council in a smooth transition from planning to implementation. The EMS Council should retain, as consultants, those individuals who worked with the task forces in technical areas such as communications, finance, and medical review.

The EMS planning document should stress that, at the point of the decision to implement the plan, the responsible entity of local government to operate the system should be designated. If this is to be a fire department, a health department, or an independent EMS department, the organizational structure should be developed immediately, with the individual responsible to manage the system either appointed or hired. From that time onward, that person works as staff to the EMS Council as its carries out the many tasks of implementation.

After the completion of the planning document, the final step is the adoption of the EMS plan by the unit of local government. The community EMS planning process does not end until the EMS system is fully operational (Fig. 20-2). The community support developed in the planning process may be the crucial difference in the decision by the unit of local government to adopt the EMS plan and take responsibility for the EMS system.

Adopting the EMS plan. The decision to establish an EMS system is both economic and political and requires strong support from the community to assure the elected officials that the plan is needed, that it is feasible, and that the community is willing to pay the price. For some communities, public responsibility for emergency medical services will be a new concept. Local government officials have been observed to go through several phases as they attempt to deal with EMS, a problem that they frequently know little about. First, there is usually a blend of puzzlement and concern as they wonder why it has suddenly become a problem with which they must deal. They will express concern as more information is made public about the magnitude of the problem and will worry publicly about the potential for suffering and loss of life in the current inadequate system. At the same time, they may become resentful that another burden is about to be placed on the taxpayer or that government is about to invade another area of private enterprise. Finally, in their reluctance to act, they may search for less expensive and less adequate alternatives or question the validity of the plan or the seriousness of the problem. The EMS plan and the persons involved in planning must be able to respond reasonably and sympathetically to the concerns that lie behind this behavior. The presentation of the EMS plan to elected officials should be scheduled as part of a regular public meeting, covered by the media. However, a well-documented package on the EMS plan should be available to every elected official and to key members of the local government administration with adequate time for study before the public presentation. At the public meeting, the presentation should be supported by the attendance of large numbers of the key community persons who were involved in the planning process.

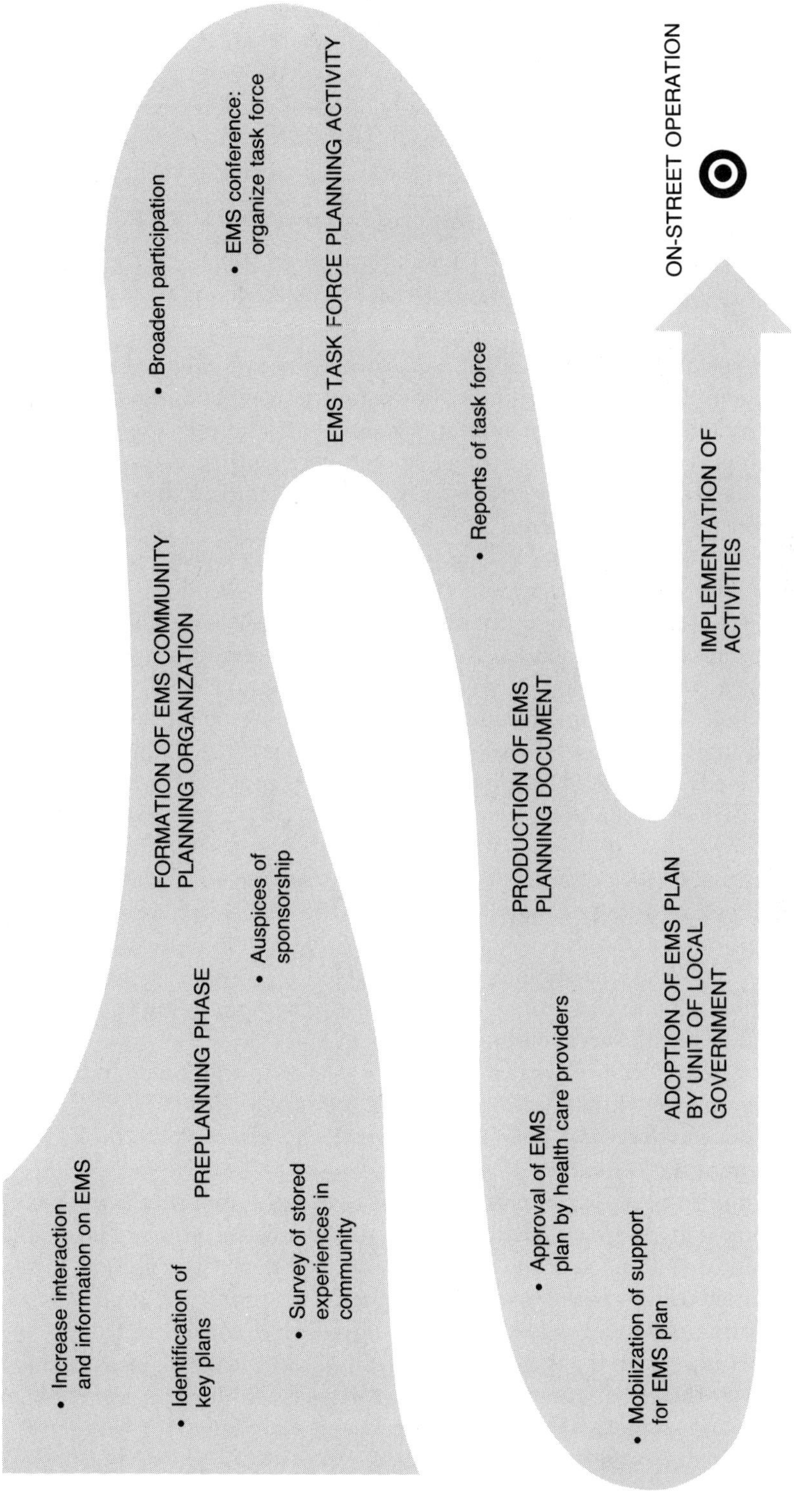

Fig. 20-2. Flow chart of EMS planning process.

PREPLANNING PHASE

- Increase interaction and information on EMS
- Identification of key plans
- Survey of stored experiences in community

FORMATION OF EMS COMMUNITY PLANNING ORGANIZATION

- Auspices of sponsorship
- Broaden participation
- EMS conference: organize task force

EMS TASK FORCE PLANNING ACTIVITY

- Reports of task force

PRODUCTION OF EMS PLANNING DOCUMENT

- Approval of EMS plan by health care providers
- Mobilization of support for EMS plan

ADOPTION OF EMS PLAN BY UNIT OF LOCAL GOVERNMENT

IMPLEMENTATION OF ACTIVITIES

ON-STREET OPERATION

The presentation should include the following:
- The *facts* that define the magnitude of the problem of emergency medical services, including mortality and morbidity rates
- The *plan*, in a brief outline form, on how to set up an EMS system that will provide a service adequate to the community need
- The *cost* of providing this type of service, broken down into start-up and annual operations costs
- The *resources* available to undertake the task, including people, agencies, and funding sources

Endorsements of the plan by health care professionals, social service agencies, community and service groups, industrial and business groups, educational institutions, and key persons in the community should be included in the planning package.

If there is reluctance on the part of local government to take responsibility for the EMS system, it is time to build on the base of participation and communication already established by the planning organization. The purpose is to create a climate of support for the elected officials, helping them to recognize that the community as a whole is ready to take what may seem to be a drastic and expensive step in setting up an excellent EMS system.[20]

The correct approach must be clearly understood by those initiating the effort to create the climate of support. They are asking the advocates of excellent emergency medical services to make direct contact with the elected officials and the administration of local government, assuring them that the community supports the plan and is willing to pay the price. This is *not* simply a public relations campaign, because support in the community must be real if an EMS system is to function successfully. However, the campaign must be carefully planned so that all involved in the effort project a consistent image and purpose. Those supporting the EMS plan should be perceived by elected officials as follows:

1. *Working with local officials to solve a serious problem:* sympathetic with the difficulties of the decision to go ahead with the EMS plan
2. *Factual and information oriented:* establishing a role as a valuable source of data and ideas on solutions
3. *Oriented solely to the task of EMS:* resisting the temptation to expand into a social or health-service reform movement
4. *Mediating and nonpolarizing:* able to deal with possible angry factions in the community without falling into the adversary mode
5. *Coalition building and nonpolitical:* broad endorsement of the EMS plan throughout the community

The community planning organization has a unique opportunity to facilitate implementation if it conducts itself properly in this critical phase. The image to be kept in mind by those involved in this phase is that of the different reactions one gets from entering water, depending on the force of entry. One can wade in gently with little resistance, or leap in with a large splash, or fall in from a height with lethal results. It is the same water in all three cases. In much the same fashion, the way that local government is approached will have a great influence on the amount and strength of the resistance.[27]

THE FUNCTIONING SYSTEM
Organization of an EMS system

An EMS system links diverse and separate activities, agencies, and institutions together to provide a quick response to the need for emergency medical care. This linkage does not replace existing organizations, agencies, or services, nor does it substitute one form of care for another. Rather, it is a way of creating a partnership of organizations and resources to provide first-class care for the duration of emergencies.

An organization must be formed within the appropriate unit of local government to be responsible for coordinating or operating the system in a designated geographic area. In addition to this organization an Emergency Medical Services Council is needed, to be composed of representatives from communities and agencies in the geographic area, which would serve as an advisory body. The EMS Council should be structured along published guidelines for establishing community councils.[12] For an EMS system to work effectively, the organization operating or coordinating it must have the administrative capability of carrying out the following functions:

1. Determine policy and administrative procedures for operating the system, establishing standards of service, and reviewing the performance of the system.
2. Coordinate the separate local governmental bodies, hospitals, and other agencies who cooperate in delivering emergency medical services.
3. Plan how emergency services will be delivered and financed, and plan for changes in the system as needs in the area change.
4. Provide community education so residents will know how to use the system; provide training in Red Cross first aid, cardiopulmonary resuscitation, and preventive medicine so that citizens will be better able to assess emergency situations and, in turn, prevent many of them.
5. Supervise and manage the EMS system, including the scheduling of EMTs and ambulances, equipment maintenance, billing and collections, payrolls, recruiting and training of EMTs, and maintaining an administrative staff.

Communications

The first contact most people have with an EMS system is its communications component. Communication provides the necessary link between the many parts of the system, making possible a coordinated, accurate, and rapid response to the need for emergency medical services.[13] The communication component should interface with other emergency and public service communications and be capable of expansion in times of major disaster. Because of the complexity of communications planning and the technical nature of the work required, ongoing monitoring by the Communications Committee of the EMS Council will be required.

Operational communication links. Operational communication is defined as the communication necessary to deliver medical care at the scene of the emergency, to provide in-transit medical care, and to coordinate available medical personnel and resources at a hospital to best serve the patient. The following four communication links illustrate the information flow in the system (Fig. 20-3).

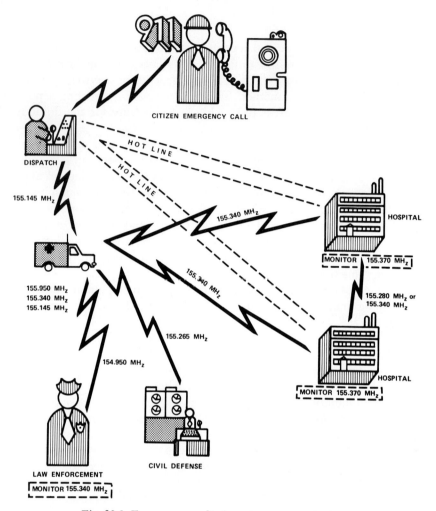

Fig. 20-3. Emergency medical services communication system.

Link 1: consumer to system. The individual in need of emergency medical services reports directly to the EMS system. Experience has indicated that the 911 emergency number is the most effective way for persons to reach the EMS system. Bell Telephone Company offers this service when communities in an area agree to be uniformly served. Although commitment to a universal number exists in most communities, implementation should be the responsibility of the EMS Council's Communications Committee.

Link 2: dispatcher to EMT and vehicle. The EMT and the vehicle are contacted by the emergency dispatcher and sent to the scene of the emergency. The responsibility of emergency dispatching requires that this position be filled with a trained EMS dispatcher. The dispatcher alerts the hospital emergency room likely to receive the patient as to the kind of problem the EMT may be facing. This allows the emergency room to have a physician standing by to supervise the

EMT at the scene. In the meantime, the dispatcher remains in communication with the vehicle, ready to contact the police or fire department if necessary, or to send additional EMTs and vehicles to the scene. If there is likely to be delay in excess of 10 minutes in the arrival of the EMT and vehicle, the dispatcher will call back to the scene and assume medical management to the degree possible. The dispatcher may be required to manage the activities of several emergencies simultaneously. With progression of the emergency run, the EMT notifies the dispatcher of the vehicle's arrival at the scene and departure from it. The dispatcher records these times on a card with a time clock so that a complete record of the run is available. Finally, the dispatcher arranges for additional coverage by alerting other designated stations to stand by in the event a second call comes from the same geographical area. As the medical care resource manager for the EMS system, the dispatcher should be at a central dispatch station. The central dispatch station should have direct one-way phone lines to the EMT, vehicle stations, and area hospitals.

Link 3: EMT and vehicle to hospital emergency room. Full utilization of EMT capabilities requires a two-way communication link with an emergency physician, which enables the EMT to perform necessary procedures for life support under medical supervision. The emergency room should be manned by a person trained in emergency communications, who will monitor the progress of the EMT's activity on the scene. This also enables the emergency room to be informed of the patient's problem and the arrival time of the vehicle.

Link 4: hospital to hospital to physician. Hospitals need to talk to each other to coordinate services and page physicians on their staff when needed. Communication between the emergency vehicle and the emergency room enables the hospital to assemble the needed manpower through its paging facilities. Physicians in the community can be reached and informed of an emergency involving one of their patients. These procedures are achieved in most cases by phone except when conditions render the phone inoperable. Although most hospitals have adequate means of paging physicians and other health care personnel, there is a need to educate hospital and ambulance personnel regarding communications procedures.

Disaster and emergency coordination. Although medical emergency communications during a disaster will continue on the established ambulance-to-hospital and hospital-to-hospital frequencies, the Civil Defense frequency may be used to dispatch additional emergency vehicles. Planning the best ways of integrating EMS communications between Civil Defense and area hospitals is an important task for the EMS Council's Communications Committee. The EMS Council should also cooperate with Civil Defense and area hospitals in assisting the mayors of local governments in disaster planning. Simulation disaster drills should be conducted to familiarize the EMS system components with disaster plans.

Personnel and training

The emergency medical technician. The EMT is the bridge between the doctor and the emergency patient. The EMT is the civilian counterpart of the skilled military paramedic and brings the emergency department closer to the patient (Fig. 20-4). The EMT may be in charge of a mobile unit that travels

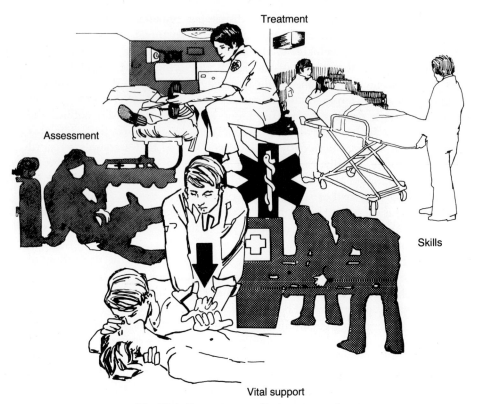

Fig. 20-4. Emergency medical service technician.

to the site of an emergency, assesses the problem, communicates with the emergency department of the hospital or with the physician in charge of emergency care, gives treatment as directed by the physician, and proceeds with the safe transport of the patient. During transport, the EMT manages the life-support systems available within the mobile unit, continuing treatment and communication with physician or other hospital emergency department personnel as necessary. When the patient enters the emergency department of a hospital, the EMT assists with care if necessary and may accompany the patient to an intensive care unit, a coronary care unit, or other care facility. Community emergency procedures vary, but the training of EMTs prepares them to function in emergency situations in all parts of the medical facility.

Recruiting, selecting, training, and supervising EMTs is a basic task of the EMS system.[4,28] Generally, qualifications for the EMT are as follows: 19 to 30 years of age, a high school education, good physical health and visual accuracy, emotional stability, leadership potential, and an ability to be trained to deal with medical emergencies. Persons with 2 years of experience in dealing with emergency medical services (rescue, first aid, and defensive driving) are given preference.

Fire department personnel and exmilitary paramedics are uniquely equipped to move quickly into the role of an EMT. The EMT position must provide competitive salaries and fringe benefits to attract capable personnel. The professional pride and job satisfaction that result from the performance of a vital public service justify the cost of setting up a stable organization to employ EMTs.

Volunteer EMTs. Some geographically isolated communities that cannot be covered in the desired response time, or those which are not able to fund a full-time EMT team, have successfully used volunteer EMTs. Volunteer EMTs with portable transceivers and a basic equipment package can be dispatched to an emergency and begin stabilization while the vehicle is en route to the scene.

Training and requirements. Currently recommended training for EMTs includes three phases: phase I, 56 hours; phase II, 120 hours; phase III, 200 hours. A regular in-service training program should be established and coordinated by the Personnel and Training Committee of the EMS Council. Training of other emergency personnel should be considered by this committee when appropriate. It is recommended that all fire-fighting personnel, selected law enforcement personnel, and other key people participate in phases I and II of EMT training. This will produce a pool of capable persons for handling large-scale disasters, as well as provide back-up during peak hours or heavy demands on the EMS system.

To operate a professional team of EMTs on a vehicle, 24 hours a day, 7 days a week, requires seven positions, thus allowing for vacation, holidays, sick leave, and training time. A volunteer corps requires 15 to 20 persons per vehicle to give continuous coverage. It is recommended that every volunteer corps employ a full-time manager who is a trained EMT and who could assist in daytime coverage during the week when volunteer responses are more difficult. In addition, this person would perform administrative duties, plan training drills, recruit for the corps, and be a link with the EMS system.

Transportation

Response time. Responsiveness is defined as the lapse of time between the receipt of a request for emergency assistance and the arrival of the EMT and vehicle at the scene of the emergency. In an EMS system, the time from dispatch to arrival at an emergency room actually increases because more time is spent by the EMT at the scene initiating treatment. From the medical viewpoint the ideal response time is less than 5 minutes—the critical time in which to begin life support procedures. For reasons of geography and population distribution, it is not always economically feasible to operate the number of vehicles and full-time EMT crews required to provide this level of responsiveness. By utilizing a mix of full-time and volunteer EMTs, however, an acceptable level of responsiveness can be achieved. The use of persons working or living in isolated areas who are trained as volunteer EMTs would help to increase the responsiveness of the system.

The response time can be shortened as more citizens are trained in emergency first aid and cardiopulmonary resuscitation. A major effort to increase citizens' awareness of their emergency needs and the ways to use the EMS system should be one of the projects of the EMS Council's Community Education Committee.

Vehicle specifications and equipment. Transportation is not the sole function of an emergency ambulance. The vehicle must be equipped with communications, life support, first aid, and rescue equipment to fully utilize the capability of the EMT.[3,21] The modular ambulance is the most economical and the only one of several types of vehicles that meets current Department of Transportation specifications without extensive modification. The modular ambulance has a box, or module, that contains emergency equipment and supplies, mounted on a 1-ton truck chassis. After sufficient mileage has accumulated, usually after 3 years, the module is removed and installed on a new chassis. This keeps the vehicle out of service for less than half a day. The emergency module is expected to last through at least three chassis changes even with the most rigorous use.

Hospital categorization and emergency room capability

Representatives of hospitals should participate in self-categorization of their emergency facilities to provide the EMS system, and in particular the dispatchers, with a clear understanding of the capabilities and limitations of the various facilities. This information is crucial in directing the vehicle to the nearest hospital capable of providing the needed care. Categorization also provides information for any group monitoring the changing needs for emergency services, and, in addition, assists the hospitals in identifying additional capabilities. The American Medical Association's Guidelines for the Categorization of Hospital Emergency Capabilities state that no hospital should refuse treatment to any patient if, in the judgment of the EMT team, transportation to a more distant hospital would cause undue suffering or loss of life.[6] A patient admitted to the hospital under these circumstances would be provided treatment until he can safely be moved to an appropriate medical facility.

Community education

Community education must be a component of the EMS system to ensure appropriate use and continued support of emergency medical services. After the EMS plan has been implemented, the public must be educated regarding what the system is, what it can and cannot do, the capabilities and limitations of an EMT, and the fee and collection policy for services.

The Community Education Committee should have continuing responsibility for initiating appropriate community education activities. Special efforts should be directed toward high-risk groups, such as the young and elderly. These efforts should be supported by educational activities in schools and hospitals using the mass media and speakers for professional associations, community, civic, and service organizations, neighborhood clubs, and house-to-house contacts by volunteer block workers. Educational materials may include EMS stickers for homes and automobiles, slide presentations, enclosures with utility bills, handouts for recreational areas, and regular newspaper communication with organizations and components of the EMS system.

One effective community education activity is fund-raising. Service organizations or a volunteer health agency could raise funds for a vehicle or purchase equipment, such as a mobile electrocardioscope. These activities can mobilize and broaden community support and communicate basic facts about emergency needs and services.

Financial planning and resources

The operation and base for emergency services should be in fire departments. Areas without fire departments could be covered by volunteer organizations. The key to the success of an EMS system is the maintenance of minimum service standards in terms of staffing, coverage, responsiveness, EMT training, vehicle specifications, and equipment. Minimum standards should be codified in ordinances by all local governments so that citizens could be assured of high standards of service even if emergency services were handled on a contract or franchise basis.

Local governments should undertake the financial responsibility for implementation and operation of the EMS system. For areas involved in regional planning for EMS systems, federal funds, appropriated for EMS systems in Public Law 93-154, could be sought for start-up equipment and implementation costs.[14,14a] However, the operational costs of an EMS system must remain a local community responsibility. Local ad valorem tax revenues and federal grants are not the only alternatives for funding an EMS system. Many communities have successfully engaged citizens in fund-raising campaigns to purchase a significant share of the equipment, thus reducing the initial costs of implementation. Local matching schemes have served as incentives for civic and service organizations to assume leadership roles in these activities.

Expanding the EMS system

An EMS system will expand as it gains increasing capability to meet emergency services needs and as public understanding increases regarding the effects of emergencies on individuals, families, and communities.

The EMS Council should continue to monitor the service and plan for new service needs. The EMS Council must be continually aware of the heterogeneous nature of the communities it serves and ensure that its membership is representative of these communities. A major function of the EMS Council will be to seek financial resources to support the expansion of the EMS system.

Continued training in communications will be necessary for persons in all components of the EMS system. Emergency and disaster simulations should be conducted at regular intervals to sharpen skills and increase system morale. Periodic evaluation of communication effectiveness should identify individuals and teams who demonstrate excellence and who should be recognized by public awards from the EMS Council.

Additional vehicles will be required when population growth exceeds the capability of present vehicles to provide the desired responsiveness. The availability of air transportation will be of concern as the EMS system expands. Helicopters could be used to (1) reach isolated areas within an acceptable response time, (2) provide immediate support to a remotely stationed volunteer EMT, (3) evacuate and transport a patient to the hospital from remote areas, and (4) move a critical patient from a less–well-equipped hospital to one where the needed care was available or pick up a patient from a recreational craft or other vessel.

Of high priority is training for all professional EMTs to advanced certification to prepare to use biomedical telemetry. Professional firemen should be scheduled into basic EMT training as a regular feature of their in-service training. An

EMT Training Center should be established to link training resources with educational institutions. With this assistance, training resources in the Red Cross and the Heart Association could focus primarily on community education and on increasing the number of volunteers who could function as a part of the EMS system.

A mechanism should be established for a periodic review of the medical effectiveness of EMTs, emergency dispatching, and all personnel and agencies dealing with emergency patients. Examination of patterns of utilization of emergency services can also identify ways of preventing the duplication of costly services.

Making emergency services more effective will require further EMT training in obstetrical, pediatric, psychiatric, and dental emergencies. Pediatric emergency planning should include the equipping of vehicles with portable incubators. EMTs and law enforcement and other public safety personnel should be trained to deal with psychiatric emergencies and with the emotional behavior of persons involved in crisis situations.

SUMMARY AND CONCLUSION

Emergency medical services have changed radically in recent years. The nation has become acutely aware that medical service to victims of trauma or serious illness before they reach the hospital represents a critical weakness in the health care system. The concept now is that of taking treatment to the patient at the scene of the emergency and stabilizing him while in communication with a physician in the emergency room.

This has been made possible by advanced design in emergency equipment and vehicles, by the application of space-age communications technology to emergency medicine, and by the emerging new profession of the emergency medical technician. It has become clear that the delivery of excellent emergency medical services requires a *system* that integrates all components necessary to provide emergency care into a flexible and coordinated arrangement.

A community that learns about the management of its own processes of change can begin to more deliberately take charge of its own future. Solving a concrete problem, such as organizing a coordinated EMS system, not only saves lives and reduces disability, but it also develops a problem-solving capability among the people of the community that can carry over to other community problems. Increasing numbers of people can begin to look at the whole community as a social system with numerous interacting components. From this perspective, many other difficult community problems will be viewed in a different light. With these tools, it can become possible to develop new strategies for community change.

REFERENCES AND RECOMMENDED READINGS

1. Accident facts, Chicago, 1972, National Safety Council.
2. Accidental death and disability: the neglected disease of modern society, Washington, D.C., 1966, National Academy of Sciences–National Research Council.
3. Ambulance design criteria, National Highway Traffic Safety Administration, National Academy of Engineering, Washington, D.C., 1971, U.S. Department of Transportation.
4. Basic training program for emergency medical technician—ambulance course guide and course coordinator orientation

program, National Highway Traffic Safety Administration, Washington, D.C., 1971, U.S. Department of Transportation.

5. Buckley, W.: Sociology and modern systems theory, Englewood Cliffs, N.J., 1967, Prentice-Hall, Inc.

6. Categorization of hospital emergency capabilities, Chicago, 1971, American Medical Association.

7. Chen, R., and Benne, K. D.: General strategies for effecting changes in human systems. In Bennis, W., et al., editors: The planning of change, New York, 1961, Holt, Rinehart & Winston.

8. Connor, D. M.: Diagnosing community problems, Ottawa, 1968, Development Press.

9. Connor, D. M.: Strategies for development, Ottawa, 1973, Development Press.

10. Connor, D. M.: Understanding your community, Ottawa, 1969, Development Press.

11. The crisis in emergency care, Medical World News, New York, 1971, McGraw-Hill Book Co.

12. Developing emergency medical services: guidelines for community councils, Commission on Emergency Medical Services, Chicago, 1970, American Medical Association.

13. Emergency medical services communications systems, Health Services and Mental Health Administration, Division of Emergency Health Services, DHEW Publication No. (HSM) 73-2003, Rockville, Md., 1972, U.S. Department of Health, Education, and Welfare.

14. Emergency Medical Services Systems Act of 1973 (Public Law 93-154), 93rd Congress, S. 2410, November 16, 1973.

14a. Emergency medical services systems: program guidelines, Health Services Administration, Bureau of Medical Services, Division of Emergency Medical Services, DHEW Publication No. (HSA) 75-2013, Rockville, Md., 1975, U.S. Department of Health, Education, and Welfare.

15. Frey, C. F., et al.: Resuscitation and survival in motor accidents, Journal of Trauma 9:292-310, 1969.

16. Hanlon, J. J.: Emergency medical care as a comprehensive system, Health Services Reports 88:579-587, 1973.

17. Laughton, C.: Community organization practice as intervention in process, Un-published doctoral dissertation, St. Louis, 1963, Washington University.

18. Likert, R.: The human organization, New York, 1967, McGraw-Hill Book Co.

19. Long, H. B., Anderson, R. C., and Blubaugh, J. A., editors: Approaches to community development, Natural University Extension Association and American College Testing Program, 1973.

20. Mann, L. D.: Studies in community decision making. In Kramer, R. M., and Specht, H., editors: Readings in community organization practice, Englewood Cliffs, N.J., 1969, Prentice-Hall, Inc.

21. Medical requirements for ambulance design and equipment, Public Health Service, Health Services and Mental Health Administration, Division of Emergency Health Services, PHS Publication No. 1071-C-3, Rockville, Md., 1970, U.S. Department of Health, Education, and Welfare.

22. Perloff, H. S.: New directions in social planning. In Kramer, R. M., and Specht, H., editors: Readings in community organization practice, Englewood Cliffs, N.J., 1969, Prentice-Hall, Inc.

23. Ross, M. G.: Case histories in community organization, New York, 1958, Harper & Brothers.

24. Rothman, J.: An analysis of goals and roles in community organization practice. In Kramer, R. M., and Specht, H., editors: Readings in community organization practice, Englewood Cliffs, N.J., 1969, Prentice-Hall, Inc.

25. Schein, E. H.: Process consultation: its role in organizational development, Reading, Mass., 1969, Addison-Wesley Publishing Co., Inc.

26. Seale, S. W., Jr.: Planning and implementing community and county emergency medical services systems, San Antonio, Tex., 1974, Southwest Research Institute.

27. Specht, H.: Disruptive tactics. In Kramer, R. M., and Specht, H., editors: Readings in community organization practice, Englewood Cliffs, N.J., 1969, Prentice-Hall, Inc.

28. Training of ambulance personnel and others responsible for emergency care of the sick and injured at the scene and during transport, Public Health Service, Health Services and Mental Health Administration, Division of Emergency Health Services, PHS Publication No.

1071-C-4, Rockville, Md., 1970, U.S. Department of Health, Education, and Welfare.

29. Warren, R. G.: The community in America, Chicago, 1963, Rand McNally & Co.

30. Warren, R. G.: Types of purposive social change at the community level. In Kramer, R. M., and Specht, H., editors: Readings in community organization practice, Englewood Cliffs, N.J., 1969, Prentice-Hall, Inc.

31. Webber, M. M.: Systems planning for social policy. In Kramer, R. M., and Specht, H., editors: Readings in community organization practice, Englewood Cliffs, N.J., 1969, Prentice-Hall, Inc.

32. Where minutes count, U.S. News & World Report, pp. 6-9, July 6, 1972.

INDEX